Peter Winn • Pamela A. Fenstemacher
Richard G. Stefanacci • R. Scott DeLong
Editors

Post-Acute and Long-Term Care Medicine

A Guide for Practitioners

Third Edition

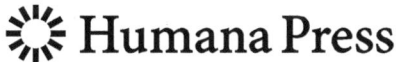 Humana Press

Editors
Peter Winn
Family and Preventive Medicine
OU Health Science Center
Oklahoma City, OK, USA

Richard G. Stefanacci
Thomas Jefferson University
Philadelphia, PA, USA

Pamela A. Fenstemacher
The University of Pennsylvania
Jenkintown, PA, USA

R. Scott DeLong
Department of Geriatrics, Penn Medicine
Lancaster General Health
Lancaster, PA, USA

ISSN 2364-1150   ISSN 2364-1169 (electronic)
Current Clinical Practice
ISBN 978-3-031-28627-8   ISBN 978-3-031-28628-5 (eBook)
https://doi.org/10.1007/978-3-031-28628-5

This Humana imprint is published by the registered company Springer Nature Switzerland AG
The registered company address is: Gewerbestrasse 11, 6330 Cham, Switzerland

Current Clinical Practice

Current Clinical Practice provides an array of practical resources for primary care clinicians. Designed for internists, family physicians, physician assistants, and nurse practitioners, the Current Clinical Practice series offers evidence-based, easy-to-read titles covering a broad range of disorders commonly presented in the primary care setting. Series editor Tommy Koonce, MD, is an Associate Professor of family medicine and Vice Chair of education at UNC School of Medicine in Chapel Hill, North Carolina.

Preface

Whether practitioners are still in training, recently graduated, or deciding to change the direction or focus of their career path, by either choice or necessity, many may find themselves immersed in the long-term care (LTC) arena. Any practitioner can be overwhelmed when confronted by an LTC system that is both complex and highly regulated, let alone taking care of patients and residents who can challenge even the most experienced among us. These patients are challenging, due to not only multiple chronic medical conditions (multimorbidities) and extensive and complicated medication regimens, but also advanced age and increasing frailty. As experienced clinicians, educators, and medical directors in LTC, the chapter authors have written this guide for practitioners with the overarching goal of improving the quality of care provided throughout the LTC continuum by updating the current knowledge in this field with the expertise they have acquired over many years of practice.

Both the Society for Post-Acute and Long-Term Care Medicine (AMDA) and its state chapters continue to work tirelessly to meet the needs of practitioners. Even the most experienced practitioners who have taken AMDA's course on medical direction have commented on how much of the information on LTC care presented in the course is neither readily available nor frequently taught. The content of this guide is aimed at filling this void. The chapters of this guide address the varied components of the LTC system as well as how to care for the patients and residents living within it.

Since the first and second editions of this guide were published, post-acute and long-term care have continued to evolve, further evident by the impact of the COVID-19 pandemic, the incorporation of zoom meetings by the interprofessional team, and the expanded use of telehealth/telemedicine. Indeed, the practice in post-acute and long-term care has itself developed into a subspecialty. The Centers for Medicare and Medicaid Services (CMS) has promulgated its Triple Aim as to the need to improve patient outcomes, to improve patient satisfaction, and to lower the cost to the healthcare system. Others have proposed a Fourth Aim (to improve healthcare workers' satisfaction and lessen burnout) and a Fifth Aim to ensure patient equitable access to health care. Accountable Care Organization (ACOs) and

Population Health Management are ongoing CMS initiatives that focus on the prevention and the early treatment of chronic medical illness.

As practitioners, we are all challenged by an ever-changing healthcare environment that entails bundling of healthcare services, value-based purchasing, transitions in care, medication reconciliation (including the CMS Quality Prescribing Initiative), HIPAA compliance (and possible audits), different electronic medical records at different healthcare settings, and EMR meaningful use. As editors of this guide, we hope that these challenges will become less daunting with the information provided in this guide.

For this third edition, the 19 chapters of the second edition have been updated and a chapter is added on COVID-19 given its impact on practice in post-acute and long-term care. The editors of this guide were approached by Springer publishing to write this third edition before the COVID-19 pandemic emerged. As such, our chapter authors became overwhelmed with providing patient care on the front lines in nursing and assisted living facilities. The editors appreciate their perseverance in updating all the chapters, several of whom are new authors. Thus, this guide update became a 2-year endeavor!

The authors are passionate about LTC with many having worked within the Society to develop AMDA's clinical practice guidelines, present at conferences, write AMDA white papers, and develop the Certified Medical Director course. We hope that you find *Post-Acute and Long-Term Care Medicine* as an invaluable resource to complement your endeavors to optimize the care and living experience of patients and residents in LTC and to enhance patient-centered care as well as patient choice, well-being, dignity, and an improved quality of life.

This guide is dedicated to Chris Laxton, Executive Director, and the office staff of the Society for Post-Acute and Long-Term Care Medicine and its cadre of professional volunteers who represent many healthcare disciplines. We also welcome two additional co-editors, Dr. Richard Stefanacci and Dr. Scott DeLong. The editors wish to acknowledge Crystal Pearson for the long hours, dedication and patience in supporting our editors in updating and editing the chapters of this guide.

Jenkintown, PA, USA   Pamela A. Fenstemacher
Oklahoma City, OK, USA   Peter Winn
Philadelphia, PA, USA   Richard G. Stefanacci
Lancaster, PA, USA   R. Scott DeLong

Contents

Contributors

David Brechtelsbauer University of South Dakota Sanford SOM, Sioux Falls, SD, USA

Brandon Cantazaro University of Texas Rio Grande Valley School of Medicine, Edinburg, TX, USA

R. Scott DeLong, MD, CMD Geriatrics at Home Program, Penn Medicine Lancaster General Health/Penn Medicine Geriatric Fellowship, Lancaster, PA, USA

Andrew Dentino Rio Grande Valley Graduate Medical Education Consortium, Edinburg, TX, USA

Debra Dobbs School of Aging Studies, College of Behavioral and Community Sciences, University of South Florida, Tampa, FL, USA

Pamela A. Fenstemacher The University of Pennsylvania, Jenkintown, PA, USA

Leonard Gelman Community Care, Ballston Spa, NY, USA

Todd H. Goldberg Department of Internal Medicine/Geriatrics, Jefferson Abington Hospital, Abington, PA, USA

Daniel Haimowitz Levittown, PA, USA

Elizabeth Hames UnitedHealth Group, Minnetonka, MN, USA

Daniela Hernandez University of Texas Rio Grande Valley School of Medicine, Edinburg, TX, USA

Randall D. Huss Department of Family Medicine and Geriatrics, Mercy Clinic, Rolla, MO, USA

Mitchell A. Kaminski Thomas Jefferson University, Jefferson College of Population Health, Philadelphia, PA, USA

Cynthia Kuttner Wilmington VA Medical Center, Wilmington VA Community Living Center, Wilmington, DE, USA

Thomas Lawrence Geriatric Medicine and Long Term Care, Main Line Health System, Main Line Health Center, Philadelphia, PA, USA

Steven A. Levenson Baltimore, MD, USA

Joel A. Levien Gastroenterology, Jackson, TN, USA

Naushira Pandya Department of Geriatrics, Nova Southeastern University, Kiran C Patel College of Osteopathic Medicine, Fort Lauderdale, FL, USA

Department of Geriatrics, Kiran C. Patel College of Osteopathic Medicine, Nova Southeastern University, Lauderdale, FL, USA

Robert C. Salinas OU Department of Family and Preventive Medicine, Oklahoma City, OK, USA

Department of Family and Preventive Medicine, The University of Oklahoma, College of Medicine, Oklahoma City, OK, USA

Verna Sellers Madison Heights, VA, USA

David A. Smith Geriatric Consultants of Central Texas, Brownwood, TX, USA

Richard G. Stefanacci Thomas Jefferson University, Jefferson College of Population Health, Philadelphia, PA, USA

Andres Suarez University of Texas Rio Grande Valley School of Medicine,, Edinburg, TX, USA

Krishna Suri University Hospitals, Cleveland, OH, USA

Keith A. Swanson Department of Pharmacy: Clinical and Administrative Sciences, OU College of Pharmacy, Oklahoma City, OK, USA

Laura Trice St. Elizabeth Healthcare, Edgewood, KY, USA

Raghuveer Vedala Department of Family and Preventive Medicine, University of Oklahoma Health Sciences Center, Oklahoma City, OK, USA

Carlyn E. Vogel School of Aging Studies, College of Behavioral and Community Sciences, University of South Florida, Tampa, FL, USA

Deborah Way Palliative Care Services, Corporal Michael J. Crescenz VA Medical Center, Philadelphia, PA, USA

Peter Winn Department of Family and Preventive Medicine, The University of Oklahoma, College of Medicine, Oklahoma City, OK, USA

Department of Family and Preventive Medicine, University of Oklahoma Health Sciences Center, Oklahoma City, OK, USA

Sheryl Zimmerman Program on Aging, Disability, and Long-Term Care, Cecil G. Sheps Center for Health Services Research, University of North Carolina at Chapel Hill, Chapel Hill, NC, USA

Post-Acute Care and Long-Term Services: Evolution to Value-Based Care

Richard G. Stefanacci and Mitchell A. Kaminski

Introduction

In the past, long-term care (LTC) meant nursing homes and there was no "post-acute care (PAC)" except for a patient going home after a lengthy hospital stay. As hospital lengths of stay shortened, the need for transitional post-acute services grew. Nursing homes stepped up, dedicating some of their beds for post-acute services. Of course, with this change, competition for profitable fee-for-service revenues developed within both the PAC and LTC space. With the move toward value-based care over the past decade, PAC and LTC providers are being forced to move from fee for service to global payment strategies. The Quadruple Aim* guides providers to deliver reductions in total cost of care, improve patient experience and population health outcomes, and reduce caregiver burden. This represents a seismic shift from LTC in the past and one that continues to evolve. This chapter discusses these changes.

Because hospitals are paid based upon Diagnosis-Related Groups (DRGs), and receive a set payment regardless of the length of stay, decreasing hospital lengths of stay has been a priority for years. Hospitals now profit through shorter lengths of stay. But, while fixed payment based upon DRGs has incentivized reduced LOS for acute payment, reducing LOS benefits organizations that take on risk for total cost of care as well. The shift in health care delivery from volume to value forces payers and providers to reconsider the site of care.

The PAC and LTC industries are faced with adapting to change arguably more than any other segment of the health care industry. Changes in the finances, delivery, and environment have forced change like never before. Financing PAC and LTSS and examples of alternative facilities and payment models are summarized in Table 1. PAC payment is shifting away from fee-for-service, which reimburses

R. G. Stefanacci (✉) · M. A. Kaminski
Thomas Jefferson University, Jefferson College of Population Health, Philadelphia, PA, USA

© The Author(s), under exclusive license to Springer Nature Switzerland AG 2023
P. Winn et al. (eds.), *Post-Acute and Long-Term Care Medicine*, Current Clinical Practice, https://doi.org/10.1007/978-3-031-28628-5_1

Table 1 Financing of PAC and LTSS

	Post-acute care (PAC)	Long-term services and supports (LTSS)
Financing	Medicare part A	Medicaid Private Pay
Nursing Home/Skilled Nursing Facility (SNF)	Subacute/SNF-short-term (ST)	SNF-long-term (LT)
Alternative facilities	Long-term acute care hospital (LTACH) Inpatient rehab facility (IRF) homecare	Assisted living facility (ALC) Continuing care retirement community (CCRC) homecare
Systems	SNF direct admissions Hospital preferred SNF network Home first promotion	Program for all-inclusive care for the elder (PACE) Special needs plans—institutional (SNP-I)

post-acute providers for what is done, without regard to necessity or clinical outcomes. PAC and LTC providers must now demonstrate true value of care to all stakeholders including payers, health systems, providers, older adults, and their families. Providers should include their quality and total cost of care when demonstrating true value of care. Many practices, which had maximized fee-for-service revenues, for example, through prolonging PAC lengths of stay and providing unnecessary services, are now unsustainable as providers are incentivized to provide value-based care.

The need for change is evident as 73% of variation in total Medicare spending occurs in PAC; it is the single-greatest driver of spending variation. According to the Medicare Payment Advisory Commission (MedPAC) in their March 2019 Report to Congress, direct spending for PAC represents 8.3% of Medicare FFS spending, and one of every 4 dollars spent by a Medicare Advantage (MA) plan. Inefficient and low-quality PAC also drives additional wasteful acute care spending. For accountable care organizations and health plans seeking savings by reducing the total cost of care, the taming of PAC costs represents a critical approach to bending the cost curve in healthcare.

In this chapter, we will review the structures of PAC and LTSS, emphasizing what providers need to know to meet the challenges posed by value-based care (VBC). Metrics such as SNF length of stay and readmission rates become a key focus. Tools provided by VBC models, such as the "3-day waiver," provide leaders new flexibility in care patterns. In addition, clinical goals that promote care coordination across all silos of care challenge leaders to understand and implement new models of care. Familiarity with the use of data and technology is required.

All of these changes promote the Quadruple Aim (improved quality, efficiency, and patient and provider experience), with a focus on patient-centered care, which in PAC is offered at the right place, at the right time, and incorporates the wishes and goals of the patient and family. In addition, there are opportunities to reduce costs and improve population health outcomes. Caregiver burden, both for formal professional caregivers and family/friends, can be addressed. Again, like never before, PAC and LTSS need to evolve to meet new requirements: to remain a critical, valued component of the health care continuum.

Long-Term Services and Supports

Skilled Nursing Facility: LT

For patients who are unable to be cared for in their own home, placement in an SNF may be needed for custodial care. The definition of SNF eligibility is increasingly critical, as this criterion applies to admission not only to an SNF, but also to an Assisted Living Community (ALC), via Medicaid waiver programs, as well as the PACE (Program for All-inclusive Care of the Elderly) program.

Custodial care is care that is primarily for the purpose of assisting the individual in meeting personal rather than medical needs, which is not a specific therapy for an illness or injury and is not skilled care. Also, custodial care serves to assist an individual in the activities of daily living, such as assistance in walking, getting in and out of bed, bathing, dressing, feeding, using the toilet, preparation of special diets, and supervision of medication that usually can be self-administered. Custodial care is maintenance care provided by health aides when an individual has reached the maximum level of physical or mental function. In determining whether an individual is receiving custodial care, the factors considered are the level of care and medical supervision required and furnished rather than the diagnosis, type of condition, degree of functional limitation, or rehabilitation potential.

Post-acute Facility-Based Care

Medicare Part A benefits cover post-acute services in primarily four care settings:

- Home Health Services
- Subacute Skilled Nursing Facility (SNF)
- Inpatient Rehabilitation Facility (IRF)
- Long-Term Acute Care Hospital (LTACH)

The four settings provide an appropriate scope of services covering a range of acuity. A comparison of key components of each setting is summarized in Table 2. With each step up from Home to LTACH comes a significant increase in cost. Because of the shift to value and greater focus on reduction of post-acute care costs with evidence questioning the need of higher acuity care setting the move has been to shift to the left toward more home and home-like settings. MedPAC has proposed Site-neutral payments [1]. Site-neutral payments reflect the Commission's position that the program should not pay more for care in one setting than in another if the

Table 2 Comparison of PAC venues

	Home health services	Subacute SNF	IRF	LTACH
Type of care provided	Part-time intermittent skilled nursing care; therapy services, limited home health aid	Short-term rehab typically following a 3-day inpatient stay	Intensive rehabilitation therapy where patient requires 3 h of therapy at least 5 days per week	Continued hospital level of care
Typical medical conditions treated	Acute and chronic conditions with skilled nursing and/ or therapy needs	CHF COPD Joint replacement Infections	Stroke Neurological disorder	Complex medical condition Complex wounds Vent weaning
Daily therapy requirements per patient	Intermittent, based upon medical need	1–1.5 h	>3 h	N/A
Average length of stay	Based upon need; recertified every 30 days	27 days	13 days	26 days
Average cost per patient	Median cost $24/h[a]	$11,000	$17,000	$38,500

[a] https://www.aplaceformom.com/caregiver-resources/articles/in-home-care-costs

POST-ACUTE CARE
The increasing slide of acuity push-down

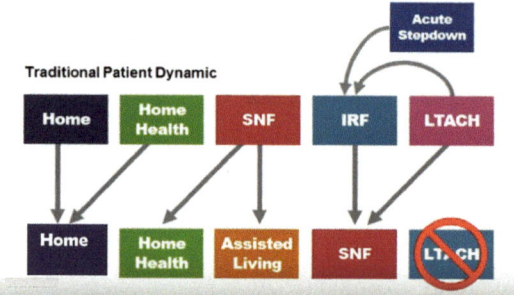

Fig. 1 Acuity push-down

care can safely and effectively be provided in a lower cost setting. This shift in acuity of care to lower-cost settings is illustrated in Fig. 1: Acuity Push-down.

The shift away from SNF to less expensive home care is also being promoted in Bundle-based care programs, for example, orthopedists are now incentivized through these programs, which reimburse based upon 90-day costs around major joint replacement, to discharge patients directly home where they receive rehabilitation services [2].

Home Health Services

Home health services represent a key strategy in providing VBC by supporting earlier acute hospital discharge in a venue that is less expensive, and usually more comfortable for the patient. CMS provides strict guidelines, which must be met for care reimbursement.

Medicare Part A (Hospital Insurance) and/or Medicare Part B (Medical Insurance) cover eligible home health services such as:

- Part-time or "intermittent" skilled nursing care
- Physical therapy
- Occupational therapy
- Speech-language pathology services
- Medical social services
- Part-time or intermittent home health aide services (personal hands-on care)
- Injectable osteoporosis drugs for women

Usually, a home health care agency coordinates the services ordered by a physician. It's important to realize that Medicare doesn't pay for:

- 24-h-a-day care at home
- Meals delivered to the home
- Homemaker services (like shopping, cleaning, and laundry), and custodial or personal care (like bathing, dressing, or using the bathroom) when this is the only care needed.

All people with Part A and/or Part B who meet all of these conditions are covered:

- They must be under the care of a doctor, and getting services under a plan of care created and reviewed regularly by a doctor.
- They must need, and a doctor must certify that they need, one or more of these:
  - Intermittent skilled nursing care (other than drawing blood)
  - Physical therapy, speech-language pathology, or continued occupational therapy services. These services are covered only when the services are specific, safe, and an effective treatment for the condition. The amount, frequency, and time period of the services needs to be reasonable, and they need to be complex or only qualified therapists can do them safely and effectively. To be eligible, either: (1) the condition must be expected to improve in a reasonable and generally predictable period of time, or (2) a skilled therapist is needed to safely and effectively develop a maintenance program for the condition, or (3) a skilled therapist is needed to safely and effectively provide maintenance

therapy for the condition. The home health agency providing the care must be approved by Medicare (Medicare certified).

- The beneficiary must be homebound, as certified by a physician.

Patients are not eligible for the home health benefit if they need more than part-time or "intermittent" skilled nursing care. They may leave home for medical treatment or short, infrequent absences for nonmedical reasons, like attending religious services. Patients can still get home health care even if they attend adult day care

Inpatient Rehabilitation Facilities (IRF)

Inpatient Rehabilitation Facilities (IRFs) provide a higher intensity of services than SNF, within a hospital setting or as free-standing facilities. Acute inpatient rehabilitation services are available for patients requiring acute rehabilitation, defined as restoration of a disabled person to self-sufficiency or maximal possible functional independence [3]. To qualify for an IRF, patients need to require an interdisciplinary, coordinated team approach that involves a minimum of 3 daily hours of rehabilitation services. Continuation of acute rehabilitation services at an IRF requires evidence of progress toward stated goals, documented by objective functional measurements [4]. In addition to hospital conditions of participation for Medicare and Medicaid patients admitted to IRFs, CMS operates under the "60 Percent Rule," [5] meaning that a designated percentage of admissions must fall within specific diagnostic categories to maintain IRF accreditation.

Postoperative acute inpatient rehabilitation at an IRF may be considered medically necessary for individuals undergoing more than one major joint replacement during a single hospitalization, but Medicare and other payers typically do not consider it to be medically necessary when a single joint is replaced. Exceptions are made when the individual has a serious comorbidity or comorbidities that result in functional deficits that necessitate an acute inpatient level of rehabilitation in order to achieve a satisfactory outcome within a reasonable time period [6].

Hip and knee replacements, also known as lower extremity joint replacements (LEJRs), are some of the most common surgeries that Medicare beneficiaries receive [7]. In an effort to control these costs, the Centers for Medicare and Medicaid Services (CMS) implemented the Comprehensive Care for Joint Replacement Model [2]. Within the model, a bundled payment is provided on the basis of a quality measurement for the complete episode of care associated with a hip or knee replacement. The Comprehensive Care for Joint Replacement Model aims to hold hospitals, physicians, and post-acute care providers financially accountable for the quality and value of the care they deliver to Medicare beneficiaries for hip and knee replacements. This financial accountability begins with surgery and continues through to recovery. Additionally, the episode of care structure encourages health care providers to increase their coordination of care.

Long-Term Acute Care Hospital (LTACH)

Care provided by an LTACH is hospital-based care, as such, admissions require documentation that patients have a complicated course of recovery that requires prolonged hospitalization.

Treatment at an LTACH may be required in the face of complex medical issues that meet the criteria of two or more medically active conditions that require:

- Three or more interventions including intravenous medications
- Continuous intravenous fluids (but not a "keep vein open" order)
- Total parenteral nutrition or peripheral parenteral nutrition, and blood products
- At least one physician visit per day
- Frequent diagnostic services
- Active participation in therapies at least 5 days per week

Beyond general complex medical issues, the other two major categories that may require LTACH level of care include complex wound/burns and mechanical ventilation weaning.

Subacute/SNF-ST

Short-term subacute care or SNF-ST is a distinct form of health care service that focuses on providing the skilled medical care needed to transition the patient to the home setting after a qualifying acute-care hospitalization. Although the qualifying hospitalization has historically required a minimum of 3 days, Medicare and managed care plans are increasingly granting waivers to this requirement in an effort to decrease the hospital length of stay. The waivers allow a patient to be directly admitted to SNF or after an acute hospital stay of less than 3 days' duration. There is further discussion of the 3-Day Rule Waiver below. The use of these waivers has also increased in response to COVID-19 with the need to avoid hospitalizations.

Subacute care may be used specifically for rehabilitation purposes for any number of conditions. In general, the rehabilitation needs of patients in these settings include fewer than three treatment modalities and most often physical therapy.

Beyond the need for physical therapy, patients can also qualify for subacute services under one of the following categories:

- Observation
- Assessment
- Monitoring of a complicated or unstable condition

  - Complex teaching services to the individual or caregiver requiring 24-h SNF setting versus intermittent home health care setting
  - Complex medication regimen
  - Initiation of tube feedings; active weaning of ventilator dependent individuals
  - Wound care (including decubitus/pressure ulcers)

Although Medicare Part A benefit covers up to 100 days of subacute services during a benefit period, most stays in subacute care facilities are much shorter than that, lasting 21 days on average. This length of stay is in part because of the Medicare benefit, which covers 100% of the first 20 days and then from days 21–100, requires a daily $185.50 coinsurance from the beneficiary [8]. There must be daily documentation of the patient's progress or complications in order to maintain coverage of subacute care.

Direct Subacute Admissions

The cost of most hospital stays exceeds $2000 per day, while SNF costs are typically less than a quarter of that. Because hospitalization represents the greater expense, care had been moving from the hospital setting to SNF. But organizations taking on risk for total cost of care will reduce costs further when patients are sent home, when appropriate, instead of to an SNF. For example, through a "Home First" strategy, providers now perform previously inpatient procedures, such as joint replacement, in outpatient settings from which the patient can go directly home. SNF rehabilitation stays are reduced. Paradoxically while hospitals are working toward fewer admissions, SNFs benefit from increased admissions and occupancy. Direct admission to SNF was not reimbursed by CMS until recently, when the 3-day waiver, discussed below, was developed for organizations participating in risk-based, value-based care models [9]. These direct admissions for other conditions will allow SNFs an alternative opportunity to increase their occupancy rate.

Direct admissions will be coming from managed care organizations, hospice, private respite, and, most recently, risk-bearing Medicare FFS ACOs, but only to those SNFs that are prepared to handle this process—a process significantly different than the traditional admission, which is a transition from the hospital. Those SNFs appropriately equipped to handle direct admissions will benefit from improved clinical and financial outcomes.

In order to avoid inappropriate use of SNF, CMS put into place the 3-Day Rule in 1965. To qualify for Skilled Nursing Facility (SNF) extended care services coverage, Medicare patients were required to meet the 3-day rule before SNF admission. The 3-day rule requires that the patient have a medically necessary 3-day-consecutive inpatient hospital stay. The 3-day-consecutive stay count doesn't include the day of discharge, or any pre-admission time spent in the ER or outpatient observation.

While Medicare Advantage programs, and risk-bearing accountable care organizations (ACOs) have been able to be granted a waiver for this requirement, the Three-Day Rule remains in place for traditional FFS Medicare beneficiaries. A temporary waiver of the 3-day rule was put into place in 2020 due to the COVID-19 Pandemic, but was expected to be reversed in 2021. This temporary waiver promoted hospital bed access for COVID-19 patients in 2020. Patients with COVID-19 could be admitted to SNFs, when medically appropriate, with the temporary 3-Day Waiver. The waiver is available if: (1) the beneficiary does not reside in a nursing home or SNF for long-term custodial care at the time of the decision to admit to a SNF; and (2) the beneficiary meets all other Centers for Medicare & Medicaid Services (CMS) criteria for SNF admission:

- Is medically stable
- Has confirmed diagnoses (e.g., does not have conditions that require further testing for proper diagnosis)
- Does not require inpatient hospital evaluation or treatment, and
- Has an identified skilled nursing or rehabilitation need that cannot be provided on an outpatient basis or through home health services

In order to achieve this, SNFs may begin to accommodate direct admissions at their facilities. In most cases, when it is determined that a patient needs to be admitted to an SNF, they are sent to the emergency department (ED) and then admitted to the hospital. Only after they have been evaluated are they sent to an SNF. This process can be stressful, costly, and time consuming. Direct admission to the SNF can remedy many of these issues and as such continues to be a growing area of focus. A SNF is required to have and maintain an overall rating of 3 Stars or higher in the CMS 5-Star Quality Rating System in order to participate in the SNF 3-day rule Waiver. A focus on initial and ongoing treatment—as well as assessment of those treatments in a timely manner—requires careful planning.

There are both clinical and financial benefits to utilizing SNFs for direct admissions. Beyond the obvious financial benefits, there are also clinical reasons, as it is commonplace for older adults to experience iatrogenic events when hospitalized. In one paper on the subject, it was found that at least one-third of all patients had some ill effect during hospitalization that was not related to the progression of any pathologic process, and 9% of patients had a major untoward event [2]. Thus, decreasing hospital admissions has both significant clinical and financial benefits that are critical in a value-based care system.

Perhaps the easiest direct admissions to SNFs are those coming from an ED, since a rapid comprehensive assessment can be completed as well as the initial treatment. In fact, our facilities, Forest and Chestnut Hill Healthcare Center in Newark and Passaic New Jersey, have developed programs where patients are sent for Rapid Assessment + Initial Treatment, a process which we affectionately refer to as RAbbIT. RAbbIT requires collaborating with the ED in advance to establish a process where patients can be rapidly assessed with initial treatment started for continuation within the SNF. Without a value-based collaborative process in pace, EDs typically admit to the hospital patients who could be directly admitted to the SNF. Besides the ED, this collaboration can be set up with ever-expanding urgent care centers. Together, EDs and urgent care can be used as the starting point for admission directly to the SNF.

For those not coming through these channels, the SNF must be prepared to have a primary care provider (PCP) make an assessment and establish the treatment plan upon admission. This availability of an admitting provider through either virtual provider access or having a dedicated advanced practice nurse at the facility is critical to managing direct admission. Increased PCP availability in an SNF can come through the establishment of a PCP community office within the SNF. This PCP community office not only allows for greater PCP time in the SNF but provides an opportunity for a community's older adults to become familiar with the SNF in a positive light.

A potential barrier to efficient direct admissions is access to medications. Onsite instant dispensing machines for medications often have mechanisms to help prevent errors, for example, the machine can require that a patient identification number be entered before a medication will be dispensed. Many dispensing machines can also interface with hospital computer systems to integrate their data with information from order entry systems and medication administration records. Dispensing machines can also issue alerts and ask whether an adverse drug event has occurred whenever the machine dispenses a common reversal agent or antidote.

Subacute/SNF-ST Reimbursement

On July 31, 2018, the Centers for Medicare & Medicaid Services (CMS) issued a final rule [CMS-1696-F] outlining fiscal year (FY) 2019 Medicare payment updates and quality program changes for skilled nursing facilities (SNFs) [10]. The final rule includes policies that continue a commitment to shift Medicare payments from volume to value via three significant changes to:

1. The case-mix classification system used under the SNF Prospective Payment System (PPS),
2. The Quality Reporting Program (QRP), and
3. The Value-Based Purchasing Program (VBP)

The final rule builds on the Improving Medicare Post-Acute Care Transformation of 2014 (IMPACT) Act. Understanding these programs and the impact the final rule has on them is important for long-term care (LTC) and SNF providers as it will affect how care is delivered and what outcomes facilities will be held accountable.

The process to modernize the SNF PPS case-mix classification system began as CMS outlined a new case-mix model called the Resident Classification System, Version I (RCS-I) that it was considering as a replacement for the existing Resource Utilization Group, Version IV (RUG-IV) case-mix model, used to classify residents in a covered Part A stay into payment groups under the SNF PPS. Through input from LTC stakeholders, CMS made significant changes to the RCS-I model, resulting in the new model called the SNF Patient-Driven Payment Model (PDPM).

Effective October 1, 2019, CMS began using PDPM, with a focus on the patient's condition and resulting care needs, rather than on the amount of care provided, in order to determine Medicare payment. This new model increases the incentives to treat the needs of the whole patient instead of focusing on volume of services, which had required substantial paperwork to track over time [11]. PDPM is a case-mix reimbursement model that will pay SNFs based on how they meet a patient's needs using ICD-10 diagnosis codes, patient characteristics, and other clinically relevant factors to classify patients [12]. CMS also significantly reduced the overall complexity of the PDPM with the final rule, as compared to the RUG reimbursement system.

Specifically, PDPM adjusts Medicare payments based on each aspect of a resident's care, most notably for non-therapy ancillary services (NTAS), which are items and services not related to the provision of therapy such as drugs and medical supplies, thereby more accurately addressing costs associated with medically complex patients. The rule also places a 25% limit on group and concurrent therapy, i.e., 75% of care needs to be individual to that patient; this is meant to ensure that SNF patients will continue to receive the highest caliber of therapy in line with their individual needs and goals rather than completely within a group session [4].

Based on changes contained within this final rule, CMS estimates that the FY 2019 aggregate impact will have been an increase of $820 million in Medicare payments to SNFs, resulting from the FY 2019 SNF market basket update required to be 2.4% by the Bipartisan Budget Act of 2018 [1]. While this may seem like a large number, it represents less than $50,000 per SNF.

Under the SNF QRP, SNFs that fail to submit the required quality data to CMS will be subject to a 2% reduction in funding [5]. CMS states that they reviewed the SNF QRP's measure set in accordance with the Meaningful Measures Initiative to identify how to move the SNF QRP forward in the least burdensome manner while continuing to incentivize improvement in the quality of care provided to patients. Specifically, the goals of the SNF QRP and the measures used in the program cover most of the Meaningful Measures Initiative priorities, including:

- Making care safer
- Strengthening person and family engagement
- Promoting coordination of care
- Promoting effective prevention and treatment
- Making care affordable

Currently, all measures adopted in the SNF QRP meet the requirements and are in satisfaction of the Improving Medicare Post-Acute Care Transformation of 2014 (IMPACT) Act. There were no new measures proposed in the final rule for the SNF QRP.

However, in the final rule, CMS did adopt an additional factor to consider when evaluating measures for removal from the SNF QRP measure set. This factor considers costs that are associated with a measure, and then weighs them against the benefit of its continued use in the program. CMS will also publicly display the four SNF QRP assessment-based quality measures and increase the number of years of data used to display two claims-based SNF QRP measures, Discharge to the Community and Medicare Spending per Beneficiary, from 1 year to 2 years.

Beginning October 1, 2018, the SNF VBP Program applied either positive or negative incentive payments to services furnished by SNFs based on their performance on the program's readmissions measure. The single claims-based all-cause 30-day hospital readmissions measure in the SNF VBP aims to improve individual outcomes through rewarding providers that take steps to limit the readmission of their patients to a hospital. This single measure does not require SNFs to report information in addition to the information they already submit as part of their claims because CMS uses existing Medicare claims information to calculate the measure.

Again, these changes likely will result in a shift to caring for medically complex patients as well as shift to value as a foundation for reimbursement. This means that the "who" we care for in a SNF will shift from those needing therapy services such as stroke and joint replacement to more medically complex patients such as those with chronic obstructive pulmonary disease (COPD) or congestive heart failure (CHF). The "how" of care delivery will also change as a result of these new types of patients, as they will require less therapy and more nursing and other specialized services like respiratory or cardiac therapy for end-stage management of COPD and CHF. SNF providers will need to think more about how to deliver care to these medically complex patients with these value-based accountability outcomes. The result will be SNFs that are better integrated into the entire care continuum, better equipped to care for medically complex patients, and better at linking patients from the hospital to the community. But this will require unique skill sets and team members that are able to keep SNF patients healthy in the community rather than requiring avoidable hospitalizations, improving both clinical and financial outcomes.

Preferred SNF Network

As health systems increase their focus on population health through care coordination, they are looking to manage their post-acute care more aggressively, especially through development of a Preferred SNF Network [13]. SNFs with higher quality scores and greater efficiency (lower 30-day readmission rate, for example) and who collaborate more effectively with health systems are preferred. The value of health system-preferred SNF networks was illustrated in a recent study in *Health Affairs* [14]. In the article, researchers studied several hospitals that had developed formal SNF networks as part of their care management efforts. These hospitals saw a relative reduction from 2009 to 2013 of 4.5% in readmission rates for patients discharged to SNFs compared to hospitals without formal networks. Overall, researchers found that establishing preferred SNF provider networks is one approach hospital administrators are using to reduce excess 30-day readmissions and avoid Medicare penalties, and to reduce beneficiaries' costs as part of value-based payment models.

By appreciating this benefit of preferred SNF networks, leaders at SNFs can better understand how to become a successful partner with health systems while improving care for their residents.

Figure 2 contains an adaptation of a letter sent by a health system, Meadow Creek Healthcare System, to an area SNF after they had evaluated the facility as a potential member of their preferred network. This correspondence illustrates the basis of selection for a preferred provider and specific areas of opportunity for improvement.

CMS Star Ratings	
Overall	
Inspection	
Staffing	
Quality Measures	
Re-Hospitalization Rate	
During SNF Stay	
Following SNF Stay	
Overall	
Surveys of Health System Discharge/Transition to SNF Team (Rating: 1 negative – 5 positive)	
Perception of Support or Challenges in dealing with facility	
Perception of Scope & Quality of Services Offered	
Desire for referral of Self or Loved One to this facility	
Average Rating	

Fig. 2 Preferred SNF evaluation report

While all health systems will have their own individual process, most will concentrate on these same critical elements when choosing a preferred network. SNF leaders can proactively ready their facility in the key areas discussed in the letter.

Once established, each health system's preferred SNF network will be deemed successful on the basis of a panel of measurable outcomes. These accountability measures will likely be centered on the following:

The measure of success of many health system's SNF network is based on clinical and financial outcomes. These accountability measures focus primarily on keeping patients safe in the SNF and community. The measures considered include those in Table 3.

Note that these measures rely heavily on each SNF being able to successfully care for patients in their facility, which includes transitioning them to their homes in the community. These efforts depend on each SNF having the resources and skilled staff to provide the level of care needed to recognize and treat issues rather than allowing them to escalate to require a hospitalization. A central component of delivering this care is having a process in place to identify opportunities to prevent avoidable emergency department (ED)/hospital utilization—one such method is use of the INTERACT tool [15].

Health systems often strongly recommend that all unplanned ED/hospitalizations undergo a thoughtful analysis to identify opportunities to prevent future occurrences. This activity typically reveals care improvement opportunities related to end-of-life planning or access to medical evaluation. Once an area is identified, a plan can then be put into place to address the perceived problem, such as maintaining physician orders for life-sustaining treatment forms for all residents, using virtual after-hour medical services, or having a dedicated advanced practical nurse available to care for all facility residents.

Also of note is the CMS Star Rating and total cost of care measures. These are a direct result of health systems increasingly taking on financial responsibility for care outside of the hospital through bundled payments, accountable care organizations (ACOs), and other risk arrangements. Thus, managing total cost of care is critical for success in these arrangements. As previously discussed, an SNF that has

Table 3 SNF measures of success

CMS star rating (must be >3)
• Overall
• Quality measures
HCQIS (QIO) Data
• Readmission rate to hospital during SNF stay
• Readmission rate to hospital after SNF stay
• Overall SNF readmission rate to hospital
CMS Star Rating
• Percentage of short-stay residents who were rehospitalized after a nursing home admission
• Percentage of short-stay residents who have had an outpatient emergency department visit
• Percentage of short-stay residents who were successfully discharged to the community
SNF total cost of care
• Average SNF stay cost
• Average SNF total cost of care

and maintains an overall rating of 3 Stars or higher in the CMS 5-Star Quality Rating System will be preferred in order to participate in the SNF 3-day rule Waiver and provide for direct SNF admissions.

Special Needs Plans

While much has been talked about regarding ACOs and bundled payments, Special Needs Plans (SNP) miss the attention of long-term care (LTC) stakeholders despite the fact that these are the most significant value-based offerings for LTC [16]. SNPs, created by Congress in 2003, are Medicare coordinated care plans (CCP) specifically designed to provide targeted care to a limited enrollment of special needs individuals. SNPs are responsible for addressing the total cost of care. There are three different types of SNPs:

1. Dual Eligible SNP (D-SNP) for dual eligible beneficiaries (2,157,682 enrollees)
2. Chronic Condition SNP (C-SNP), serving an individual with a severe or disabling chronic condition, as specified by the Centers for Medicare & Medicaid Services (CMS) (345,951 enrollees)
3. Institutional SNP (I-SNP) for an institutionalized individual (71,474 enrollees)

Obviously the I-SNP has direct application to LTC stakeholders, as it is specific to skilled nursing facilities (SNFs). But the other SNPs, C-SNP and D-SNP, also have LTC application, as those individuals will be served in the SNF subacute setting as well as after transitioning. A detail even more significant for LTC stakeholders is that, as LTC shifts from facility-based SNFs to the community, older individuals in need of LTC can be better served through these SNPs.

Again, these models provide LTC providers opportunities to better coordinate care and provide services beyond those covered by Medicare or Medicaid, such as needs related to social determinants of health.

I-SNPs are SNPs that restrict enrollment to MA eligible individuals who, for 90 days or longer, have had or are expected to need the level of services provided in an LTC/SNF, an LTC nursing facility (NF), a SNF/NF, an intermediate care facility for individuals with intellectual disabilities, or an inpatient psychiatric facility. A complete list of acceptable types of institutions can be found online.

An I-SNP may operate either single or as multiple facilities; CMS may allow establishment of a county-based service area, as long as the I-SNP includes at least one LTC facility that can accept enrollment and is accessible to county residents. "As with all MA plans, CMS will monitor the plan's marketing/enrollment practices and LTC facility contracts to confirm that there is no discriminatory impact."

The below conditions must be met for an I-SNP to enroll MA eligible individuals living in the community but requiring an institutional level of care (LOC):

1. "A determination of institutional LOC that is based on the use of a state assessment tool. The assessment tool used for persons living in the community must be the same as that used for individuals residing in an institution. In states and territories without a specific tool, I-SNPs must use the same LOC determination methodology used in the respective state or territory in which the I-SNP is authorized to enroll eligible individuals."
2. "The I-SNP must arrange to have the LOC assessment administered by an independent, impartial party (i.e., an entity other than the respective I-SNP) with the requisite professional knowledge to identify accurately the institutional LOC needs. Importantly, the I-SNP cannot own or control the entity."

These "at-risk" models administered through an SNP, through investment in clinical management in the nursing home setting, have the potential to allow individuals to receive care on-site and avoid costly inpatient transfers.

Given the high need for flexibility beyond FFS, successful SNPs should focus their attention on wellness, caregivers, coordination, prescription/medication management, end-of-life care, social determinants of health, and mental health. Of these, one of the most critical is medication management. Medication management is meant to assist individuals in taking their medications on time, at the proper time, and consistently, while helping prevent incorrect medication administration and the resulting potential harms.

Learnings from COVID-19

Almost 1 month prior to being declared a worldwide pandemic, a case of coronavirus disease (COVID-19) was identified in a resident of a long-term care skilled facility in King Country, Washington. It was among the earliest reported in the USA. As of June 2021, 4% of COVID-19 infections but 31% of deaths (at least 184,000) were reported in USA nursing homes. At one point, 43% of deaths were attributed to LTC facilities. The rate has declined dramatically with the COVID-19 vaccine rollouts. The Pandemic underscored the vulnerability of the frail geriatric population residing in LTC facilities. The enclosed, congregate living settings that nursing homes represent, the volume of outside visitors, and staff members, many paid low-wages with multiple jobs at other LTCFs caring for the residents, augmented the risk of infection for the vulnerable elderly residents.

The response by nursing homes mitigated the risk of transmission of COVID-19, but also highlighted key strategies to maximize residents' and staff members' safety. These involve some key insights that lead to "best practices":

- Reinforce basic infection transmission precautions such as consistent handwashing, and mask wearing for residents or staff with respiratory symptoms. Staff, resident, and visitor education is necessary.
- Promote successful immunization campaigns for residents and staff of facilities.
- Realize that National and Global infectious disease trends will ultimately invade long-term care facilities. Keep abreast of public health information.
- Promote an organized team response for consistent, successful program management. Nursing facilities are required, as part of the Pandemic response, to designate one or more individual(s) as the Infection Preventionist(s) (IPs) who are responsible for the facility's Infection Prevention Control Program (IPCP).
- Assure adequate Personal Protective Equipment (PPE) inventory for infection breakouts. Funding and inventory processes need to be in place
- Screen and limit outside visitors during epidemics or pandemics.
- Avoid staff turnover and employment of outside temporary staff members as much as is feasible.
- Reduce outside visitors through use of automated dispensing pharmacy services instead of manual delivery of pharmaceuticals.
- Encourage physicians and other provider staff, who often visit other facilities, to conduct rounds and patient visits virtually/remotely.

Providers who are in leadership positions can help promote nursing facility safety:

- Gain credibility and apply pressure for response with leadership, including communication with Board members.
- Work for buy-in of your residents, families, and staff; communicate with them regularly.
- Make PPE and the protection of your residents and staff the top priority. Control the environment as much as possible.
- Rely on the basics of process development and management.
- Work with a lead for policy development, tracking, and education.
- Partner with your workforce to achieve the common goal of safety; make expectations clear.

COVID-19 demonstrated much about skilled nursing facilities from the vulnerability to the need to share information on the dangers and appropriate management of an infectious disease. COVID-19 demonstrated much about skilled nursing facilities from the vulnerability to the need to share information on the dangers and appropriate management of an infectious disease.

The Interdisciplinary Team

An interdisciplinary team of health care professionals who provide both a comprehensive and coordinated assessment and management of each resident's medical, psychological, social, and functional needs is essential for resident well-being in LTC (Table 4). This in fact is mandated in nursing facilities but is also a practical approach to provide care for the elderly in the assisted living facility and home as well.

Summary

In this chapter, we have reviewed how evolving payment models are impacting providers of Post-Acute Care and Long-term Support Services. While previously based on simple fee-for-service payment, new value-based payment strategies are increasingly holding providers accountable for the total cost of care. This requires the coordination of care across all care venues, including the patients' homes. Higher value SNFs and Home Care service providers will be rewarded through designations in preferred networks. Success requires evolving to a model of care involving close collaboration across teams of providers that continually deliver value care.

Table 4 The interdisciplinary care team in nursing facilities

Title	Scope of practice	Education
Certified nurses aids (CNA)	Work under the supervision of a nurse and provide assistance to patients with daily living tasks	In addition to a high school diploma or GED, completion of a 6- to 12-week CNA certificate program at a community college or medical facility
Licensed practical nurse (LPN)	Provide the patient care on a very personal level. They usually report directly to physicians and RNs, and are usually responsible for taking vitals and monitoring in-and-out volumes, treating common conditions like pressure sores, and preparing or performing several procedures such as dressing wounds, bathing and dressing, and giving enemas. In some, but not all, states LPNs and LVNs may administer prescribed medicines or start IV fluids	Required to pass a licensing examination, known as the NCLEX-PN, after completing a State-approved practical nursing program. A high school diploma or its equivalent usually is required for entry

(continued)

Table 4 (continued)

Title	Scope of practice	Education
Registered nurse (RN)	Work directly with patients and their families. They are the primary point of contact between the patient and the world of health care, both at the bedside and in outpatient settings. RNs perform frequent patient evaluations, including monitoring and tracking vital signs, performing procedures such as IV placement, phlebotomy, and administering medications. Because the RN has much more regular contact with patients than physicians, the RN is usually first to notice problems or raise concerns about patient progress	The three major educational paths to registered nursing are a bachelor's degree, an associate degree, and a diploma from an approved nursing program. Nurses most commonly enter the occupation by completing an associate degree or bachelor's degree program. Individuals then must complete a national licensing examination in order to obtain a nursing license
Registered Nurse Assessment Coordinator (RNAC)	The Registered Nurse Assessment Coordinator (RNAC) will assist the Director of Nursing (DON) with ensuring that documentation in the center meets Federal State and Certification guidelines. The RNAC will coordinate RAI process assuring the accuracy timeliness and completeness of the MDS RAPS and Interdisciplinary Care Plan. The Registered Nurse Assessment Coordinator (RNAC) conducts the nursing process—Assessment Planning Implementation and Evaluation—under the state's Nurse Practice Act for Registered Nurse Licensure	
Director of Nursing (DON)	The Director of Nursing has the responsibility of overseeing the standards of nursing practices for the organization's nursing services. The DON participates with other members of Nursing Services and Administration in the development of patient care programs, policies, and procedures to meet all requirements including ethical and legal concerns	
Social worker	Assist people by helping them cope with issues in their everyday lives, deal with their relationships, and solve personal and family problems	All States and the District of Columbia have licensing, certification, or registration requirements regarding social work practice and the use of professional titles. Although standards for licensing vary by State, a growing number of States are placing greater emphasis on communications skills, professional ethics, and sensitivity to cultural diversity issues. Most States require 2 years (3000 h) of supervised clinical experience for licensure of clinical social workers

Table 4 (continued)

Title	Scope of practice	Education
Dietitian	Plan food and nutrition programs, supervise meal preparation, and oversee the serving of meals. They prevent and treat illnesses by promoting healthy eating habits and recommending dietary modifications. They perform nutrition screenings for their clients and offer advice on diet-related concerns such as weight loss and cholesterol reduction	At least a bachelor's degree. Licensure, certification, or registration requirements vary by State
Physical therapist	Physical therapists provide a variety of medical services to help individuals who have been injured or physically affected by illness to recover or improve function. A physical therapist must be able to evaluate a patient's condition and devise a customized physical rehabilitation and treatment plan to enhance strength, flexibility, range of motion, motor control, and reduce any pain, discomfort, and swelling the patient is experiencing	Graduate from a physical therapist educational program with a master's or doctoral degree
Occupational therapist	Occupational therapists help patients improve their ability to perform tasks in living and working environments. They work with individuals who suffer from a mentally, physically, developmentally, or emotionally disabling condition. Occupational therapists use treatments to develop, recover, or maintain the daily living and work skills of their patients. The therapist helps clients not only to improve their basic motor functions and reasoning abilities, but also to compensate for permanent loss of function. The goal is to help clients have independent, productive, and satisfying lives	A master's degree or higher in occupational therapy is the minimum requirement for entry into the field
Recreational therapist	Recreational therapists devise programs in art, music, dance, sports, games, and crafts for individuals with disabilities or illnesses. These activities help to prevent or to alleviate physical, mental, and social problems	Bachelor's degree with some additional training is usually required for this field
Attending primary care physician	Responsibility for initial patient care, and support discharges and transfers. Also make periodic, pertinent on-site visits to patients and insure adequate ongoing coverage (see chapter "The Role of Practitioners and the Medical Director")	In addition to 4 years of medical school most nursing home attending physicians complete a primary residency, which is typically 1–3 years. Some go on to complete a geriatric fellowship as well

(continued)

Table 4 (continued)

Title	Scope of practice	Education
Medical director	Roles and responsibilities of the medical director in the nursing home can be divided into four areas: physician leadership, patient care–clinical leadership, quality of care, and education. Nursing facilities are required to have a medical director as outlined in OBRA 87 (see chapter "The Role of Practitioners and the Medical Director")	Currently Maryland is the only State that requires Medical Directors to be a Certified Medical Director (CMD) in Long-Term Care or have similar training. CMD was established by the American Medical Directors Association to professionalize the field of medical direction
Nurse practitioner (NP)	Advanced practice nurses provide high-quality health care services similar to those of a doctor. NPs diagnose and treat a wide range of health problems. They have a unique approach and stress both care and cure. Besides clinical care, NPs focus on health promotion, disease prevention, health education, and counseling (see chapter "Nurse Practitioners, Clinical Nurse Specialists and Physician Assistants")	The entry-level training for NPs is a graduate degree. At this time, NPs complete a master's or doctoral degree program. This means that NPs earn a bachelor's degree in nursing (4 years of education), then their graduate NP degree (2–4 years of education)
Consultant pharmacists	Focuses on reviewing and managing the medication regimens of patients, particularly those in institutional settings such as nursing homes. Consultant pharmacists ensure their patients' medications are appropriate, effective, as safe as possible and used correctly; and identify, resolve, and prevent medication-related problems that may interfere with the goals of therapy	The Doctorate of Pharmacy (Pharm.D.) is the only professional Pharmacy degree, and the 5-year Bachelors of Science in Pharmacy is being phased out as a professional degree. Since this program traditionally follows 2 years of pre-pharmacy education, students typically take 6 years of post-secondary education to obtain their Pharm.D
Nursing home administers	Responsibility as the managing officer of the facility to plan, organize, direct, and control the day-to-day functions of a facility and to maintain the facility's compliance with applicable laws, rules, and regulations The administrator shall be vested with adequate authority to comply with the laws, rules, and regulations relating to the management of the facility	Typically, a certificate program of about 120 h is required before sitting for a licensing examination. Most are required to have completed a bachelor's degree program as well as preceptor training as an NHA

[a] Part-time position

References

1. http://www.medpac.gov/docs/default-source/reports/chapter-6-site-neutral-payments-for-select-conditions-treated-in-inpatient-rehabilitation-facilities.pdf.
2. https://www.managedhealthcareconnect.com/articles/admission-criteria-facility-based-post-acute-services.
3. Brault MW. Americans with disabilities: 2010. Washington, DC: US Census Bureau; 2012. www.census.gov/prod/2012pubs/p70-131.pdf.
4. Feinberg L, Reinhard SC, Houser A, Choula R. Valuing the invaluable: 2011 update the growing contributions and costs of family caregiving. http://assets.aarp.org/rgcenter/ppi/ltc/i51-caregiving.pdf.
5. O'Shaughnessy CV; National Health Policy Forum. National spending for Long-Term Services and Supports (LTSS), 2012. Basics_LTSS_03-27-14.pdf.
6. https://www.cms.gov/Outreach-and-Education/Medicare-Learning-Network-MLN/MLNProducts/Downloads/InpatRehabPaymtfctsht09-508.pdf.
7. https://www.prolianceorthopedicassociates.com/dr-barrett-blog/the-results-of-the-2020-american-joint-replacement-registry.
8. https://www.medicare.gov/coverage/skilled-nursing-facility-snf-care.
9. https://www.managedhealthcareconnect.com/articles/direct-admissions-skilled-nursing-facilities-are-you-ready.
10. https://www.managedhealthcareconnect.com/articles/how-reimbursement-changes-long-term-care-will-impact-who-and-how-we-care.
11. LaPointe J. AHA finds flaws with the patient-driven payment model for SNFs. RevCycleIntelligence.com. https://revcycleintelligence.com/news/aha-finds-flaws-with-the-patient-driven-payment-model-for-snfs
12. Centers for Medicare and Medicaid Services (CMS). Skilled Nursing Facilities Patient-Driven Payment Model Technical Report. cms.gov website. https://www.cms.gov/Medicare/Medicare-Fee-for-Service-Payment/SNFPPS/Downloads/PDPM_Technical_Report_508.pdf. Published April 2018
13. Stefanacci RG. How to Be Included in a Health System's Preferred SNF Network. Ann Longterm Care. 2017;25(5):24–6.
14. McHugh JP, Foster A, Mor V, et al. Reducing hospital readmissions through preferred networks of skilled nursing facilities. Health Aff. 2017;36(9):1591–8.
15. Pathway Health Services. Quality improvement tool for review of acute care transfers-INTERACT version 4.0 tool. Pathway Health website. http://www.pathway-interact.com/wp-content/uploads/2017/04/148604-QI_Tool-for-Review-Acute-Care-Transf_AL.pdf
16. https://www.managedhealthcareconnect.com/articles/special-needs-plans-are-special-long-term-care

Home Health Care

Robert C. Salinas

Introduction

It is estimated that by the year 2050, the number of people age 65 and over in the USA will increase from 46 million to 90 million, representing the fastest growing segment of our population. Although this age group makes up 16% of the current population, it disproportionately accounts for approximately 36% of all health care-related expenditures [1]. As older Americans have a strong desire to remain in their homes (or in an independent or assisted living facility) and age in place, this trend will continue to increase the need for community-based home care services. Many are afflicted with multiple chronic conditions (multi-morbidities), homebound, and experience difficulty in accessing timely and needed health care services. As a result, many receive fragmented and inadequate medical care.

With hospital-based care shifting more to community-based care, a dramatic paradigm shift is occurring [2]. In addition to "urgent care at home" programs, telemedicine, remote patient monitoring, palliative, and home-based primary care programs, "hospital at home" programs are being developed that enable patients to receive acute care at home. Hospital at home programs have proven effective in reducing complications while cutting the cost of care by 30% or more, leading to entrepreneurial efforts to promote their use. Thus, a combination of "high tech and high touch" programs are making home-based care a viable option for patients who are in need of acute care or hospital post-acute care.

The elderly often require emergency room evaluation for acute illness, unintended injuries, and exacerbation of chronic conditions such as congestive heart failure, chronic obstructive pulmonary disease, and diabetes [3]. These patients experience shorter lengths of stay in the hospital setting [4]. Many need post-acute

R. C. Salinas (✉)
OU Department of Family and Preventive Medicine, Oklahoma City, OK, USA

P. Winn et al. (eds.), *Post-Acute and Long-Term Care Medicine*, Current Clinical
Practice, https://doi.org/10.1007/978-3-031-28628-5_2

care to regain their premorbid functional status and to remain safe in the community [5]. Distant monitoring technology, changes in clinician reimbursement, and more intersystem communication can prevent hospital admissions and readmissions. Accordingly, home-based care has become a vital part of the health care system. Further expansion and integration of home-based care can help meet the needs of an overburdened health care system for persons who are homebound [6]. Home-based care has the potential to decrease the costs of care, improve patient outcomes, and improve patient, family, and health care workers' satisfaction. This chapter reviews the delivery of medical care in the home, practitioner home visits, and services provided by home health and hospice care agencies.

Home Care

Home care is defined as the provision of health care-related services and durable medical equipment to patients at home for the purpose of restoring and maintaining his or her maximal level of function, independence, comfort, and health [6, 7]. This entails a clinician coordinated interdisciplinary approach and the use of therapeutic, diagnostic, and social support services. Generally, the patients' goals of care determine the plan of care and the level of services needed. This can include house calls by a physician, nurse practitioner, or physician assistant in collaboration with the services provided by the home health care agency. Home care services are eligible for patients who have intermittent skilled needs subsequent to a decline in functional status due to an exacerbation of a chronic condition, acute illness, or injury, or who transition to home upon discharge from a hospital, rehab facility, or a skilled nursing facility (SNF).

The Physician House Call

Despite wanting to "age in place" at home, some older adults may opt to move into an assisted living facility (ALF), a personal care home or group home, or an independent living facility (ILF). *Contrary to common belief, patients are **not** required to be homebound in order for a practitioner to provide a house call and to be reimbursed for the medical service they provide.* However, there **are** homebound requirements for patients who require services provided by a home health agency. Situations under which a practitioner can justify a home visit include:

- An acute care visit when the patient is unable to travel to an outpatient clinic or emergency room.
- Ongoing management of a progressive and debilitating chronic condition.
- Need to gather more information about the environmental and social conditions of a patient, for example, who continues to experience recurrent falls and injuries or if there is a suspicion for abuse or neglect.

- Recurrent ER visits and/or hospital admissions.
- Provision of palliative care and discussion of end-of-life care preferences, including hospice care [8].

Some physicians have established their practice exclusively in home care. Home-based primary care (HBPC) can be a viable alternative for some practices, and has been shown to potentially reduce overall cost of care for patients diagnosed with serious illness [9]. The Veterans Hospital Administration has had a well-established HBPC program for over 30 years.

Preparing for the House Call

In preparation for a home visit, it is important to anticipate the purpose and goals of the visit in order to better determine the patient's care plan. This requires advance notice of the visit to the patient, family members, and/or caregivers, as well as the home health agency or hospice and the patient's community-based caseworker (if the patient has one) who is responsible for coordination of the patient's care. Planning ahead can ascertain what procedural instruments and supplies may be required such as toenail clippers or supplies for injections (Table 1).

During the home visit:

- Address the patient's medical condition.
- Review all medications including those prescribed, over-the-counter, and any herbal supplements, and the reason for each.
- Assess the patient's functional status, memory and cognitive ability, and level of independence (Basic ADL's and Instrumental ADL's).
- For patients with physical limitations, identify the need for adaptive or durable medical equipment to maximize safety and independence. Assistive devices and durable medical equipment such as a walker or bedside commode can aide a person in remaining independent in the home and delay institutionalization.

Table 1 The doctor's bag

Stethoscope	Examination gloves (latex free)
Blood pressure cuff	Syringes and needles
Thermometer	Sharps container
Pen light	Scissors/forceps/toenail clippers
Pulse oximeter	Laptop EMR
Prescription pad	Guaiac Cards/developer
Pharmacopeia	Hand wipes
Reflex Hammer	Band-aides/Ace Bandages

Table 2 Assessment in the home

Patient overall assessment
Functional assessment (BADLs, IADLs, falls)
Mental/cognitive assessment
Nutritional assessment/food availability
Medication use and compliance
Advance care planning
Assessment of caregiving burden
Assessment of the caregiver
Environmental assessment
Safety in the home/outside
Needs for durable medical equipment (DME)
Community assessment
Safety of neighborhood for health care providers
Availability of community resources

Table 3 Medicare part B reimbursement 2021

New patients		Established patients	
Code	Reimbursement[a]	Code	Reimbursement[a]
99341	$51.98	99347	$52.24
99342	$73.73	99348	$79.94
99343	$121.95	99349	$122.90
99344	$172.85	99350	$170.25

[a] Reimbursement will vary from state to state

- *Identify the environmental need for home adaptation*, remodeling, or retrofitting that can improve home access, safety, and mobility.
- *Caregiver assessment* is also important in determining if a plan of care can be successfully implemented in the home (Table 2 lists important aspects of a home assessment).
- To recognize and address caregiver burnout.

Billing for Services

Under current Medicare rules, any licensed physician, nurse practitioner, or physician assistant can perform a house call and bill for services rendered using the appropriate CPT code for the level of service provided [7]. Most third party payers follow the rates and guidelines for billing set forth by Medicare and Medicaid. Practitioners are also allowed to bill based on the amount of time directly spent with and in counseling the patient. It is important that each component of the patient encounter be appropriately documented for the level of service coded as to history, examination, and medical decision-making complexity (see Table 3). Note that

Table 4 Members of the home health care team

Skilled nurse
Physical therapist
Speech therapist
Occupational therapist
Home health care aide
Social worker
Case manager
Wound care nurse
Medical Director[a]

[a] Some home health care agencies or corporate entity may have either a medical director or corporate medical director

practitioners are **not** allowed to bill for travel time associated with making a house call. Numerous versions of mobile-capable electronic health records (EHR) have the ability to document and to facilitate the exchange of patient information such as medication reconciliation, laboratory results, and diagnostic studies.

Agency Home Health Care

Under current Medicare guidelines, beneficiaries who have a documented need for episodic care may be eligible for home health care. The purpose of home health care is to have an interdisciplinary team of qualified health care providers (see Table 4) to provide assistance in the home for a person who requires skilled nursing care, physical therapy, speech therapy, and other services. Often a referral is made when a physician or an advance practice provider notes a patient's decline in health and level of function that places the patient at risk for falls, hospitalization, or institutionalization [6]. At other times, home health care can assist in delivery of palliative care in seriously ill patients who are ineligible for hospice or have chosen not to enroll in hospice [10].

Members of the Team

Delivering effective home health care depends on each member of the health care team using their skill set aimed at restoring health based on the patient needs [11], while negotiating health care goals with the patient and family and then developing a plan of care that can sustain efforts to attain and maintain these goals. The home health team must have regular contact with the patient and the patient's family and be able to ascertain whether the plan of care can be successfully implemented in the home (or elsewhere).

Skilled Nursing

A licensed practice nurse (LPN) or registered nurse (RN) can provide skilled-level care to patients in the home that may include:

- Educating patients and caregivers on acute and chronic medical conditions.
- Instructing on how/when to administer medication.
- Obtaining laboratory specimens and reporting results.
- Coordinating home X-ray studies, home infusion of medication and IV therapy.
- Providing wound care.
- Administering vaccinations.

The nurse's admission assessment should include functional, memory and cognitive status, and medication reconciliation of prescribed and all over-the-counter medications [12–15]. Most home health care agencies now use a software program to screen for potential drug–drug interactions with this report subsequently sent to the patient's physician for review.

Nurses usually provide services one to two times a week, but can be more frequent at the start of care (front loaded visits) in order to meet patient needs. Nurses often identify other medical conditions that need to be brought to the attention of the practitioner and also recognize barriers to the delivery of care, such as caregiver stress or financial burdens. The role of the home health nurse continues to expand and can include the promotion, monitoring, and maintenance of health [16].

Physical Therapist

Home health physical therapists provide therapy to improve lower extremity strength and conditioning. Patients often have a history of falls or have become deconditioned following hospitalization. Referrals for home physical therapy frequently are for patients who have suffered a stroke or had lower extremity orthopedic surgery [17, 18]. Physical therapists assist in educating the patient's caregivers on how to improve patient function, safety, and independence and provide recommendations for durable medical equipment (DME) such as canes, walkers, shower chairs, and suggestions for retrofitting bathrooms.

Speech Therapist

Under the current Medicare home health care guidelines, a physician can request a referral for home health care solely for the purpose of providing speech therapy in the home. The speech therapist can also perform an initial screen for swallowing that may subsequently necessitate a formal swallowing study in order to more adequately assess dysphagia and make recommendations as to diet consistency.

Occupational Therapist

Home health occupational therapists often work in tandem with physical therapists to promote better function of the upper extremities and self-care of the basic ADLs. The occupational therapist may also recommend adaptive equipment or DME that can assist the patient. Some therapists may have acquired skills in assessing a patient's swallowing.

Social Worker

Most home health care agencies have medical social workers on staff, or if not, will out contract this service. Medical social workers can play an important role in the care of patients with complex psychosocial needs. This may include to help identify caregivers (paid and informal), to address caregiver stress, and to make inquiries and suggestions to alleviate financial hardship.

Home Care Aide

Based on necessity, home health care agencies can provide nurse aides to assist patients in their ADLs such as bathing and dressing and to provide light housework if a patient is too weak to do so. They can supplement the personal care provided by family members and other caregivers who may be in the home less frequently than needed. *Use of an aide to provide services is contingent upon the need for skilled nursing for the patient.*

Requirements for Agency Home Health Care

There are several requirements that must be met for a physician to order home health care for a (Medicare) beneficiary. **First**, as of April 2020, a physician, an Advance Practice Nurse, Clinical Nurse Specialist, or Physician Assistant must determine that the patient meets the requirement for "homebound" status and **secondly** that the patient has a need for episodic skilled nursing care, physical therapy, or speech therapy.

The definition and interpretation of homebound status often leads to confusion. This is reviewed in Table 5.

For the *initial Home Health certification*, the Affordable Care Act (ACA) now requires that the certifying physician or advance practice provider, document a *face-to-face encounter* with the patient. This encounter *must have addressed the medical condition for which this episode of home health care is being ordered. The*

Table 5 Definition of homebound status

For a patient to be eligible to receive covered home health services under both Medicare Part A (by the home health agency) and Part B (by the practitioner), the law requires that a physician or allowed practitioner certify in all cases that the patient is confined to his/her home. For purposes of the statute, an individual shall be considered "confined to the home" (homebound) if the following two criteria are met:
1. Criterion One:
The patient must either:
• Because of illness or injury, need the aid of supportive devices such as crutches, canes, wheelchairs, and walkers; the use of special transportation; or the assistance of another person in order to leave their place of residence
OR
• Have a condition such that leaving his or her home is medically contraindicated
If the patient meets one of the Criterion One conditions, then the patient must **ALSO** meet two additional requirements defined in Criterion Two
2. Criterion Two:
• There must exist a normal inability to leave home
AND
• Leaving home must require a considerable and taxing effort.

documentation of a face-to-face encounter must occur within 90 days prior to the start date of home health care or within 30 days after the start of care. This encounter is only required for the initial certification period and not recertification. The face-to-face can be done via telemedicine. The documentation for necessity includes the name of the certifying physician or advance practice provider, date of the face-to face encounter, the patient's homebound status, the need for skilled services, and a signature and date from the ordering physician or other provider. The face-to-face encounter can be performed by a resident physician in training under the supervision of the teaching physician. The face-to-face documentation can be included in the certification document, a separate standardized form or via tele-health [19].

Not infrequently, the home setting may not be the best venue to provide and coordinate complex care, especially for frail patients who have multiple health care needs. In such cases, options may include admission to a rehabilitation center, a long-term acute care hospital (LTACH) or a skilled nursing facility. Any physician involved with the patient's care may order home health. *Many patients now leave the hospital with a referral for home health care services in an attempt to reduce readmission to the hospital within 30 days and thus avoid financial penalties to the hospital.*

Home health care can improve care transitions through medication reconciliation, patient and caregiver education related to a recent hospitalization, symptoms that warrant medical attention and notification, and ensuring timely practitioner follow-up [20]. Multiple health care providers and family members are often involved in the patient's care as the patient transitions from one health care setting to another. Effective communication among providers during these "transitions in care" is paramount to ensuring that providers and families are informed of the need to change the patient's plan of care [21–23].

A physician or advance care provider can provide either a **written or verbal** order to the home health agency to begin services. The referral should include information on the patient's overall functional status as well as the primary reason for the referral while respecting the patient's preferences and goals of care. Background information regarding the caregivers in the home and any concerns should be shared with the home health agency to help clarify potential barriers that may affect the patient's outcome.

Physician Reimbursement for Home Health Care Services

Certification/Recertification Codes

Physicians or advance practice providers who order home health care from a qualified Medicare agency are eligible to receive payment for reviewing the home health care agency plan of care. Once a referral to home health has been made, the physician or advance practice provider will receive an *initial certification form (Form 485)*, to review and agree with the plan of care, and to return the signed and dated form to the home health care agency. The face-to-face necessity documentation is only required for the **initial** certification. Upon review and completion of the Form 485, *the physician or advance practice provider can bill for the initial certification period/initial plan of care (G01800), as well as subsequent recertification (G0179)*. Note that each certification period is for 60 days. Speak to your billing department to ensure that your documentation to support these codes meets the criteria to bill for completing this form.

Care Plan Oversight Code

If a physician or advance practice provider spends a minimum of 30 min in a 30-day period providing oversight and directing services during an episode of home health, he or she is allowed to bill for Care Plan Oversight (CPO) using code (G0181). When billing for CPO the time involved must be documented throughout the 30-day period (Table 6). One important caveat is that surgeons are not allowed to bill for CPO as it is already bundled into the fee for postoperative care. Table 7 lists the G codes for home health care. Physicians are encouraged to document and bill for CPO; however physicians *are not allowed to concurrently bill for Transitional Care Management Services* or *Chronic Care Coordination* during a CPO 30-day period unless they decide not to bill for CPO.

Table 6 Billing for home health care services

	Initial certification	Recertification	CPO
Licensed doctor (M.D./D.O.)	Yes	Yes	Yes
Resident doctor (in-training)	No	No	No
Non-physician practitioner (NP/PA)	Yes	Yes	Yes

Table 7 Certification, recertification, CPO codes

Code	Description
G0180-certification	Initial home health certification, also known as reviewing and signing the initial plan of care (Form 485)
G0179-recertification	Recertification of the plan of care: if the patient's care continues for an additional 60 days, the physician must review and sign recertification plan of care (Form 485)
G0181-care plan oversight	Indicated for the supervision of a patient under the care of a Medicare-certified home health care agency (patient not present). Oversight is indicated for the patient whose care is complex and involves multiple disciplines, therapy that requires regular physician/NP/PA contact

Summary: The Future of Home Health Care

Due to the projected growth in the number of people living with chronic illness and the likelihood for escalating medical expenditures, the provision of medical care in the home continues to evolve as a viable option for clinicians and their practice. Home-based medical care can help lessen the cost associated for caring for patients with serious illnesses. As such, the Centers for Medicare and Medicaid (CMS) is exploring various innovative and alternative health care delivery models in an attempt to contain future costs. For example, new technological advances that allow distance monitoring of vital signs in the home of patients with heart failure in order to identify exacerbations early and to prevent costly hospitalization have been used with great success [24]. Telemedicine technology not only allows home health nurses to monitor a patient's vital signs and daily weight from a distance, but also to share this information with practitioners. Other models of care such as the "hospital at home" programs can reduce the high costs associated with hospitalization while still obtaining as good a health outcome for patients who opt to receive such treatment at home, are promising [25, 26].

Pearls for the Practitioner
- Many frail elderly are homebound and experience great difficulty in accessing timely and needed health care services, including regular visits to a physician's office.
- Home care is defined as the provision of health care-related services and durable medical equipment to patients in the home for the purpose of restoring and maintaining his or her maximal level of function, comfort, and health.

- Home health care provides an interdisciplinary team of qualified professionals that strives to maximize outcomes for patients.
- Home health care services are best delivered by determining both **health care** and **life goals** with the patient and family and then developing a plan of care that can sustain the efforts in reaching those goals.
- Only licensed physicians working with a qualified Medicare agency are eligible to receive payment for reviewing and signing the home health care agency plan of care (Form 485). But physician assistants and advanced practice nurses are allowed to bill for Care Plan Oversight.
- During a home visit clinicians should not only assess the patient's medical conditions, but also assess the patient's functional status, cognitive ability, and level of independence/dependence.
- Patients are **not** required to be homebound in order for a physician to visit and to submit billing for the house call.
- The documentation of a face-to-face encounter must occur either within **90 days prior** to the start date of home health care **or within 30 days after the start of care** and is only required for initial certification and not recertification. Each certification period is 60 days.
- The face-to-face encounter form should include the name of the certifying physician, date of encounter, the patient's homebound status, the need for skilled services, signature, and date of the ordering physician.

References

1. Census Bureau releases comprehensive analysis of fast-growing 90-and-older population. https://www.census.gov/newsroom/releases/archives/aging_population/cb11-194.html. Accessed 16 June 2015.
2. Holtz-Eakin D. High-cost medicare beneficiaries. Congressional Budget Office. 2005. p. 1–12. http://www.cbo.gov/ftpdocs/63xx/doc6332/05-03-MediSpending.pdf.
3. Roberts DC, McKay MP, Shaffer A. Increasing rates of emergency department visits for elderly patients in the United States, 1993 to 2003. Ann Emerg Med. 2008;51(6):769–74.
4. Baker DW, Einstadter D, Husak SS, Cebul RD. Trends in postdischarge mortality and readmissions: has length of stay declined too far? Arch Intern Med. 2004;164(5):538–44.
5. Kane RL. Finding the right level of posthospital care: "we didn't realize there was any other option for him". JAMA. 2011;305(3):284–93.
6. Murkofsky RL, Alston K. The past, present, and future of skilled home health agency care. Clin Geriatr Med. 2009;25(1):1–17.
7. Levine SA, Boal J, Boling PA. Home care. JAMA. 2003;290(9):1203–7.
8. Lukas L, Foltz C, Paxton H. Hospital outcomes for a home-based palliative medicine consulting service. J Palliat Med. 2013;16(2):179–84.
9. De Jonge KE, Jamshed N, Gilden D, Kubisiak J, Bruce SR, Taler G. Effects of home-based primary care on Medicare costs in high-risk elders. J Am Geriatr Soc. 2014;62(10):1825–31.
10. Labson MC, Sacco MM, Weissman DE, Gornet B, Stuart B. Innovative models of home-based palliative care. Cleve Clin J Med. 2013;80(Electronic Suppl 1):eS30.
11. Toto P. Success through teamwork in the home health setting: the role of occupational therapy. Home Health Care Manag Pract. 2006;19(1):31–7.

12. Mager DR. Medication errors and the home care patient. Home Healthc Nurse. 2007;25(3):151–5.
13. Forster AJ, Murff HJ, Peterson JF, Gandhi TK, Bates DW. The incidence and severity of adverse events affecting patients after discharge from the hospital. Ann Intern Med. 2003;138(3):161–7.
14. Meredith S, Feldman P, Frey D, Giammarco L, Hall K, Arnold K, et al. Improving medication use in newly admitted home healthcare patients: a randomized controlled trial. J Am Geriatr Soc. 2002;50(9):1484–91.
15. Coleman EA, Smith JD, Raha D, Min SJ. Posthospital medication discrepancies: prevalence and contributing factors. Arch Intern Med. 2005;165(16):1842–7.
16. Boult C, Reider L, Frey K, et al. Early effects of "guided care" on the quality of health care for multimorbid older persons: a cluster randomized control trial. J Gerontol A Biol Sci Med Sci. 2008;63A(3):321–32.
17. Stevens JA, Thomas K, Teh L, Greenspan AI. Unintentional fall injuries associated with walkers and canes in older adults treated in U.S. emergency departments. J Am Geriatr Soc. 2009;57(8):1464–9.
18. Fortinsky RH, Baker D, Gottschalk M, King M, Trella P, Tinetti ME. Extent of implementation of evidence-based fall prevention practices for older patients in home health care. J Am Geriatr Soc. 2008;56(4):737–43.
19. Medicare Benefit Policy Manual. Chapter 7 home health service. http://www.cms.gov/Regulations-and-Guidance/Guidance/Manuals/downloads/bp102c07.pdf. Accessed 16 June 2015.
20. Gorodeski EZ, Chlad S, Vilensky S. Home-based care for heart failure: Cleveland Clinic's "Heart Care at Home" transitional care program. Cleve Clin J Med. 2013;80(Electronic Suppl 1):eS20–6.
21. Coleman EA, Berenson RA. Lost in transition: challenges and opportunities for improving the quality of transitional care. Ann Intern Med. 2004;141(7):533–6.
22. Kripalani S, LeFevre F, Phillips CO, Williams MV, Basaviah P, Baker DW. Deficits in communication and information transfer between hospital-based and primary care physicians: implications for patient safety and continuity of care. JAMA. 2007;297(8):831–41.
23. Kuo YF, Sharma G, Freeman JL, Goodwin JS. Growth in the care of older patients by hospitalists in the United States. N Engl J Med. 2009;360(11):1102–12.
24. Boling PA, Chandekar RV, Hungate B, Purvis M, Selby-Penczak R, Abbey LJ. Improving outcomes and lowering costs by applying advanced models of in-home care. Cleve Clin J Med. 2013;80(Electronic Suppl 1):eS7–14.
25. Leff B, Burton L, Mader SL, et al. Hospital at home: feasibility and outcomes of a program to provide hospital-level care at home for acutely ill older patients. Ann Intern Med. 2005;143(11):798–808.
26. Sheppard S, Doll H, Angus R, et al. Avoiding hospital admission through provision of hospital care at home: a systematic review and meta-analysis of individual patient data. Can Med Assoc J. 2009;80(2):175–82.

Assisted Living and Residential Care

Debra Dobbs, Carlyn E. Vogel, Daniel Haimowitz, and Sheryl Zimmerman

Introduction

Assisted living has become an integral component of LTC for persons who neither require nor choose to avail themselves of nursing home services in preference for a less institutionalized care setting. AL is usually less expensive than the cost of long-term nursing home care (though its cost may vary considerably both within a state or from state to state). AL aspires **to optimize resident autonomy, privacy, and dignity.** Due to a variety of factors that includes a resident's desire to "age in place," and to remain as independent as long as possible, together with shorter hospital stays and the provision of more acute care in AL/RC, many residents eventually experience an increase in functional dependence and healthcare needs similar to nursing home residents of 20–30 years ago.

This chapter will provide an overview of AL—its history, definition, facility and resident characteristics, resident rights, financing, and staffing. As well as disaster preparedness and COVID-19, the provision of medical care, medication management, the clinician's role (be it physician or mid-level practitioner), models of care,

D. Dobbs (✉) · C. E. Vogel
School of Aging Studies, College of Behavioral and Community Sciences, University of South Florida, Tampa, FL, USA

D. Haimowitz
Levittown, PA, USA

S. Zimmerman
Program on Aging, Disability, and Long-Term Care, Cecil G. Sheps Center for Health Services Research, University of North Carolina at Chapel Hill, Chapel Hill, NC, USA

© The Author(s), under exclusive license to Springer Nature Switzerland AG 2023
P. Winn et al. (eds.), *Post-Acute and Long-Term Care Medicine*, Current Clinical Practice, https://doi.org/10.1007/978-3-031-28628-5_3

communication and care coordination, medical direction, and practitioner billing. It concludes with a discussion on the future of AL and clinical suggestions for practitioners.

Assisted Living

History

The AL *industry* has experienced rapid growth over the past 15–20 years in response to the needs of older adults who can no longer live independently nor be cared for at home by family. Core values of AL include resident autonomy, choice, privacy, dignity, and to age in a home-like environment. In comparison to nursing homes, the availability of AL has increased dramatically because of the increase in the older adult population, the need for supportive care, and States' limits on the number of certified nursing home beds. A wide variety of AL communities exist, ranging from small "mom and pop" homes with as few as four beds to large AL communities housing several hundred residents. Many are for-profit. There is a multitude of names for AL nationally (Table 1), which will be hereafter referred to as Assisted Living Communities (ALCs). Both the varied needs of consumers and the variety of service options drive the AL *market.*

There has been controversy as to whether AL is a social or medical model of care. Although these models often coexist, many stakeholders and owners emphasize the social model perspective to stress the home-like intent of AL and oppose requirements for increased medical oversight and increased State regulation. However, over time, and in recognition of instances of elder neglect and abuse that has occurred, the need for increased regulatory oversight became evident. This varies from state-to-state.

Given the variability of quality in AL, the National Assisted Living Workgroup was established in 2003 at the request of the US Senate Special Committee on Aging. Subsequently this workgroup submitted 110 recommendations aimed at improving quality in AL—one of which was the establishment of the Center for Excellence in Assisted Living (CEAL), an informational clearinghouse, promoting research, best practices, and policy review. CEAL has stressed the importance of *person-centered care*, defined as *"a comprehensive and on-going process of*

Table 1 Various names for Assisted Living Communities (ALCs)

Adult congregate living care, adult foster care, adult homes, adult living communities, basic care communities, board and care, catered living services, community-based retirement communities, community residence communities, community residential care communities, congregate care, domiciliary care, elder care homes, enhanced care, enhanced living, home for the aged, old-age homes, personal care, residential care communities for the elderly, residential communities for groups, retirement residences, service-enriched housing, shared housing establishments, sheltered housing, supportive care, and supported living *transforming an entity's culture and operation into a nurturing, empowering one that promotes purpose and meaning and supports well-being for individuals in a relationship-based home environment"* [1]. CEAL has developed a Toolkit on Person-Centered Practices in Assisted Living (PC-PAL)[2]. Through resident and staff questionnaires the toolkit focuses on measuring an ALC's person-centeredness with the goal of promoting ongoing quality improvement.

Definition

Variation among different ALCs makes it challenging to establish a uniform definition of AL. The AL Workgroup has developed the following definition:

Assisted living is a state regulated and monitored residential LTC option. Assisted living provides or coordinates oversight and services to meet the residents' individualized scheduled needs, based on residents' assessments and service plans, and their unscheduled needs as they arise [2].

Services required by state law and regulation must include but not limited to:

- 24-h *awake* staff to provide oversight and meet scheduled and unscheduled resident needs
- Provision and oversight of personal and supportive services (assistance with physical, i.e., basic activities of daily living)
- Health-related services (e.g., medication management)
- Social services
- Recreational activities
- Meals
- Housekeeping and laundry services
- Transportation service

Community Characteristics

One of the key differences between nursing homes and AL communities is that there are **no federal regulations for AL.** Accordingly, each state has developed its own regulations. Some advocates propose that there could be potential benefit to federal oversight in order to establish more clear and uniform standards that promote *quality resident care* and *safety*.

Due to varied State regulations, ALCs differ widely in size, levels of care, and philosophy. The adage "if you've seen one AL community you've seen one AL community" applies. Many are freestanding communities, while others may be part of a continuing care retirement community (CCRC). Sixty-five percent of ALCs serve up to 25 residents, 31% have 26–100 beds, while 4% have greater than 100 beds. More than 50% of residents dwell in ALCs of 26 or more beds [3]. Rooms are typically a private or semiprivate studio and a one- or two-bedroom apartment. Proponents of AL usually admonish against shared rooms unless by choice. There are many corporate AL chains, 81% being for-profit, 18% nonprofit, and 1% government/other [3]. In 2020, the largest were Brookdale Senior Living, Sunrise Senior Living, Five Star Senior Living, Enlivant and Atria Senior Living [4]. Most Western and Midwestern states have a higher number of ALCs than the national average. In the West there is a comparable number of ALC and nursing home beds per 1000 persons aged 65 and over, whereas nursing home beds outnumber ALC beds in other regions of the country [3].

Staffing

Staffing in ALCs can vary widely. There is no requirement for a nurse to be on site, although more than half of facilities do have a RN or LPN on staff [5]. Half provide social work services [3], and activities/recreational staff are more frequent in larger communities. Documentation and charting will vary with *state-specific regulations* and *scope of practice* such as whether AL staff are able to take verbal orders from physicians and other healthcare professionals. State regulations and community-specific policies also may vary as to which medical conditions would preclude admission or give cause for a resident to be discharged from an ALC. Ventilator dependency, stage IV pressure injuries, the need for intravenous fluids, and communicable airborne infections that would require resident isolation would usually prohibit admission to AL. However, ALCs may choose to admit residents who need a moderate level of physical assistance such as with transfers to a wheelchair.

A special license or certification to provide *dementia care* in ALCs is required in 40 states, and research has shown the need for state regulation to promulgate requirements to ensure appropriate dementia care [5]. State regulators have begun to focus on dementia care especially related to resident safety, staff training, and provision of dementia-friendly activities [5]. Organizations such as the National Alzheimer's Association have developed guidance for dementia care for ALC staff [6]. In 2016, 14% of ALCs had a dementia care unit and 9% of facilities served only adults living with dementia [3].

Resident Characteristics

Resident characteristics often reflect facility admission and discharge policies, state regulation, and affordability for resident families. In 2016, 29% of residents needed assistance with transfer [3]. Though the level of ADL dependency is not as extensive as that seen in nursing home residents, it does exceed that of community-dwelling older adults. Residents generally need assistance with at least two ADLs and have a median length of stay of 22 months [7].

Residents with dementia usually require more social and behavioral support, and less medical care. Overall, 42% of residents have Alzheimer dementia or other age-related dementia [3]. Prevalence rates of *dementia* range from 24 to 47% while rates of *cognitive impairment* can range as high as 90% [5, 8]. Residents are typically non-Hispanic white, female, and age 85 or older [7]. Recently there has been a slight increase in non-white residents [9], with more having multiple medical conditions. Hypertension and dementia are the most prevalent [10]; while other common conditions include heart disease, depression, arthritis, and osteoporosis [11]. *Multiple medication use* is a major concern. Residents take an average of 12–14 medications, and 78% require assistance taking their medication [12, 13]. Thus, *polypharmacy* and *medication management* are important issues that need to be addressed by facility staff and practitioners. While some residents are either entirely or partially responsible for making the decision to move into an ALC, for other residents, their spouse, adult children, or other family member often make this decision. More than 70% of residents move into an ALC from their own home or apartment, and 60% relocate within 10 miles of their previous permanent residence [6]. Overall, 60–90% of residents are satisfied with the care they receive. The two main reasons residents leave an ALC are a change in health status or unfortunately, death. About 60% of residents eventually need to transition to a long-term nursing facility after a stay of 22 months [7] while others either move back home or to a relative's home, or transfer to a different ALC. Understanding facility resident admission and discharge criteria can facilitate clinicians/ practitioners discussions with residents and families who decide on what is best to meet a resident's care needs during their anticipated illness trajectory.

Residents' Rights

A resident has the right to choose and receive services that promote dignity, autonomy, independence, and quality of life. Needed and requested services should be agreed upon in the contract between the ALC and resident. While AL does not generally provide ongoing skilled nursing, residents are *eligible to receive home health services on an intermittent basis* to meet skilled nursing needs. Residents are also entitled to receive hospice services if the plan of care at the AL is able to accommodate the needs of the resident within the policies of the community.

An ongoing concern is that residents and families are often unaware of ALC level of services (often tiered) and its costs. Marketing information should be transparent and disclose all ALC fees and services to the resident/family prior to signing the admission contract. The ALC needs to inform residents and families on its transfer and discharge policies including the appeals process. The AL Workgroup recommendations regarding resident rights and ALC responsibilities are listed in Tables 2 and 3, respectively.

Table 2 Resident rights

Within the boundaries set by law, residents have the right to …
• Be shown consideration and respect
• Be treated with dignity
• Exercise autonomy
• Exercise civil and religious rights and liberties
• Be free from chemical and physical restraints
• Be free from physical, mental, fiduciary, sexual and verbal abuse, and neglect
• Have free reciprocal communication with and access to the LTC ombudsmen program
• Voice concerns and complaints to the ALC orally and in writing without reprisal
• Review and obtain copies of their own records that the ALC maintains
• Receive and send mail promptly and unopened
• Private unrestricted communication with other
• Privacy for phone calls and right to access a phone
• Privacy for couples and for visitors
• Privacy in treatment and caring for personal needs
• Manage their own financial affairs
• Confidentiality concerning financial, medical, and personal affairs
• Guide the development and implementation of their service plans
• Participate in and appeal the discharge (move-out) planning process
• Involve family members in making decisions about services
• Arrange for third-party services at their own expense[a]
• Accept or refuse services
• Choose their own physicians, dentists, pharmacists, and other health professionals
• Choose to execute advance directives
• Exercise choice about end-of-life care
• Participate or refuse to participate in social, spiritual, or community activities
• Arise and retire at times of their own choosing
• Form and participate in resident councils
• Furnish their own rooms and use and retain personal clothing and possessions
• Exercise choice and lifestyle as long as it does not interfere with other residents' rights
• Unrestricted contact with visitors and others as long as that does not infringe on other residents' rights
• Come and go rights that one would enjoy in their own home
• In addition, residents' family members have the right to form and participate in family councils

[a] An ALC may require that providers of third-party services ensure that they and their employees have passed criminal background checks, are free from communicable diseases, and are qualified to perform the duties they are hired to perform

Table 3 ALC responsibilities

In the context of resident rights, the ALC has a responsibility to …
• Promote an environment of civility, good manners, and mutual consideration by requiring staff, and encouraging residents, to speak to one another in a respectful manner
• Provide all services for the resident or the resident's family that have been contracted for by the resident and the provider as well as those services that are required by law
• Obtain accurate information from residents that is sufficient to make an informed decision regarding admission and the services to be provided
• Maintain an environment free of illegal weapons and illegal drugs
• Obtain notification from residents of any third-party services they are receiving and establish reasonable policies and procedures related to third-party services
• Report information regarding resident welfare to state agencies or other authorities as required by law
• Establish reasonable house rules in coordination with the resident council
• Involve staff and other providers in the development of resident service plans
• Maintain an environment that is free from physical, mental, fiduciary, sexual and verbal abuse, and neglect

Financing

Costs for assisted living tend to be significantly lower than those for nursing home care and are usually private pay. Infrequently, LTC insurance is the payment source. Costs vary widely depending on AL type, resident care needs, and geographic region. The median annual cost for a private room is $51,600 compared to $105,850 for a private nursing home room. Annual costs are lowest in Missouri ($36,000) and highest in Delaware ($80,280) [14]. Costs usually include monthly rent, meals, and basic services. Unlike skilled nursing facilities, there is no Medicare reimbursement to ALCs, but 44 states have a *Medicaid waiver program* under the Centers for Medicare & Medicaid Services (CMS) to cover personal and skilled care for *qualified low-income residents*. In 2016 Medicaid covered some services for 17% of residents [3]. These waivers are only available when a resident meets *both* the state's criteria for being "nursing home eligible" *and* meet the Medicaid financial eligibility requirement. However, residents often experience a long delay before receiving such a waiver. ALC providers often report inadequate reimbursement under these waiver programs. As of 2020, 25 states administer Medicaid through *managed care* in order to better coordinate care and to contain costs for Medicaid recipients with complex healthcare needs [15]. The lack of public funding for AL makes affordability a major concern for the future viability of the AL industry. Another concern is "a la carte" pricing policies by many ALCs, with additional changes when residents need increased assistance. As many residents have limited funds, families may be reluctant or unable to pay the increased fees, resulting in substandard care. Despite concerns about affordability, only 6% of residents move out of an ALC due to financial reasons [6].

Staff Training

Both a sufficient number **and** sufficiently trained staff **and** 24-h staffing should be available at the ALC. Staff should be familiar with the changes that occur with normal aging and be trained in the basics of medication management and the recognition and assessment of medical and social problems that commonly occur in older adults. When staff lack education and training in basic geriatric principles, nor recognize a resident change in condition, emerging conditions may go undetected and result in increased morbidity and unnecessary hospitalization.

Ideally, staff should be able to determine when to contact a family member and/or the resident's assigned practitioner when a significant *change of condition* occurs. State regulations now require more rigorous staff and administrative training. Most states require *dementia care training* for direct care staff [10]. As a majority of ALCs admit and retain residents near the end of life, *palliative and end-of-life care* education are increasingly important for nursing and direct care staff [16]. End-of-life training for staff has been associated with a greater utilization of hospice and more engagement with family and residents in advance care planning [17].

Studies have shown that the most common resident/family complaints and survey deficiencies cited are related to medication administration (48%), staffing and staff qualifications (41%), and services insufficient to meet resident needs (36%) [18]. A report in 2020 found similar results with the two most common cited deficiencies among Florida ALCs related to staffing requirements and lack of staff in-service training [19].

Disaster Preparedness and COVID-19

Disaster preparedness and response, including that to the recent COVID-19 pandemic, require an *all-hazards approach*, whereby disaster planning incorporates common principles that can be readily adapted to a specific event, such as a hurricane, wildfire, earthquake, or pandemic [20]. Although most states require ALCs to have a disaster plan, these plans are not as prescriptive as those for nursing facilities [21]. As a case in point, less than 10% of ALCs in Florida reported having a pandemic emergency plan separate from an infection control plan [20].

Despite accounting for less than 1% of the US population, LTC settings have disproportionately contributed to 5% of COVID-19 cases [22]. As of March 2021, the "Atlantic COVID-19 Tracker" project reported that 1 out of every 12 COVID deaths in the USA occurred in residents of LTC facilities (including nursing homes and ALCs) [23]. Most of the federal guidance recommendations for COVID-19 are related nursing facilities and do not take into consideration the unique situation of ALCs (such as the designation of as "essential," workers who care for residents with dementia). Common strategies that facilitate family visitation during COVID-19 included use of technology such as face-time via Skype and Google Hangouts, window visits, and outdoor socially distanced visits. COVID-19 testing in ALCs has also been a challenge. In order to meet this need, some communities have contracted a physician to serve as their "Director of Laboratory" in order to meet CLIA requirements.

Decisions made by ALC administrators *before, during*, and *after* hazard events are varied. Among 143 ALCs that were affected by hurricanes in 2004 and 2005, three-quarters sheltered residents in place, while 23% evacuated during at least one hurricane [24]. For Hurricane Irma (2017), administrators who had worked for at least 10 years in ALCs felt more prepared and had increased confidence in the decision to either evacuate or shelter in place [21]. **Also vital is collaboration with local emergency operation centers and state agencies.** During both Hurricane Irma and the COVID-19 pandemic, administrators in ALCs with more than 25 beds and part of a corporate chain were more satisfied with the level of collaboration with state agencies compared to others who were not [20]. The availability of corporate resources of larger ALCs can have an essential role in the coordination of the needs of the ALC. The establishment of state healthcare coalitions can bring together private and public organizations to share emergency response responsibilities [20].

Medical Care

The clinician's role in AL has been largely undefined, due in part to the industry's history of distinguishing between the "medical" vs. "social" models of care, and the concern that involvement of medical providers may result in "medicalization" and higher costs [25, 26]. AMDA—The Society for Post-Acute and LTC Medicine has stressed the importance of medical care in AL, and convened a consensus conference to address the needs and issues related to ALCs. Four concerns were identified: medication management, the clinician's role, communication and care coordination, and clinical direction [27].

Medication Management

Medication management is a major concern. As in other settings, it entails evidence-based prescribing, e-prescribing, and administration. Healthcare providers should be knowledgeable about the basic tenets of geriatric prescribing (see the chapter "Medication Management in Long-Term Care" for a more detailed review). These tenets include the five "Rs"—the **R**ight medication, at the **R**ight time, the **R**ight dose, and the **R**ight route of administration for the **R**ight patient. The Beers Criteria of *potentially inappropriate* medications for older adults is a useful guide [28]. Unlike skilled nursing facilities, there is no federal requirement for a consultant pharmacist to perform a monthly medication review. However, consultant pharmacists do provide medication review and monitoring at 84% of ALCs [10]. The over-prescribing of medication [29] is an issue that consultant pharmacists can address, particularly for those who have advanced qualifications in geriatric pharmacy patient care.

Administration of medication can result in errors if unskilled non-licensed staff have had inadequate training and/or supervision. However, sufficiently trained medication aides in ALCs do **not** commit more errors than LPNs [30]. Requirements for the extent of staff training and oversight of medication administration do vary among states, as does allowing nurse delegation [31]. In addition, staff may lack assessment skills, and result in medication-related adverse side effects being unrecognized. Furthermore, unlike in nursing homes, medical providers may not be notified when a resident has refused to take his/her medication. Also challenging is allowing residents to self-administer medication, which over time may become unsafe. Adding to the complexity is the use of over-the-counter medication and alternative and herbal therapies, and those brought to the resident by family members.

Other medication issues include diverse record keeping and untimely medication delivery and storage. Order changes, inadequate medication monitoring, and multiple provider prescribing, all challenge safe medication management. Although **medical practitioners** may have no influence on a particular ALC's structure, staff competency, ongoing quality improvement processes, or accountability in regard to medication administration and management, **they can offer expertise in medication management.**

When applying the basic principles of medication management in older adults, careful consideration must be given to the fact that any medication can cause side effects. Because staff may have limited training, common geriatric syndromes potentially caused by medication (e.g., falls, incontinence, change in appetite, new or worsened mental status) may be unrecognized. Without well-established notification channels, the attending clinician may be unaware when new medications are prescribed or doses changed by another practitioner. In addition, as in nursing homes, medications are often prescribed without a face-to-face visit by the practitioner.

Because the federal government categorizes an AL resident the same as a community-dwelling person in regard to Medicare Part D (the benefit for medication coverage), residents and their families may be presented with higher pharmacy costs when reaching the "donut hole," at which time the increased costs, combined with other AL fees, can result in significant financial hardship for the resident and family.

Clinician's Role and Models of Care

Residents often require an initial assessment by a practitioner prior to move-in, with the assessment varying by state and facility. Toward that end, one of the recommendations of the AMDA consensus conference was to develop standard assessment tools and clinical protocols to help improve clinical care [27]. Unlike a formal mandatory plan of care in a nursing home, the ALC may develop a **"service plan,"** which is similar in nature. Some service plans, however, may *not* incorporate a healthcare plan.

Unlike nursing homes where there are mandatory medical visits every 60 days, *ALC residents are required to be seen at least annually.* Follow-up care can be provided by private community-based clinicians. As previously noted, ALCs can use contract services from home health and hospice agencies. It is important to recognize that residents typically receive care by clinicians who are neither geriatricians nor specialty trained in geriatrics or long-term care medicine. These clinicians may have an age bias and not recognize the special challenges and needs of the aging ALC resident, and not be cognizant of the risks inherent to hospitalization (e.g., delirium, pressure injuries, inappropriate prescribing, and nosocomial infections).

Many residents continue to receive routine medical care in a medical office/clinic outside the ALC, by the providers who had treated them prior to their move into the facility. However, there is an increasing use of models of care where physicians either alone or in combination with nurse practitioners and/or physician assistants, visit residents at the ALC on a regular basis. One study has shown that 50% of physicians visited an AL setting *once a year or less*, while only 20% visited weekly or more [32]. Another study using CMS 2017 claims data found that fewer than 0.001% of clinicians who care for ALC residents had more than 80% of their billing attributed to care to residents in ALCs. Though this number is minute, it is 56% increase from 2014 [33]. Many ALCs have recognized the benefit of medical care being provided on-site (see Table 4).

Table 4 Benefits of medical care providers performing on-site care at an ALC

• Learns about ALC capabilities
• Sees resident in their own environment
• Improved communication with AL staff
• Increased reimbursement from Center for Medicaid and Medicare for domiciliary codes
• No need for community transportation/escort costs
• No need for family transport time/costs
• More efficient use of clinician and staff time
• Increased resident/family/community satisfaction
• Potential for more patients for the clinician
• Potential for improved resident care
• Potential for reduced medical errors
• Better marketing/public relations for community

Communication and Care Coordination

Effective communication and care coordination is essential to healthcare in all settings. There is a need to develop professional and respectful relationships between the ALCs staff and the residents' medical providers that can facilitate clear and timely communication, especially as it relates to medication management and ongoing documentation of resident health status [26]. However, poor communication can occur at multiple levels. Staff may have no formalized "sign out" between shifts, insufficient assessment skills, nor when and how to contact providers. Practitioners may not receive accurate information from staff (especially after hours), nor be aware of the ALC's capabilities. Many clinicians who practice only in the hospital and/or the community are unaware of the differences in the provision of care and services available between ALCs and nursing homes. This lack of awareness is problematic when a resident returns from the emergency department or hospital to the ALC that lacks the ability to provide needed monitoring and treatment, or when a resident, who remains at the ALC is no longer able to receive the level of care needed. For this reason, some suggest the development of a medical provider education packet that describes the health and medical services that the ALC is capable to provide to residents [26].

Care Coordination and Care Transitions

Lapses in care and commination commonly occur when older adults are either newly admitted to an ALC or readmitted from the hospital. The "National Transitions of Care Coalition" website includes information and tools for consumers, facilities, and healthcare professionals to facilitate transitions of residents between healthcare facilities. It is important for practitioners to assure that residents are transferred back to the ALC when safe to do so. Additional services provided by a home care agency may be necessary. To ensure a safe, appropriate, and timely transition of care, staff should be encouraged *to evaluate the resident prior to their return from the hospital or skilled nursing facility.*

Care Coordination and Technology

While most ALCs lag behind hospitals and nursing homes in the use of technology, advances have been made. As of 2016, 26% of ALCs used some form of electronic health records [34]. High-tech sensor devices and other innovations are already in use in ALCs to better monitor residents, as are various tool, such as medication reminders, fall detection systems, and technologies to help residents to stay engaged and connected with friends and family [35]. Smart home technology is being increasingly used, such as the TabSafe In-Home Medication Dispensing System that can assist older adults with medication management and allows providers both to make medication adjustments and to monitor as-needed (PRN) medication use. Smart toilets and bladder scanners are already available to monitor residents in some ALCs. In addition, assistive robots can help older adults overcome physical limitations and to safely engage in daily activities. Cost savings may be possible if robot "companions" enable ALC corporations to virtually visit communities while telemedicine can enable clinicians to promptly assess residents in remote regions. With the COVID-19 pandemic, more frequent use of telemedicine will continue for non-pandemic care.

Care Coordination and Accountable Care Organizations

As part of the Affordable Care Act, Accountable Care Organizations (ACOs) were enacted in 2012 to serve as *provider networks to share financial responsibility and risk* for providing care to a defined Medicare fee-for-service population. Under the law, an ACO must be responsible for at least 5000 Medicare beneficiaries for at least 3 years [36]. If the ACO is able to provide better care as defined by certain quality metrics, and the care results in cost savings to Medicare via fewer days spent in the hospital, then providers who are part of the ACO will share in the Medicare savings. Nursing homes have played a key role in post-acute care as providers in ACOs. If nursing homes can provide quality care and avoid readmission to hospitals, this can result in considerable cost savings to the ACO. Four tenets (see below) are needed for AL providers to participate in a ACO provider network [37]. Due to a lack of necessary resources ALCs with less than 25 beds and those *not* part of a large corporate-owned chain have less leverage for contracting with an ACO.

- ALCs should assess both their ability and intent to keep residents out of the hospital; if the AL does not see itself as a network partner who is able to reduce hospital admissions, then being part of the ACO is not a good idea because of the financial penalties associated with frequent resident hospitalizations.
- ALCs should have strong care coordination programs. Lack of care coordination between care settings can lead to costly mistakes and not only frequent hospitalizations, but also medication errors [38].
- ALCs need to build coalitions with quality post-acute and LTC providers.
- ALCs need to measure and maintain partnerships, and to electronically track hospital admission rates and resident transitions: key data points that align with other ACO providers.

Clinical Direction (i.e., Medical Director or Not!)

Clinician confidence in staff has been shown to increase in smaller ALCs, when there is an increased presence of nursing staff and if the facility has established the position of a physician Medical Director [29]. Though there is no federal mandate that requires an ALC to have a Medical Director or Physician Advisor, some facilities have established this position. The AL Workgroup did not reach a majority consensus to support a recommendation that ALCs have a Medical Director, but did agree that an "external professional consultant" should be contracted. Not unsurprisingly, the need for increased "on site" medical oversight and coordination of care in AL become necessary during the COVID-19 pandemic [39].

Clinical Direction and Hospice

In 2016, hospice services were available in 81% of nursing homes and 68% of ALCs [3]. The addition of hospice care may allow residents to stay in the ALC during their final days of life. The Medicare hospice benefit provides an all-inclusive daily payment for hospice services based upon four levels of care: (1) routine home care, (2) general inpatient care, (3) inpatient respite care, and (4) continuous home care. Residents who receive hospice can receive routine home care (least expensive) or continuous home care (most expensive). Sixty percent of Medicare beneficiaries who received hospice in ALCs had an ill-defined condition, dementia, or Alzheimer's disease as their terminal diagnosis. Ill-defined conditions included, adult failure to thrive, senility without psychosis, and unspecified debility [40]. However, Medicare no longer accepts these nonspecific diagnoses.

The federal government has been scrutinizing hospice payments in ALCs. The US Department of Health and Human Services Office of Inspector General (OIG) released a report in 2015 entitled "Medicare Hospices Have Financial Incentives to Provide Care in Assisted Living Communities" as part of a mandate to reform the hospice payment system as directed by the Patient Protection and Affordable Care Act. The median length of stay on hospice per beneficiary is 98 days in ALCs, compared to 50 days in nursing homes, 30 days in skilled nursing, and 45 days in the home. The OIG concluded that hospices are incentivized to target ALCs because they offer the greatest financial gain to the hospice agency. Targeted reviews, adoption of claims-based measures of care, and making hospice data available to beneficiaries are subsequent recommendations. The entire report is available at www.oig. hhs.gov. In general, in all settings, the federal government is more closely scrutinizing the level of care at which a hospice is billing [40].

Practitioner Billing E/M Codes

The appropriate and correct use of billing codes is essential for practitioners. **Note as of January 1, 2023 assisted living visits should use the home visit E/M codes 99341, 99342, 99344, and 99345 for new patient visits and 99347, 99348, 99349, and 99350 for established patient visits.**

AL uses *Place of Service Code 13*. Reimbursement for AL medical services is generally higher than equivalent codes for other sites of service, such as the office and nursing home. This can serve as an incentive for clinicians to include AL resident visits in their practice.

The Future of Assisted Living

The increased number of AL beds, rising resident acuity, and concerns about the quality of care have resulted in increased scrutiny of the *AL industry*. Over time, state regulations have increased and more attention has been given to affordability. In 2014, CEAL convened a roundtable entitled "The Future of Assisted Living: Consumer Preferences and the Era of Healthcare Reform." At that time, the three main factors driving change in AL were increased resident medical acuity, the provision of healthcare transitions from traditional settings to non-institutional community settings through ACOs, and the increased expectations of baby boomers due to a higher level of education, more work experience and use of technology. The CEAL identified 14 major themes (Table 5), with key areas of focus being personnel, data, state regulations, and affordability.

In 2021, a diverse group of stakeholders came together through AMDA-The Society for Post-Acute and Long-Term Care to foresee the future of AL. They identified current issues related to *models of AL* (e.g., noting that the combination of services and housing limited consumer choice), *regulations* (e.g., while intended to improve quality, they often are outdated or ineffective), *financing* (e.g., AL costs are too expensive and so inaccessible to most consumers), *residents* (e.g., rising acuity necessitates a need for proficient healthcare), and the *nurse and direct care workforce* (e.g., insufficient numbers, training, and opportunities that limit the quality of care) [41]. Implications on future practice and policy and research were delineated.

The AL industry will likely follow nursing home trends toward quality improvement. The American Health Care Association and National Center for Assisted Living (AHCA/NCAL) have established *The Quality Initiative for AL*, which focuses on four core areas with measurable goals.

Table 5 Important themes in AL (asterisk indicates key themes)

• Aging in place
• Diverse models
• Future market
• Assisted living without walls
• Value proposition
• State regulations*
• Data*
• Technology in AL
• Personnel*
• Keeping the "home" in AL
• Risks and choice
• Affordability*
• Consumer education
• Flexibility

- Safely reducing hospital readmissions
- Reducing the off-label use of antipsychotics
- Increasing staff stability and
- Increasing customer satisfaction

Measurement tools and demonstrative cases can be downloaded from the NCAL website (NCAL.gov). ALCs are encouraged to use these tools to measure and track progress related to each core area. Practitioner leadership can greatly assist these initiatives.

By way of example, INTERACT (Interventions to Reduce Acute Care Transfers), a quality improvement program that was developed for nursing homes, has also been adapted for AL. INTERACT focuses on the *management of acute change* in a resident's condition. It includes validated clinical and educational tools and strategies for use in daily practice to improve the early identification, management, documentation, and communication of acute changes in resident condition, with the goal to prevent avoidable hospitalizations. The program has expanded to include tools specifically for AL providers and tested through support of a CMS Innovation Grant. Pilot communities assessed and provided feedback on the four categories of *INTERACT tools (quality improvement, communication, decision support,* and *advance care planning*) to help finalize the Assisted Living Version 1.0 tools, now publicly available at the INTERACT website http://interact2.net.

Clinical Suggestions for Practitioners

This section provides suggestions for healthcare providers aimed at optimizing their practice in AL. Some of the suggestions may be easier to accomplish if a Medical Director position has been established.

Adapt Already Established and Evidence-Based Policies and Procedures for AL

Many healthcare practitioners familiar with the workings of nursing homes also take care of AL residents. Nursing home residents are required to be seen at a minimum of every 60 days, and with the increasing acuity and frailty of ALC residents, it behooves clinicians to establish regular on-site visits for AL residents at least quarterly and more often if medically necessary. Pertinent guidelines can be adapted for use in ALCs, such as falls prevention, notification protocols, and reduction of antipsychotic medication. Use of a consultant pharmacist for monthly or quarterly medication reviews is encouraged. Suggestions for efficient time management in LTC are also applicable to clinician care in AL (Table 6) [42].

Table 6 Time management guidelines

• Limit practice to only 1–2 ALCs you know well
• Use a midlevel practitioner for management of routine problems
• Have a regular day for seeing residents at a particular community
• See the sickest patients first
• Develop protocols for common problems such as constipation, weight loss, falls, behavioral problems, and fever
• Train staff to limit after-hour telephone calls to urgent problems and provide mechanisms for staff to address nonurgent problems (such as daily telephone calls, regularly checked message lines or e-mails, and regular rounds by the healthcare practitioner)
• Speak with residents and families about advance directives shortly after admission and with major status changes; document these discussions clearly
• Anticipate future events and discuss expectations with the family in advance to aid in decision-making and the adjustment process
• Learn as much as possible about family dynamics to eliminate any surprises when healthcare decisions need to be made; communicate your expectations through discussions with staff, standing orders, and in-service programs
• Educate yourself about assisted living regulations, especially those affecting provision of medical and nursing services
• Work as a partner with the staff and care providers

Meet Regularly with the ALC Administrator

Getting buy-in from the administrator is an important strategy that can help improve resident care. The clinician may initiate topics for discussion and ask the administrator how clinician involvement can help with state survey compliance and ALC marketing. Improvement in mutual communication and medical documentation is generally an area of concern. Scheduled meetings can vary, from monthly to less often. Minutes from previous meetings should be kept, and it is recommended that the focus on an identified area of concern be continued until the problem is resolved, prior to addressing another area. If the administrator is unable to attend meetings, clinicians should at least keep in regular contact with whoever in the AL is the liaison for medical care. A clinician could also have opportunity to participate as a member of an "advisory committee" for overseeing the care being provided to residents by the rehabilitation, hospice, and home healthcare agencies that visit the facility.

Provide In-Service Training to Staff, Residents, and Family Members

A well-educated staff is a critical component to providing high quality care. For example, a clinician or a mid-level practitioner can present educational sessions to frontline staff on such topics as geriatric principles, medication administration and adverse drug effects, best practices in communication, the *Choosing Wisely* campaign(s), and common illnesses in older adults (e.g., dementia, hypertension, diabetes, stroke, mental health disorders). There are AL-specific articles in nursing journals that can benefit staff. In addition, residents and families are often eager to learn about common geriatric conditions, advance directives, and medication issues. Some ALCs have "family nights" at which clinician-led "Q and A" or "Ask the Doc" sessions can be invaluable. Many communities have resident and/or family councils. Clinician attendance at these councils can be of great value to improve education and communication and to help to identify other issues of concern within the community.

Ensure Effective Communication

Clinicians can help communities establish a process for timely notification when there is a change in patient status, a medication error, or a questionable treatment ordered by a consultant. The community should convey timely and accurate information whenever a resident leaves the community to see a different clinician (Table 7), and during an urgent or emergency transfer. It is vitally important to include the current medication regimen and *copies* of any advance directives for healthcare. As such, clinicians can help ALCs develop a packet of information for each resident that would be available in an emergency, including copies of items such as insurance information, family contact numbers, activity, diet, and treatment orders as well as past medical history, pertinent consultant reports, and lab results. Developing relationships and communicating with local emergency department providers and emergency medical services can be helpful, as inappropriate use of these resources can lead to unnecessary transfers, hospitalizations, patient/family stress, and excess costs [43]. In addition, transferred residents should be clearly identified that they reside in an ALC (and not a nursing home).

If an ALC does not have a resident medical chart, clinicians can share their office chart with the ALC. Use of a communication book can be useful to leave messages for and from the ALC staff. If there is a chart, the clinician should request a separate section for medical progress notes. Copying or scanning the ALC note into the office EMR or faxing the ALC note to the medical office can keep office records updated.

Providers have a responsibility to return telephone calls promptly and professionally. A major concern is the poor response time from primary care providers. Providers should establish a protocol so that the ALC knows how to contact their office for nonurgent and emergent calls. Having a system to contact the ALC is

Table 7 Standard information recommended for AL transfer/communication forms

Community name and phone and fax numbers	Attending physician name and information
Reason for transfer/consultation	Patient Name, DOB
Up-to-date medication list	Family contact information
Relevant H&P/progress notes/labs/X-rays	

essential, as well as identification of the point person to contact. Consider calling regularly at a specific time of day. Returning a call during the same staff shift can help limit miscommunication between shifts at the assisted living.

Communication with families on a regular basis is important and can prevent problems and misunderstanding and improve resident, family, and staff satisfaction. Family should be contacted whenever there is a change in resident status and when a resident is transferred out of the ALC. Discussing family expectations upon resident admission can help identify any that are unrealistic. Medication issues and medication costs are a frequent resident/family concern and should be addressed with the family at appropriate intervals.

Focus on High-Risk Medications and Medical Problems

Common geriatric disease states are often conducive to risk reduction strategies. As in nursing homes, special attention must be given to the prevention of falls and decubitus ulcers, diabetes management (especially hypoglycemia), and resident elopement. Some medications have more potential for significant harm than others, such as anticoagulants (e.g., warfarin), diabetic drugs (both oral and injectable), opioids, and antipsychotics. Many of the materials related to the *CMS National Partnership to Improve Dementia Care* and the reduction of antipsychotic use are applicable to AL (and referred in the 2015 GAO report "Antipsychotic Drug Use: HHS Initiatives to Reduce Use in Older Adults in Nursing Homes, but Should Expand Efforts to Other Settings"). The AMDA *Medicine Quality Prescribing Campaign* (based on an IOM report to prevent medication errors and promote safe prescribing) and more recently the AMDA "Drive to Deprescribe" initiative, offer additional information and guidance.

Initiate Discussions on Advance Directives for Healthcare

Many ALC residents either have no advance healthcare directive or have one that will not be applicable in an emergency situation. The importance of this was evident during the COVID-19 pandemic. Encouraging their use, as well as resident and staff education, can be instrumental in clarifying residents' preferences for care and for life. It is recommended that tools such as the POLST (Physician Orders for Life Sustaining Treatment) be used. The format of the POLST may differ from one state to another.

Encourage Preventive Medicine and Person-Centered Care

The importance of *health promotion, disease prevention,* and *wellness services* for AL residents is well recognized. ALCs present opportunities for treatment and management of chronic conditions, with potential resident benefit [27]. Examples include screening for cancer, Alzheimer's disease, hypercholesterolemia, and osteoporosis, as well as using immunization protocols and promoting exercise programs.

Person-centered care has been recognized as an important component of quality of life for AL residents, yet measures have only been developed recently to describe, quantify, and ultimately improve person-centered care. The Person-Centered Practices in AL (PC-PAL) has developed questionnaires to improve person-centeredness by measuring care from the perspectives of residents and staff, and is supported by multiple national organizations [44]. *Medical leadership* can help bring this material to the attention of ALC administration and encourage its use.

Urge Hiring of a Medical Director

The ALC administration or corporation may be unaware of the advantages of contracting a clinician as a Medical Director and may be concerned about its extra financial cost. It is important to recognize that appropriate medical direction may improve resident care, communication and marketing, lower liability risk, and prevent avoidable ER transfers and hospitalization.

As most ALCs do not have written policies or procedures for quality improvement related to medication management, drug regimen review, and monitoring for adverse drug events [45], such an initiative would be an opportune focus for Medical Director leadership. AMDA's *Position Statement on Assisted Living* lists some potential roles and responsibilities of an AL Medical Director (see Table 8). The challenge to the clinician is conveying the significant benefits this position can provide. There is evidence that having a full-time clinician at the ALC by itself can improve care, as one study showed a statistically significant decrease in hospitalizations and hospital days, and a suggestion of a decrease in falls [46]. ALCs might consider having a Medical Director *on retainer*, not as a dedicated position, but as

Table 8 Potential roles and responsibilities of AL medical director

Practitioner services
• Assist the ALC in ensuring that residents have appropriate physician coverage and ensure the provision of physician and healthcare practitioner services
• Assist the ALC in developing a process for reviewing physician and healthcare practitioners' credentials
• Provide specific guidance for physician and healthcare practitioner performance expectations
• Assist the ALC in ensuring that a system is in place for monitoring the performance of healthcare practitioners
• Facilitate feedback to physicians and other healthcare practitioners on performance and practices
• Assist the ALC with resident assessment and development of the clinical component of the service plan, when necessary

Table 8 (continued)

Clinical care
• Participate in administrative decision making and the development of policies and procedures related to resident care and medication management
• Participate in administrative decision making on staffing levels, coverage, licensing, and training requirements for resident-care staff
• Assist in developing, approving, and implementing specific clinical practices for the ALC to incorporate into care-related policies and procedures, including areas required by laws and regulations
• Review, respond to, and participate in federal, state, local, and other external inspections
• Assist in reviewing policies and procedures regarding the adequate protection of residents' rights, advance care planning, and other ethical issues

Quality of care
• Assist the ALC in establishing systems and methods for reviewing the quality and appropriateness of clinical care, medication management, and other health-related services and provide appropriate feedback
• Participate in the ALC's quality improvement process
• Advise on infection control issues and approve specific infection control policies to be incorporated into ALC policies and procedures
• Assist the ALC in providing a safe and caring environment with optimal levels of family and community involvement
• Assist in the promotion of employee health and safety
• Assist in the development and implementation of employee health policies and programs

Education, information, and communication
• Promote a learning culture within the community by educating, informing, and communicating
• Assist the ALC in developing medical information and communication systems with staff, residents, families, and others
• Assist in establishing appropriate relationships with other healthcare professionals

an administrative position to be available as needed. As some ALCs may have a clinician who sees a majority of their residents, he/she may become a sort of "de facto" Medical Director or consultant. Although, as such, this position does not provide coverage for administrative liability, the provider may be empowered to suggest or enact changes beneficial for resident care.

Guide Families and Colleagues to Available Resources

Clinicians often play an important role when older adults are no longer able to be cared for at home. Several organizations offer information and guides to choosing an ALC (e.g., National Center for Assisted Living, AARP, Assisted Living Federation of America). Hospital case managers may not be aware of these resources, including CEAL and AL consumer groups. Some areas of the country have literature available to families that list housing options including AL, such as SourceBook: Guide to Retirement Living for several eastern states.

Champion State "Mini-AL Workgroups"

One of the recommendations from the national AL Workgroup was to establish state-level public meetings to review its recommendations. Virginia has already convened such a meeting. Wisconsin has developed an innovative collaborative called the Wisconsin Coalition for Collaborative Excellence in Assisted Living (WCCEAL), which includes regulatory and public funding agencies, the state ombudsman's program, as well as state AL and residential care provider associations. This Collaborative has developed performance measures and satisfaction surveys that can be voluntarily used by Wisconsin AL providers as quality improvement tools. A clinician interested and involved in AL may have the opportunity to spearhead a "mini-AL Workgroup" or similar collaborative in their state.

Clinical Leadership in Quality Assurance/Performance Improvement (QAPI)

As data collection and analysis to improve resident outcomes is increasingly important, QAPI meetings are occurring more frequently in ALCs. The basic elements of QAPI are Design and Scope; Governance and Leadership; Feedback, Data Systems and Monitoring; Performance Improvement Projects (PIPs); and Systematic Analysis and Systemic Action. Data to assist ALCs in their relationships with ACOs can be tracked and evaluated through the QAPI process. The AHCA/NCAL *Quality Initiative for AL* also features QAPI principles. QAPI is mandated in nursing homes, and physician leadership should ideally take the lead to guide AL communities in adopting similar initiatives.

Summary

Physicians, nurse practitioners, and physician assistants play an essential role in the treatment of residents who live in ALCs. The trend of increasing resident medical acuity and recognition of the importance of healthcare providers in AL makes this an exciting time to practice in AL. Once understanding the capabilities of the ALC, the potential for clinician collaboration in establishing seamless community-based care, promotion of preventive care and wellness, early identification of sentinel events, and contribution to quality-of-life outcomes shows great promise [47]. Ideally, the clinician can be a "middle man" advocating for resident care and helping to establish a safety net for patient care [27] while understanding ALC concerns and striving to maintain affordability for residents and their families.

Pearls for the Practitioner
- ALCs are regulated by state agencies, which leads to significant state-to-state variability in rules, requirements, and terminology.

- ALCs vary significantly in size, resident characteristics, philosophy, staff, and resident care capabilities.
- Staff number, availability, training, and capabilities can vary greatly by state and location, leading to potential challenges with communication, medication management, and overall resident care.
- Treating residents in the ALC has benefits for residents, families, the staff, the faculty and practitioners.
- Many barriers to quality care may be addressed by increased clinician involvement in ALC. Promote the position of a physician consultant or medical director.
- In the wake of COVID-19, and future epidemics/pandemics, the need for oversight in infection control is pivotal.

Acknowledgments We want to acknowledge Kathryn Hyer, who made immense contributions to the field of assisted living before her untimely death in January 2021.

References

1. Toolkit for person-centeredness in assisted living. UNC & CEAL. 2014.
2. The Assisted Living Workgroup. Assuring quality in assisted living: guidelines for federal and state policy, state regulation and operations. A report to the US Senate Special Committee on Aging. 2003.
3. Harris-Kojetin L, Sengupta M, Lendon JP, et al. Long-term care providers and services users in the United States, 2015–2016. National Center for Health Statistics. Vital Health Stat 3. 2019.
4. Argentum. 2020 largest providers report.
5. Zimmerman S, Sloane PD, Reed D. Dementia prevalence and care in assisted living. Health Aff (Millwood). 2014;33(4):658–66.
6. Alzheimer's Association Campaign for Quality Residential Care. Dementia care practice: recommendations for assisted living residences and nursing homes.
7. Facts & Figures. AHCA & NCAL. 2020.
8. Thomas KS, Zhang W, Cornell PY, et al. State variability in the prevalence and healthcare utilization of assisted living residents with dementia. J Am Geriatr Soc. 2020;68(7):1504–11.
9. Toth M, Palmer L, Bercaw L, et al. Trends in the use of residential settings among older adults. J Gerontol B Psychol Sci Soc Sci. 2022;77(2):424–8.
10. Carder P, O'Keeffe J, O'Keeffe C. Compendium of residential care and assisted living regulation and policy: 2015 edition. Washington, DC: U.S. Department of Health & Human Services, Office of the Assistant Secretary for Planning and Evaluation; 2015.
11. Caffrey C. Residents living in residential care communities: United States, 2010. NCHS data brief no 91. Hyattsville: National Center for Health Statistics; 2012.
12. PharMerica. Medication management issues in assisted living. 2020.
13. The MacIntosh Company. Medication management in assisted living. 2019.
14. Genworth. Genworth cost of care survey 2020. https://pro.genworth.com/riiproweb/productinfo/pdf/282102.pdf. Accessed 24 Aug 2021.
15. Managed long-term services and supports. Medicaid and CHIP Payment and Access Commission.
16. Travis LJ, Thomas KS, Clark MA, et al. Organizational characteristics of assisted living communities with policies supportive of admitting the retaining residents in need of end-of-life care. Am J Hosp Palliat Med. 2021;38(8):947–53.
17. Dobbs D, Kaufman S, Meng H. The association between assisted living direct care worker end-of-life training and hospice use patterns. Gerontol Geriatr Med. 2018;4:2333721418765522.

18. U.S. Department of Health and Human Services. State residential care and assisted living policy: 2004. 2005.
19. June JW, Meng H, Dobbs D, et al. Using deficiency data to measure quality in assisted living communities: a Florida statewide study. J Aging Social Policy. 2020;32(2):125–40.
20. Dobbs D, June J Dosa D, Peterson LJ, Hyer K. Protecting frail older adults: long-term care administrators' satisfaction with public emergency management organizations during hurricane Irma and COVID-19. Public Policy and Aging Report, 2021;31(4):145–150.
21. Peterson LJ, June J, Sakib N, Dobbs D, Dosa DM, Thomas KS, Jester DJ, Hyer K. Assisted living communities during Hurricane Irma: the decision to evacuate or shelter in place and resident acuity. J Am Med Dir Assoc. 2020;21(8):1148–52.
22. Zimmerman S, Katz P, Kunze M, O'Neil K, Resnick B. The need to include assisted living in responding to the COVID-19 pandemic. J Am Med Dir Assoc. 2020;21(5):572–3.
23. Curiskis A, Kelly C, Kissane E, Oehler K. What we know—and what we don't know—about the impact of the pandemic on our most vulnerable community: the Atlantic Tracker Project. 2021. https://covidtracking.com/analysis-updates/what-we-know-about-the-impact-of-the-pandemic-on-our-most-vulnerable-community. Accessed 11 Sept 2021.
24. Brown LM, Christensen JJ, Ialynytchev A, et al. Experiences of assisted living facility staff in evacuating and sheltering residents during hurricanes. Curr Psychol. 2015;34:506–14. https://doi.org/10.1007/s12144-015-9361-7.
25. Utz R. Assisted living: the philosophical challenges of everyday practice. J Appl Gerontol. 2003;22:379–404.
26. Schumacher J. Assisted living communities and medical care providers: establishing proactive relationships. Seniors Hous Care J. 2005;13(1):35–48.
27. Vance J. Proceedings of the AMDA assisted living consensus conference, Washington, DC October 24, 2006. J Am Med Dir Assoc. 2008;9(6):378–82.
28. AGS 2012 Beers Criteria Update Expert Panel. AGS updated beers criteria for potentially inappropriate medication use in older adults. J Am Geriatr Soc. 2012;60:616–31.
29. Sloane PD, et al. Medication undertreatment in assisted living settings. Arch Intern Med. 2004;164:2031–7.
30. Zimmerman S, Love K, Sloane PD, Cohen LW, Reed D, Carder PC, Center for Excellence in Assisted Living-University of North Carolina Collaborative. Medication administration errors in assisted living: scope, characteristics, and the importance of staff training. J Am Geriatr Soc. 2011;59(6):1060–8.
31. Beeber AS, Zimmerman S, Madeline Mitchell C, Reed D. Staffing and service availability in assisted living: the importance of nurse delegation policies. J Am Geriatr Soc. 2018;66(11):2158–66.
32. Sloane P, et al. Physician perspectives on medical care delivery in assisted living. J Am Geriatr Soc. 2011;59:2326–31.
33. Unruh MA, Qian Y, Casalino LP, Katz PR, Ryskina KL, Jung HY. The prevalence and characteristics of clinicians who provide care in assisted living facilities, 2014–2017. J Gen Intern Med. 2021;36(8):2514–6.
34. Caffrey C, Cairns C, Rome V. Trends in electronic health record use among residential care communities: United States, 2012, 2014, and 2016. National Health Statistics Reports; no 140. Hyattsville: National Center for Health Statistics. 2020.
35. Rashidi P, Mihailidis A. A survey on ambient-assisted living tools for older adults. IEEE J Biomed Health Informatics. 2012;17(3):579–90.
36. ACOs and long-term care: don't get left behind. Duane Morris LLP & Affiliates. 2012.
37. Baxter A. 4 steps assisted living can take toward ACO status. Senior Housing News. 2016.
38. James JT. A new, evidence-based estimate of patient harms associated with hospital care. J Patient Saf. 2013;9(3):122–8.
39. Vipperman A, Zimmerman S, Sloane PD. COVID-19 recommendations for assisted living: implications for the future. J Am Med Dir Assoc. 2021;22(5):933–938.e5. https://doi.org/10.1016/j.jamda.2021.02.021. Epub 2021 Feb 25. PMID: 33773962; PMCID: PMC7904515.

40. Medicare hospice provider compliance audit: suncoast hospice. U.S. Department of Health & Human Services. Report. No. A-02-18-01001.
41. Zimmerman S, Carder P, Schwartz L, Silbersack J, Temkin-Greener H, Thomas KS, Ward K, Jenkens R, Jensen L, Johnson AC, Johnson J, Johnston T, Kaes L, Katz P, Holt Klinger J, Lieblich C, Mace B, O'Neil K, Pace DP, Scales K, Stone RI, Thomas S, Williams PJ, Williams KB. The imperative to reimagine assisted living. J Am Med Dir Assoc. 2022;23(2):225–34.
42. Anderson EG. Nursing home practice: 10 tips to simplify patient care. Geriatrics. 1993;48:61–3.
43. Schumacher J. Examining the physician's role with assisted living residents. J Am Med Dir Assoc. 2006;7(6):377–82.
44. Zimmerman S, et al. A measure of person-centered practices in assisted living: the PC-PAL. J Am Med Dir Assoc. 2015;16:132–7.
45. Mitty E. Medication management in assisted living: a national survey of policies and practices. J Am Med Dir Assoc. 2009;10(2):107–14.
46. Pruchnicki A. Full time primary care in an assisted living community. AMDA poster submission, annual symposium. 2005.
47. Schumacher J. Physicians and their assisted living residents: adventures in falls (mis) communication. AMDA annual symposium presentation, 2009.

PACE

Verna Sellers and Laura Trice

Introduction

Effective and value-based healthcare for older people is becoming increasingly important as the number of older adults who require high quality long-term care for chronic illness continues to increase. How can healthcare providers best serve the needs of those who are both frail and elderly? Models of care must incorporate cost containment without compromising participants' quality of care or quality of life. Though frail elders say they want to remain at home in their community, frequently, complex medical conditions and lack of financial and community resources may make nursing home placement the only option [1].

PACE is a unique healthcare delivery system that strives to successfully integrate a full spectrum of services for frail persons 55 years of age and older. PACE organizations deliver a combination of primary, specialist, acute, long-term, and home-based care as well as palliative care to its enrollees. Use of interdisciplinary team care, managed care services, and care coordination result in improved health outcomes and reduced expense over time.

The average PACE enrollee is 77 years old, has an average of eight acute and chronic medical conditions, and three limitations in activities of daily living (ADLs). Over 95% of PACE participants continue to live in the community [2]. Comparing this to the data for older adults living in Assisted Living Facilities, who require assistance with two or more ADLs and average three chronic medical conditions, the PACE member population is frailer.

V. Sellers (✉)
Madison Heights, VA, USA

L. Trice
St. Elizabeth Healthcare, Edgewood, KY, USA

© The Author(s), under exclusive license to Springer Nature
Switzerland AG 2023
P. Winn et al. (eds.), *Post-Acute and Long-Term Care Medicine*, Current Clinical
Practice, https://doi.org/10.1007/978-3-031-28628-5_4

61

Pace History

Program of All-inclusive Care for the Elderly (PACE) originated in 1971 in San Francisco's Chinatown, with a $2000 federal grant to the Chinatown-North Beach Health Care Planning and Development Corporation (later renamed On Lok Senior Health Services). Marie-Louise Ansak, a Swiss social worker, developed a long-term care model for an elderly Chinese population that considered nursing home placement culturally unacceptable. Ansak developed the concept for the original PACE site out of the British Day Hospital's model, which offered therapeutic and minor medical services, with patients returning home at the end of the day. The American version, "On Lok" (Cantonese for peaceful abode) expanded these provisions, thereby creating a global approach to managing patient cases, which included offering housing, a full range of medical and social services, and therapies.

On Lok continued to succeed and grow in the 1970s, and by the 1980s On Loc had received waivers from Medicare and Medicaid to pilot a new financing system that allowed the PACE programs to provide full medical services for a fixed monthly payment for each enrollee in the program [3]. In 1986, federal legislation allowed for other PACE sites and in 1997, PACE received permanent Medicare and Medicaid provider status under the Balanced Budget Act. Alexian Brothers Community Services in St. Louis became the first PACE site to become a permanently recognized part of the Medicare and Medicaid programs. When the Federal Interim Regulation for PACE was published in 1999 there were 30 programs in 19 states. PACE organizations became subject to both Federal and State regulation and surveys in a manner similar to those of long-term care facilities.

PACE expansion to rural markets was initiated by a 2005 Deficit Reduction Act with $7.5 million in funding. There are currently over 137 PACE programs in 31 states with more than 53,000 enrollees.

The National PACE Association (NPA) was founded in 1994 to support PACE programs. NPA provides education resources, communication forums, and collects *benchmarking data* to compare participant characteristics and service delivery across sites. NPA works closely with members of Congress, senior administration officials, and state policy-makers to educate and to promote a reimbursement and regulatory environment that enables PACE programs to provide high-quality, individualized, and innovative care. The NPA Primary Care Committee develops resources to assist PACE clinicians, serves as a clinical resource to the NPA Board of Directors, and promotes PACE to the wider medical community.

Financing

PACE offers an innovative financing model that integrates capitated Medicare and Medicaid dollars per enrollee. Once enrolled, PACE becomes the participant's sole source of Medicare- and Medicaid-covered services, including coverage of medications. Most PACE participants are dually eligible, i.e., have both Medicare and Medicaid, but do have the option to pay privately if they do not. Medicare rates are calculated for each participant using a risk-adjusted payment methodology similar to Medicare Advantage plans. Medicaid rates are negotiated between each PACE organization and the state agency administering the Medicaid program. PACE organizations assume all financial risk for delivering all healthcare services that would normally be covered under Medicare Parts A, B, D and Medicaid. PACE programs are considered Medicare Advantage Programs and are funded under Medicare Part C. PACE is in a unique position as both payor and provider of services that allows for payment flexibility, creativity, and innovation. In 2015 the US Secretary of the Department of Health and Human Services authorized for-profit entities to also operate PACE with the goal of reaching more people. This is contingent on their ability to demonstrate that they can provide care that is similar to nonprofit PACE with regard to access to care, quality of care, and cost-effectiveness [4].

Outcomes

Although there are limited outcome studies on PACE, the results are generally positive: PACE has been shown to improve functional status and quality of life, and decrease mortality [5–7]. Findings also suggest that the very old (80–90 years), those living alone, using ambulation aids, cognitively impaired, and requiring assistance to perform instrumental activities of daily living (IADLs) benefit the most from a noninstitutional long-term care approach such as PACE [8].

Rates of hospitalization, readmission, and potentially avoidable hospitalization (PAH) are lower for PACE enrollees than for comparable Medicaid nursing home residents [7, 9, 10–12]. The variation in study results across PACE sites reflects their heterogeneity in case mix, longevity, and experience of the interdisciplinary team (IDT). The programs availability of transitional housing, contracts, and agreements with local hospitals and skilled nursing facilities, as well as the local medical culture also caused the programs results to vary [7, 11 12]. In the PACE community an adage frequently used to describe the diversity of the programs is, "if you have seen one PACE program, you have seen one PACE program."

A Day at the PACE Day Health Center (DHC)

The IDT
- Primary care provider (may be a Physician or Physician Assistant or Nurse Practitioner as defined by state laws with regard to oversight, practice authority, and prescriptive authority)
- Registered nurse
- Master's-level social worker
- Physical therapist
- Occupational therapist
- Recreational therapist or activities coordinator
- Dietician
- PACE center manager
- Home care coordinator
- Personal care attendant or his or her representative
- Driver or his or her representative

Case Scenario
Like other PACE enrollees, Anna enjoys attending the DHC an average of three times a week. Her home health aide (HHA) arrives at Anna's home early to prepare Anna for the day. Anna's daughter welcomes the aide into their small apartment. Anna depends on PACE HHAs for her daily personal care since a stroke left her wheelchair bound. Bathed and dressed, Anna waits in the living room for the PACE driver to pick her up for the trip to the DHC. Meanwhile in the kitchen, her daughter shares a list of concerns with the aide, which include financial and medical, as well as equipment and supply issues for her mother. The aide assures her daughter that everything will be addressed at the IDT meeting later in the morning. Her driver arrives to transport Anna to the DHC. A PACE driver for many years, he is very familiar with all the people on his route and Anna greets him like an old friend.

When Anna enters the DHC, the staff greets her, while giving her a nametag. Her arrival time is entered into the electronic medical record, alerting clinical staff that plans to see her during the day. The DHC serves as the main medical center as well as the social services base for PACE participants. There is a full schedule of recreational activities that Anna may attend but she first heads for the therapy department. She had completed skilled therapy after a stroke 2 years ago, but like many PACE participants, benefits from an ongoing restorative therapy program.

Meanwhile, Anna's IDT is meeting in a conference room nearby. The IDT is responsible for the initial assessment, periodic reassessment, plan of care, and coordination of 24 h care delivery as written in the Code of Federal Regulation (42 CFR:460.104). Medical care is coordinated by the PACE IDT assigned to each participant. The IDT's members include physicians, nurse practitioners, behavioral health specialists, nurses, social workers, therapists, van drivers, aides, and other staff. This group meets regularly as the status of a PACE participant evolves.

The HHA has reported Anna's daughter's concerns to the home care coordinator, to be discussed at the IDT meeting. Problems with increased knee pain, questions about a new medication, issues with a defective wheelchair and difficulties paying the rent are all discussed. Agreeing to a plan, IDT members will address these issues and concerns in the next few days.

Anna then arrives at the PACE clinic for an acute visit with her PACE primary care provider (PCP) who routinely sees Anna every 3 months alternating between reassessment and wellness visits. Because the clinic is physically part of the DHC, acute visits are flexible and frequent. Frontline staff, HHAs, and drivers are often the "eyes and ears" of a PACE program, often identifying changes in condition well ahead of clinic staff. The PCP was informed about Anna's new onset of left knee pain during the IDT meeting, that her daughter has noticed a decrease in her mobility and that the therapy staff also noticed decreased range of motion during the morning restorative exercises. After ordering conservative treatment measures, the physician reassures Anna she'll see her again on a subsequent DHC visit.

Working at a PACE is a "dream job" for the PCP. With a small patient panel, typically 100 or less, there is the opportunity to manage complex social and medical conditions of each enrollee and to see positive outcomes.

Anna's nurse, telephones to update her daughter, reassures her that her mother's vital signs and weight are stable, answers questions about any new medication, and explains the plan of care for her mother's knee condition. Her occupational therapist has ordered a new part to fix her wheelchair and the social worker will schedule a meeting with her landlord.

During the next month at the DHC, Anna has the opportunity to see several PACE in-house specialists from podiatry, optometry, dentistry, and behavioral health.* (In-house services vary from center to center.) PACE also schedules and provides transportation for any other specialist appointments approved by the IDT. Several times a year PACE admits Anna to a contracted nursing home for respite allowing her daughter to visit family in another state. Should Anna ever need a hospital or skilled nursing facility (SNF) stay, PACE clinical staff will continue to follow her at the SNF with the IDT authorizing and overseeing all care.

In the late afternoon, Anna leaves the DHC for her trip home. The driver will deliver all her medications, frozen meals, and incontinence products when he drops her off. Anna knows there is a PACE nurse and provider on call 24/7 should any issues arise at home during the night or on the weekends.

Tired but happy, Anna is already looking forward to her next DHC visit!

In 2020 PACE programs throughout the country were faced with the COVID-19 pandemic. PACE programs showed success in mounting a COVID-19 response that upheld safety, promoted the physical and mental well-being of participants, and responded to the needs of family caregivers, while facing many challenges that required major changes in care provision. Administrators in a North Carolina study felt that, after the pandemic, the PACE service model is likely to remain more home-based and less reliant on the day center than in the past. As a result, PACE may have changed for the better and be well-positioned to play an expanded role in our evolving long-term care system [13].

PACE Model Practice

Beginning in 2006, the NPA Primary Care Committee began developing *Model Practices* as guides for key chronic conditions often seen in PACE participants. These model practices direct care along one of *three pathways* according to the directives and priorities of each participant: *achieving longevity, maintaining function,* or *receiving palliative care* [14]. Current Model Practices include the following:

- Atrial Fibrillation (2018)
- Diabetes Mellitus (revised 2014)
- Dementia (2014)
- Coronary Artery Disease (2020)
- Chronic Heart Failure (revised 2018)
- Chronic Kidney Disease (revised 2016)
- Chronic Obstructive Pulmonary Disease (2013)
- Preventive Care Guideline (2010)

NPA encourages the use of these model practices. NPA members may obtain the documents at *Members Only/Primary Care Resources/Model Practices.* Nonmember clinicians or organizations may not use, reproduce, or modify the model practices without the expressed written consent of the National PACE Association. To obtain permission, inquire at email info@npaonline.org.

Role of the Medical Director in PACE

My inspiration and continued passion for geriatric healthcare are a direct result of a most challenging but rewarding position I held as a PACE Medical Director.

42CFR:460.60 *The organization must employ a medical director who is responsible for the delivery of participant care, for clinical outcomes, and for the implementation, as well as oversight, of the quality assessment, and performance program.*

A PACE Medical Director operates as both a director of diverse clinical services and an administrator of a health plan. The need to move from a provider to a payor role during the work day can be very challenging that includes reviewing and enrollees' charts and financial reports. Medical Directors who come to PACE with a long-term care background usually have a good understanding of federal and state regulatory compliance while those with a primary care practice background often better understand staffing and balance sheet issues.

Medical Directors must assure that participants receive quality geriatric care in every setting including the PACE clinic, hospital, SNF, and home. Since PACE providers often provide all these direct services, the Medical Director has the opportunity to closely supervise all the clinical care the participants receive while monitoring the quality of contracted provider services. While clinical responsibilities are key, the Medical Director must also work closely with the Site manager and other administrative staff to manage the financial risk of the program and plan for expansion of the program.

Although PACE sites endeavor to recruit geriatricians for both the Medical Director and Primary Care Physician (PCP) roles, there is not always a supply to meet the need. Finding practitioners that have a passion for elderly care is always the priority. The typical PACE program is small, with an average of 300 participants; so many Medical Directors also function as the PCP in addition to their administrative duties. Recruiting, training, and retaining PCPs are key responsibilities. The PACE PCP must be able to care for medically complex elderly using sound geriatric medicine principles. Working collaboratively as an IDT member is often a new experience for a PACE PCP and usually requires 6 months to become proficient in the role. Many PACE sites also successfully use nonphysician providers such as nurse practitioners and physician assistants to serve as PCP and be a member of the IDT.

The Medical Director must also recruit and contract with a provider network that include specialists, hospitals, SNFs, pharmacy, and all ancillary services such as home care and durable medical equipment suppliers. While the program director will oversee and maintain contracts with each network member, the Medical Director must ensure that the network is educated about PACE and provides quality care.

Oversight of the Quality Assessment and Performance Improvement (QAPI) plan includes making sure that utilization of services, caregiver and participant satisfaction, safety, and clinical outcome measures are addressed. Similar to the functions of a nursing home quality committee, wound care, infections, and falls are routinely reviewed. Additional QAPI responsibilities include oversight of staff competency and tracking participant grievances.

There is great opportunity for the Medical Director to educate, mentor, and participate in research. PACE sites often become centers of geriatric excellence for sponsoring healthcare organization, with fellows, residents, medical students, and nursing students routinely rotating with PACE clinical staff.

The Primary Care Committee of the National PACE Association (NPA) provides excellent training resources for all Medical Directors regardless of experience level or background. Education sessions are offered during the summer and fall. NPA conferences and online resources are available for NPA member Medical Directors on the NPA website.

PACE in the Nursing Home

Although the goal of PACE is to care for nursing home eligible people in the community, about 10% of PACE participants require skilled or custodial nursing care. Like all other contracted services, PACE sites must ensure that contracted nursing facilities are educated about PACE and provide quality care. Ideally, PACE sites contract with an adequate number of nursing homes to be able to offer enough geographic choice to meet participant and family preferences. PACE and nursing facility administrative and clinical teams need to collaborate to ensure that documentation and care plans are integrated. It is helpful to attend the Quality Assurance meetings at all contracted nursing facilities, as well as communicating frequently with the facility administrator, medical director, and director of nursing. CMS requires a comprehensive medical record at the PACE site even if the participant resides in a nursing facility.

The Future of PACE

Operational challenges have limited growth for PACE despite its attractive features [15]. Significant human and financial resources are required to run what is essentially a small health plan. Substantial "back-office" overhead costs to process Part A and B claims as well as Part D data requirements and federal and state reporting requirements mean less dollars for patient care [16]. Hiring qualified staff especially primary care physicians and geriatricians can be challenging.

Expanding PACE organizations is often limited by federal regulation that has not kept up with modern innovations [17]. NPA is working with Congress to support more operational flexibility, growth, and innovation. Issues to explore and address include expansion of service areas, revision of the age and HF eligibility requirement, utilization of alternative care settings, and unbundling of services.

Pearls for the Practitioner
- Nursing home eligible participants that are age 55 or older can continue living in their homes with comprehensive services through PACE.
- PACE is a unique model that delivers a full continuum of care.
- With capitated Medicare and Medicaid payments, PACE serves as a model for value-based care and payment innovation.

Websites
- National PACE Association. www.npaonline.org.
- Medicare.gov. http://www.medicare.gov/your-medicare-costs/help-paying-costs/pace/pace.html.
- Medicaid.gov. http://www.medicaid.gov/Medicaid-CHIP-Program-Information/By-Topics/Long-Term-Services-and-Supports/Integrating-Care/Program-of-All-Inclusive-Care-for-the-Elderly-PACE/Program-of-All-Inclusive-Care-for-the-Elderly-PACE.html.

References

1. Trice L. PACE: a model for providing comprehensive healthcare for frail elders. Generations. 2006:90–2.
2. National PACE Association. www.npaonline.org.

3. Eng C, Pedulla J, Eleazer GP, McCann R, Fox N. Program of All-inclusive care for the Elderly (PACE): an innovative model of integrated geriatric care and financing. J Am Geriatric Soc. 1997;45:223–32.
4. Gonzalez L. A focus on the Program of All-Inclusive Care of the Elderly (PACE). J Aging Soc Policy. 2017;29(5):475–90.
5. White AJ, Abel Y, Kidder D. Evaluation of the program of all-inclusive care for the elderly (PACE) demonstration. A comparison of the PACE capitation rates to projected costs in the first year of enrollment. Baltimore: Abt Associates; 2000.
6. Mancuso D, Yamashiro G, Filver B. PACE an evaluation. Olympia: Department of Social and Health Services, Research and Data Analysis Division; 2005.
7. Weiland D, Boland R, Baskins J, Kinosian B. Five year survival in PACE compared with alternative institutional and home and community based care. J Gerontol A Biol Sci Med Sci. 2010;65(7):721–6.
8. Branch LG, Coulam RF, Zimmerman YA. The PACE evaluation: initial findings. Gerontologist. 1995;35:349–59.
9. Chatterji P, Burstein NR, Kidder D, White AJ. Evaluations of the Program of All-Inclusive Care for the Elderly (PACE)—demonstration the impact of PACE on participant outcomes. Boston: Abt Associates; 2003.
10. Meret-Hanke LA. Effects of the Program of All-Inclusive Care of the Elderly on hospital use. Gerontologist. 2011;51:774–85.
11. Beauchamp J, Cheh V, Schmitz R, Kemper R, Hall J. The effects of the program of all-inclusive care for the elderly (PACE) on quality. Princeton: Mathematica Policy Research; 2008.
12. Segelman M, Szydlowski J, Kinosian B, Mcnabney M, et al. Hospitalization in the Program of All-Inclusive Care for the Elderly. J Am Geriatric Soc. 2014;62:320–4.
13. Schamp RO. A day in the life of a PACE medical director. Caring for the Ages. 2011;
14. Aggarwal N, Sloane PD, Zimmerman S, Ward K, Horsford C. Impact of Covid-19 on structure and function of Program of All-Inclusive Care for the Elderly sites in North Carolina. J Am Med Dir Assoc. 2022;23:1109–13.
15. Boult C, Wieland DG. Comprehensive primary care for older patients with multiple chronic conditions "Nobody Rushes You Through". J Am Med Assoc. 2010;304:1936–43.
16. Hirth V, Baskins J, Dever-Bumba M. Program of All-Inclusive Care (PACE): past, present, and future. J Am Med Dir Assoc. 2009;10:155–60.
17. Bloom S. PACE has shown path to improved elder care. Modern Healthcare. 2014.

Department of Veterans Affairs Options for Long-Term Care

Deborah Way

Introduction

The Department of Veterans Affairs (VA) has developed several options for long-term care from traditional institutional care to innovative programs for community-based long-term and post-acute care. Similar to the triple aims of the Centers for Medicare and Medicaid Services, the VA is focused on providing cost-effective care using community-based services aimed at reducing hospitalizations and preventing institutionalization. These VA services include Hospital in Home, Home-Based Primary Care, Clinical Video Telehealth (CVT), Telehealth, and Homemaker Home Health Aide Care. End-of-life care including hospice may be available to Veterans based on clinical need. Also, Veterans may receive nursing facility (NF) care based on military service-connected status, level of disability, and income requirements. This would be available either at an inpatient VA facility called a Community Living Center (CLC) or at a VA contracted nursing facility.

D. Way (✉)
Palliative Care Services, Corporal Michael J. Crescenz VA Medical Center, Philadelphia, PA, USA

© The Author(s), under exclusive license to Springer Nature Switzerland AG 2023
P. Winn et al. (eds.), *Post-Acute and Long-Term Care Medicine*, Current Clinical Practice, https://doi.org/10.1007/978-3-031-28628-5_5

Community-Based Care

Hospital in Home

The VA has been a pioneer in the innovation of health care by discharging inpatients to return home to complete treatment at home. " Hospital in Home" is currently operational in approximately eight VA Medical Centers with ongoing expansion of this program. Under this program Veterans receive hospital level services that can provide parenteral infusions. In addition, Veterans receive daily visits from a medical practitioner/clinician and skilled nursing with visit of physical therapists and nurse aides as needed. In this model, Veterans can even be directly transferred to home from the Emergency Department avoiding hospitalization. Most programs are staffed solely by VA employees, although in a "partnership" model, the VA provides the medical care and DME needs, such as oxygen, while a partner home health agency and infusion pharmacy provide skilled nursing and infusion services. A small study has demonstrated a reduction in both the cost of care and the nursing home 30-day admission rate post hospital discharge [1].

Home-Based Primary Care

Home-Based Primary Care (HBPC) is a comprehensive program that serves veterans with chronic, disabling conditions and complex psychosocial needs. The goal of this program is to maximize the Veteran's independence at home and to reduce preventable emergency room visits, hospitalizations, and admissions to a long-term care facility. The success of this program stems from team-based care with attention to both the medical and psychosocial factors that affect each veteran [2]. The VA interdisciplinary team (IDT) includes a physician, nurse, social worker, rehabilitation therapist, dietitian, psychologist, and pharmacist. The team may also include other disciplines such as a nurse practitioner, physician assistant, chaplain, respiratory therapist, and recreational therapist. HBPC provides primary care in the homes of Veterans for whom clinic-based care has been ineffective [3]. In addition, the team may also coordinate care, provide palliative care, rehabilitation services, and disease management.

Veterans receive on average 2–3 "contacts" a month from various team members, in addition to a primary care visit every 4–6 weeks. Frequency of visits and intensity of care varies according to the needs of the Veteran. If a Veteran lives outside the coverage area of the team (often designated by driving time) or HBPC is unable to provide the care needed, the VA may contract with a community-based agency to provide care [2]. The Veteran may also receive additional skilled services through Medicare if he/she is a Medicare beneficiary. Overall reduction of more than 10% has been shown in Veterans who are dually eligible for VA and Medicare benefits [2]. Enrollment in HPBC has been associated with decreased hospital bed days of care, decreased nursing home bed days of care, and a decreased hospital readmission rates [4].

Clinical Video Telehealth (CVT)

The VA has a robust telehealth program. In fiscal 2019, over 909,000 Veterans received a portion of their VA care through telehealth, and over 60% of VA's primary and mental health care practitioners provided one or more Clinical Video Telehealth (CVT) appointments to a Veteran's home [5].

Telehealth

Telehealth technologies can collect and send a Veteran's *health data*, like vital signs, to the VA care team that can then use this information to remotely manage a Veteran's care. A nurse is usually the point of contact. The VA provides veteran training on the use of the home telehealth system. One study on telehealth has shown a reduction in hospital length of stay, reduction in cost of care, and an increase in patient satisfaction [6].

Homemaker Home Health Aide Care

The Homemaker Home Health Aide program provides homemakers and home health aide services to Veterans who need assistance with basic activities of daily living (BADLs) and/or instrumental activities of daily living (IADLs). The VA allows these services to be provided concurrently with other community-based services with the goal to avoid or delay admission to a nursing facility.

Nursing Facility Care

Community Nursing Facilities and Community Living Center

The VA contracts with community nursing facilities to provide care to eligible Veterans. VA funding for care is based on service-connected status, level of disability, and income. If a Veteran does not meet these requirements, then the Veteran would either private pay or be enrolled in Medicaid if indigent.

Community Living Centers (CLCs) are nursing facilities owned and operated by the VA. The structure and services are comparable to those in community

NFs. Eligibility for a CLC is also based on service-connected status, level of disability, and income.

End-of-Life Care

VA policy requires the presence of an interdisciplinary *Palliative Care consult team* at each VA facility. Hospice and Palliative Care services are part of the Veterans Health Administration Standard Medical Benefits Package. All enrolled Veterans are eligible for these services if they meet clinical need. The VA collaborates with community hospice agencies for palliative and hospice services and the Veteran has the choice between using their VA benefit or Medicare benefit to fund these services. There is no VA policy at this time that prevents Veterans from receiving hospice services in addition to other care that is palliative in nature (such as whole brain irradiation, radiation to treat painful or bleeding metastatic disease, or palliative chemotherapy/immunotherapy) *as long as* the VA is not funding duplicate care. Currently, this dual model of care is subject to acceptance by the community-based hospice.

Pearls for the Practitioner
- Ask your patient if he/she is are a Veteran. They may be entitled to care funded by the VA. The Military History Checklist will help you gather some of the information needed. https://www.wehonorveterans.org/wp-content/uploads/2020/02/Veterans_Military_History_Checklist.pdf.
- Ask to join the local Veteran Community Partnership. https://www.va.gov/healthpartnerships/vcp.asp.
- Contact your local VA. www.va.gov/geriatrics/.

Videos
- HBPC. https://www.youtube.com/watch?v=FQxGBb_mxJI.
- Geriatrics HBPC. https://www.youtube.com/watch?v=ZOQ9jTzg4qI.

Websites
- https://www.va.gov/GERIATRICS/pages/Home_Based_Primary_Care.asp.
- https://www.va.gov/health-care/about-va-health-benefits/long-term-care/.
- https://www.va.gov/GERIATRICS/pages/Paying_for_Long_Term_Care.asp.
- https://www.va.gov/GERIATRICS/pages/VA_Community_Living_Centers.asp.

References

1. Cai S, Grubbs A, Makineni R, Kinosian B, Phibbs C, Intrator O. Evaluation of the Cincinnati Veterans Affairs Medical Center hospital-in-home program. J Am Geriatr Soc. 2018;66:1392–8.
2. Edes T, Kinosian B, Vuckovic N, Nichols L, Becker M, Hossain M. Better access, quality, and cost for clinically complex veterans with home-based primary care. J Am Geriatr Soc. 2014;62:1954–61.

3. Home-Based Primary Care Program. Department of Veterans Affairs. Veterans Health Administration Handbook 1411, Revised 20 Sept. 2017 (online).

4. Leff B, Weston C, Garriguea S, Patel K, Ritchie C. Home based primary care practices in the United States: current state and quality improvement approaches. J Am Geriatr Soc. 2015;63:963–9.

5. Johnston R, Kobb RF, Marty C, McVeigh P. VA video telehealth and training programs during the COVID-19 response. Telehealth and Medicine Today. 2021;6(1).

6. Messina W. Decreasing congestive heart failure readmission rates within 30 days at the Tampa VA. Nurs Admin Q. 2016;40(2):146–52.

The Role of Practitioners and the Medical Director

Steven A. Levenson

Introduction

The role of nursing facilities continues to change within the US health care system. Traditionally, nursing facilities primarily provided personal and nursing care to the physically, cognitively and functionally impaired elderly. Today, while nursing facilities continue to provide residential and custodial care, they now admit medically complex patients, discharged from acute can and specialty hospitals. Both long-term care residents and post-acute care patients can be medically complex and have multi-morbidities and risk factors for geriatric syndromes such as pressure injuries, anorexia, and falls. Managing these patients requires proficient clinical reasoning and problem-solving skills. Accordingly, nursing facilities require more physician and nonphysician practitioner involvement in assessing and managing patients [1].

Persons who live in nursing facilities are commonly referred to as **residents**; while those who are primarily admitted to receive short-term medical and skilled care are referred to as **patients**. *Long-term residents* often need acute care in addition to ongoing chronic medical care. *Short-stay patients* often have chronic medical conditions as well as the need for both acute and post-acute medical care. Some post-acute patients may have an extended stay or need to transition to a long-term bed.

S. A. Levenson (✉)
Baltimore, MD, USA

P. Winn et al. (eds.), *Post-Acute and Long-Term Care Medicine*, Current Clinical Practice, https://doi.org/10.1007/978-3-031-28628-5_6

Physicians and nonphysician practitioners have a vital role in providing nursing facility care, while medical directors provide a crucial role in organizing, oversee-ing, and improving the overall care in the facility and assisting with challenging patient situations. Attending physicians are primarily responsible for managing individual patient medical care and can facilitate effective collaboration among the interdisciplinary team [2].

While a medical director can also serve as an attending physician, the roles and functions of a medical director are separate from those of an attending physician. The attending physician provides direct resident care; the medical director oversees, coordinates, and helps improve the facility's overall medical care and services.

Although concern over physician performance and practice is ongoing, there are mixed opinions about how to improve performance and practice [3]. In the early 2000s, Maryland implemented substantial state regulations regarding expectation for the medical director and physicians [4]. Over 20 years later, this approach has had limited success in most other states.

The Role of the Medical Practitioner

Regulations that originated from the Omnibus Budget Reconciliation Act of 1987 (OBRA '87), required every nursing facility resident or patient to have an attending physician to supervise and coordinate medical care [5]. "Supervising the care" means participating in the assessment and management of patients, monitoring changes in their medical status, and providing consultation or treatment when needed. It also includes performing regulatory visits and possibly supervising nurse practitioners or physician assistants. Table 1 describes the basic physician functions and tasks based on the Federal OBRA '87 requirements. Currently nurse practitio-ners are permitted to serve as the "attending practitioner" for hospice patients.

While many physicians provide high quality care and clinical leadership, others have little interest in chronic care medicine and been unwilling to attend at LTC facilities [6]. Some of them may lack the knowledge and skills on the care of chronic illness, the frail elderly patient, and post-acute and long-term medical care. Remember that multiple symptoms may have a common cause and multiple causes can be related to a specific symptom. Others are challenged by the practice environ-ment in nursing homes and may feel overburdened by regulatory requirements.

Increasingly, more intensive physician involvement in long-term and post-acute care is needed. Active involvement is essential to assess and manage patients, to avoid unnecessary hospitalization, and to address many issues such as ensuring accurate diagnosis, management of behavior and psychiatric symptoms, delirium, and to prevent medication-related adverse effects. AMDA—The Society for Post-Acute and Long-Term Care Medicine has developed a curriculum and certification program for medical directors and a curriculum for attending physicians covering diverse areas of physician competency, in order to promote a more uniform standard of practitioner knowledge and skills.

Table 1 Attending physician functions and tasks in the nursing facility based on Federal OBRA'87 regulations

Roles	Related functions and tasks
Supervise individual resident care	• Approve a resident's admission to the facility, e.g., this may be done by giving and approving orders upon admission • Be familiar with, and contribute to, a patient's assessment and care planning; e.g., by clarifying their medical history and underlying causes of impaired function and significant condition changes • Take an active role in supervising their patients' care; i.e., be aware of the impact of what others are doing medically with their patient and ensure that it is coordinated and appropriate

Make resident visits	• At the time of each visit:
	  – Review the total program of care, including medications and treatments rendered by other disciplines
	  – Write, sign, and date a progress note
	  – Sign and date all orders except immunization orders that may be periodic without a new order
	  – Evaluate the resident's condition and continued appropriateness of the current medical regimen

Make timely visits	• See a patient at least once every 30 days for the first 90 days after admission, and at least once every 60 thereafter (the next scheduled regulatory visit date should be determined by the admission date, not by the actual date that the last visit occurred; a visit is timely if it occurs not later than 10 days after the date it was required). Daily visits are allowed but must be medically necessary • Make all required physician visits (required visits after the initial visit may alternate between visits by the attending physician and visits by a physician assistant, nurse practitioner, or clinical nurse specialist under the physician's supervision) • Respond appropriately and in a timely manner when notified of an acute change of condition
Arrange for provision of emergency services	• Ensure that there is backup medical coverage (e.g., individual physician, physician group, or advance practice nurse) if the attending physician is unavailable. Virtual visits may be allowable
Delegate tasks appropriately	• Delegate tasks to physician assistants, nurse practitioners, or clinical nurse specialists consistent with OBRA'87 requirements and state requirements related to licensure and scope of practice • Be aware of the role of consultants in managing a patient and intervene when care is inadequate, problematic, or not pertinent (e.g., hospice, pain management, or prescribing that is causing adverse consequences)

As the health care system changes, hospitals are now partnering with long-term and post-acute care facilities to develop integrated models of care, (see chapters "Behind the Scenes at Nursing Facilities" and "Preventing Hospital Admissions and Readmissions" for further discussion). As such, more hospitalists are now paying attention to these nonhospital settings.

Practitioners must collaborate with the facility's management, clinical leadership, and direct care staff to provide competent care and to handle conflicts or problems that arise. Table 2 identifies practitioner responsibilities that are integral to high quality resident care [7].

Table 2 Practitioner's roles and related functions and tasks

Practitioner's role	Related functions and tasks
Accept responsibility for resident care	• Assess new admissions in a timely fashion • Seek, provide, and analyze information regarding a patient's current status, recent history, medications, and treatments • Sign monthly orders, interim orders, lab and test results and review the facility consultant pharmacist recommendations • Provide information and documentation that helps staff determine appropriate level of care for a new admission • Identify and authorize admission orders in a manner that enables the facility to provide safe, appropriate, and timely care
Support discharges and transfers	• Guide as needed, transfers of acutely ill or unstable patients from the facility • Provide necessary documentation and other information needed at the time of transfer to enable care continuity • Provide a pertinent discharge summary within 30 days of patient discharge or transfer from the nursing facility • If pending transfer to another practitioner, continue to provide all necessary medical care and services until another physician takes over the care
Make periodic, pertinent resident visits	• Make timely patient visits, based on their needs and on regulatory requirements, including an alternate visit schedule as appropriate • Provide pertinent progress notes that cover a patient's condition (including medical and psychiatric stability), current status, prognosis, and goals • Review and validate specific treatments and a patient's overall care approaches • Address relevant clinical issues • Provide timely. legible, and pertinent progress notes
Provide adequate ongoing coverage	• Designate alternate coverage • Inform the facility about communicating with his/her practice and designated alternate coverage • Guide alternate coverage as needed to ensure adequate and timely support • Notify the facility of any extended absence and related coverage arrangements
Provide appropriate resident care	• Perform accurate, timely, and relevant medical assessments • Define significance of resident symptoms and problems, clarify and verify diagnoses, and help establish prognosis and realistic care goals • Help determine appropriate and medically necessary treatments and services for each patient, consistent with relevant practice standards and regulatory requirements • Respond appropriately to emergency and routine notification by staff • Analyze and address laboratory and other diagnostic test results • Assess and promptly manage significant acute changes in a patient's condition • Guide ethics-related decisions (for example, options for life-sustaining treatments) • Order appropriate comfort and supportive measures as needed • Periodically review continued relevance of all prescribed medications for patients and identify and address medication-related adverse consequences

Table 2 (continued)

Practitioner's role	Related functions and tasks
Provide appropriate and timely medical orders	• Provide timely and legible medical orders • Sign and verify the accuracy of verbal orders
Provide appropriate, timely, and pertinent documentation	• Document pertinent rationale for medical decisions, consistent with meeting clinical, legal, and regulatory requirements • Complete all physician information required on death certificates in a timely manner
Perform and act appropriately	• Abide by pertinent policies and procedures • Collaborate with the medical director/facility leadership to support provision of high-quality care • Notify the medical director/facility leadership about issues and concerns • Keep the well-being of patients in mind in all situations • Be alert to any observed or suspected violations of resident rights, including abuse or neglect • Interact in a courteous, professional manner with facility staff, patients/residents, family/significant others, facility employees, and management • Inform the medical director/facility leadership of disputes or problems with other parties (e.g., staff, patients, or other practitioners) that the physician cannot readily resolve

Clinical Reasoning and Diagnostic Quality

Practitioners can favorably impact the quality of care in PA and LTC facilities by means of their clinical performance, practice, and expertise in medical decision making and problem identification in the facility.

Diverse disciplines (e.g., therapists, nurses, and dieticians) in long-term and post-acute care must collaborate to address patient and facility problems. However, decisions are often made elsewhere; e.g., prior to resident admission. Staff, patients, and families need to review and validate these decisions.

The care delivery process is key to providing safe, effective, efficient, patient-centered, equitable, and timely evidence-based care. Using the care delivery process of recognition/assessment, cause identification/diagnosis, management, and monitoring of response to an intervention is critical. The medical practitioner's role is to clarify patient issues and risks that contribute to resident illness and impairment. Patient-centered care require a thorough and thoughtful differential diagnosis of symptoms.

Key steps in developing and implementing a patient-centered medical plan include to:

1. Clarify relevant medical issues (including physical and psychiatric conditions as well as patient prognosis).
2. Determine decision-making capacity of the resident.
3. Identify the primary or proxy/surrogate decision maker.
4. Look at the "big picture."

5. Review an individual's values, wishes, preferences, goals.
6. Reconcile patient goals of life and goals of medical care.
7. Order appropriate interventions, where benefit outweighs risk.
8. Monitor and adjust interventions, as indicated.

Facility staff and practitioners must jointly support a culture of effective and consistent care and competent clinical reasoning and problem solving. *Diagnostic quality* involves minimizing and recognizing diagnostic errors that contribute to undesirable outcomes. Facilities and practitioners should review care processes and identify diagnostic and thinking errors that can result in inappropriate or harmful treatment [8].

The Role of the Medical Director

Medical directors often serve in various settings, including hospitals, insurance companies, specialty programs or services (e.g., dialysis, hospice, wound care, PACE), and in some assisted living facilities. Medical director practice in nursing facilities is required by federal regulations, which define the medical director as "a physician who oversees the medical care and other designated care and services in a health care organization or facility" [9].

Medical Director Characteristics

The background, characteristics, and performance expectations of medical directors has been researched over the years [10, 11] and promulgated by AMDA: The Society for Post-Acute and Long-Term Care Medicine (formerly known as the American Medical Directors Association). In nursing homes, most medical directors have an internal medicine or family medicine background, and approximately one in four are also trained geriatricians [12]. A medical director may cover one or several facilities. While many medical directors also serve as an attending physician, a significant number act solely in the role as a medical director with no attending physician responsibilities.

Origins of the Medical Director Role

The need for a nursing facility medical director evolved out of a government investigations stemming from a 1970 salmonella outbreak in a Maryland nursing facility [13, 14]. In the 1970s, the American Medical Association's Committee on Aging suggested the roles and functions of a medical director and recommended educating physicians on basic roles and responsibilities [15]. By 1974, skilled nursing facilities (those certified to provide skilled nursing services to Medicare beneficiaries) were required to retain a full- or part-time medical director [16].

The 1987 Omnibus Budget Reconciliation Act (OBRA) and its related regulations expanded the medical director requirements to include residential as well as skilled portions of nursing facilities. For regulatory purposes, both skilled and non-skilled facilities are referred to as "nursing facilities." Subsequently, surveyor guidance (as written in 42 CFR 483.75(i) Medical Director [F501] and recently updated as F841) has clarified CMS expectations. Beginning in the late 1980s and early 1990s, physicians serving as medical directors [17, 18] and their representative organization (AMDA) [19] have reviewed and defined the role and tasks of the medical director. In 2001, the Institute of Medicine recommended that nursing facility medical directors be given greater authority and that structures and processes be developed to enable and support and require a more focused and dedicated physician participation [20].

Key Medical Director Responsibilities

Over several decades, regulatory agencies and professional organizations have further developed the *medical director's roles and responsibilities*. There have been efforts to try to make these requirements more consistent throughout the USA. For example, AMDA has developed a program to certify medical directors as having specific administrative and medical knowledge. In contrast, requirements for medical direction in assisted living facilities vary among states. As of 2022, requirements for medical directors in assisted living facilities were minimal.

Regulatory Foundation

Federal regulations require every nursing facility in the USA to retain a physician to serve as its medical director. The primary resource of medical director regulations is OBRA '87 and the State Operations Manual on surveyor guidance. In addition, *there are some individual State regulations regarding medical director responsibilities* [21]. Federal nursing facility regulations divide requirements into several discrete segments called "F-Tags," related to one or more specific regulatory requirements used for State and Federal surveys.

A specific section of federal regulations (F-Tag 841) covers the roles and responsibilities of the medical director. The regulations regarding medical direction require that the *medical director is responsible for (1) implementation of resident care policies and (2) coordination of medical care in the facility.* Surveyor guidance provides additional information and instructions on how to survey a facility for compliance with federal regulations, including that of the medical director (F-Tag 841) (Table 3) [22]. A nursing facility can be cited for a deficiency if it does not have a medical director who is fulfilling these requirements. However, most citations of F-Tag 841 usually must relate to another F-Tag deficiency. Table 3 summarizes the guidance for surveyors to interpret whether facilities meet the requirements of F-Tag 841.

Other sections of the State Operations Manual review *whether care is consistent with current standards of practice.* The guidance defines "current standards of practice" as "approaches to care, procedures, techniques, treatments, etc., that are based on research and/or expert consensus and that are contained in current manuals, textbooks, or publications, or that are accepted, adopted or promulgated by recognized professional organizations or national accrediting bodies" [22]. *The facility is expected to obtain the medical director's input into all clinical*

Table 3 Medical director responsibilities based on F-Tag 841

Roles	Related functions and tasks
Coordination of medical care	• Be knowledgeable about current professional standards of practice in caring for long-term care residents, and about how to coordinate and oversee other practitioners • Organize and coordinate physician services and services provided by other professionals as they relate to resident care • Help the facility develop a process to review basic physician and health care practitioner credentials (e.g., licensure and pertinent background) • Help the facility develop systems to ensure that other licensed practitioners (e.g., nurse practitioners) who may perform physician-delegated tasks act appropriately and consistent with clinical standards of practice • Help the facility ensure that residents have adequate primary attending and backup physician coverage • Advise on availability, qualifications, and clinical performance of staff necessary to meet resident care needs
Implementation of resident care policies	• Have meaningful input into the development, review, approval, and implementation of resident care policies • Collaborate with facility leadership, staff, and other practitioners and consultants to help develop and implement resident care policies and procedures that reflect current standards of practice • Cooperate with facility staff to establish policies for assuring that the rights of individuals (residents, staff members, and community members) are respected • Provide clinical leadership to evaluate and update as needed treatments, practices, and approaches to care • Support and promote person-directed care such as the formation of advance directives, end-of-life care, and provisions that enhance resident decision making, including choice regarding medical care options

Table 3 (continued)

Roles	Related functions and tasks
Support for improving quality of care	• Help coordinate and evaluate the medical and all clinical care within the facility • Participate in a meaningful way in the Quality Assessment and Assurance (QAA) committee or assign and oversee a designee to represent him/her • Help the facility evaluate and address issues related to the quality of care and quality of life of residents • Collaborate with the facility to develop and implement policies and procedures related to surveillance and Infection Control • Identify performance expectations and facilitate feedback to physicians and other health care practitioners regarding their performance and practices • If the medical director is also an attending physician, have a process to address any concerns with the individual's performance as a physician • Discuss and intervene, as appropriate, with a health care practitioner regarding medical care that is inconsistent with current standards of care • Help develop systems to monitor the performance of the health care practitioners including mechanisms for communicating and resolving issues related to medical care and ensuring that other licensed practitioners (e.g., nurse practitioners) who may perform physician-delegated tasks act within the regulatory requirements and within the scope of practice as defined by State law • Help the facility identify, evaluate, and address/resolve medical and clinical concerns and issues that affect resident care, medical care, or quality of life and that are related to the provision of services by physicians and other licensed health care practitioners
Survey-related support	• Respond to surveyors on survey-related issues, including individual resident cases, physician participation, and the facility's clinical practices • Help the facility analyze its deficiencies and identify areas for improvement

policies and procedures, including services provided by other health care disciplines.

Professional Organizations and the Medical Director Role

Medical director responsibilities have been based on recommendations of professional associations. AMDA—The Society for Post-Acute and Long-Term Care Medicine is a national organization that represents long-term care medical directors and other practitioners and has written consensus statements on many topics including the medical director role and related functions and tasks (Table 4) [23]. These recommendations include additional aspects of medical direction that go beyond regulatory requirements.

Table 4 Medical director responsibilities as identified by AMDA

Role	Related functions and tasks
Physician leadership	• Help ensure appropriate physician coverage and provision of medical services • Help develop a process for reviewing practitioner credentials • Give the practitioners expectations for performance and practice • Help develop and implement a system to monitor practitioner performance and give the practitioners feedback • Ensure that residents have primary attending and backup physician coverage
Patient care/clinical leadership	• Help develop policies and procedures related to resident care • Help the facility identify and implement care-related policies Obtain physician and other health care practitioner services to help residents attain and maintain their highest practicable level of functioning, consistent with regulatory requirements • Help guide staff about interacting with practitioners and the medical director • Review and consider consultant recommendations that are related to resident care • Help protect resident rights, including advance care planning and other ethical issues • Help the facility address issues related to continuity of care and transfer of medical information and patients between the facility and other care settings
Quality of care	• Review and be available for external surveys and inspections • Participate in quality improvement processes • Advise on infection control issues, approve specific infection control policies, and evaluate infection control practices • Help the facility provide a safe and caring environment • Help promote employee health and safety, including implementation of employee health policies and programs
Education, information, and communication	• Promote a learning culture within the facility • Guide the facility to provide care consistent with current clinical standards of practice • Help develop and optimize medical information and communication systems • Represent the facility to the professional and lay community on medical and resident care issues • Be aware of social, regulatory, political, and economic factors that affect medical and health services of long-term care residents and short-stay patients • Help establish appropriate relationships with other health care organizations

Medical Director Relationship with Practitioners

The medical director is responsible for the coordination of medical care in the facility. As identified in the surveyor guidance for F-Tag 841, the medical director helps the facility provide care that is consistent with current standards of practice, and helps the facility meet its regulatory requirements" [22].

According to the OBRA'87 surveyor guidance, *practitioners are responsible to the medical director for their performance and practice.* As with the medical director, physicians and nonphysician practitioners may also be accountable to others, such as a program director in academia or an administrator of a group practice. The medical director must clarify practitioner responsibilities and performance expectations; such as regulatory requirements for frequency of patient visits, facility policies, and clinical standards of practice. In addition to other responsibilities, the medical director is expected to help the facility develop a process to review basic physician and health care practitioner credentials (e.g., licensure and pertinent background) and address and resolve concerns and issues between physicians, health care practitioners, and facility staff.

Practitioner Responsibilities

As with any supervisory or oversight position, the medical director clarifies practitioner responsibilities by:

- Setting expectations
- Explaining how to fulfill those expectations
- Establishing criteria for satisfactory performance
- Determining whether those expectations are being met
- Giving practitioners feedback on their performance and practice.

The needs of the general population and the specific requirements of each patient practice setting affect practitioner responsibilities. Long-term care medicine also includes a hybrid of ambulatory, office-based, and hospital-based practice. Individuals of other disciplines are often intermediaries between the patient and the physician; e.g., assessment and monitoring, identifying and defining problems, and conveying concerns to the physician. While residents of Assisted Living may have comparable clinical and behavioral issues, Assisted Living facilities typically have a less organized structure and fewer direct care staff than do nursing homes.

The medical director has an obligation to educate practitioners about providing care in the proper context. Medical care must identify and address risk factors (e.g., impaired nutrition, fall risk) and understand clinical decisions that can impact outcomes (e.g., decisions not to hospitalize, choice of medications and treatments).

The medical director can help the facility educate and inform the staff on appropriate clinical practice. Appropriate clinical practices for the long-term care population have been identified and discussed in the literature for several decades [24]. Practitioners should try to minimize complications (secondary and tertiary prevention), including those related to iatrogenic illness [25].

The medical director can guide staff and practitioners to better identify and address issues such as adverse drug events (ADEs), common causes of acute changes in condition, falls, altered mental status, and decline in function. The medical director's clinical knowledge and understanding of a *facility's case mix* can help the facility develop relevant policies and procedures. Both the medical director and attending physicians are essential to promoting diagnostic quality in the facility and to effectively diagnose causes of symptoms in patients [26–28].

The Medical Director's Relationship with the Facility

The administrator, director of nursing, and medical director are the key management leadership team in the nursing facility. They are ultimately responsible for the successful implementation of the facility's care processes and practices. Unlike a medical staff president or chief of staff, who primarily represents the physicians in a facility or organization, a medical director in LTC fulfills a pivotal role for the facility and its practitioners.

A facility's leadership—principally, the administrator and Director of Nursing—must know the role of the medical director as based on regulatory requirements and relevant professional society recommendations. Across the country, medical director performance varies considerably. Many facilities are still challenged to find qualified and competent attending physicians and medical directors. Some medical directors are stymied in trying to assert themselves to improve facility practice and hold practitioners accountable for the care they provide.

The OBRA '87 surveyor guidance does not specify how a nursing facility must establish medical director services. It requires that the medical director be currently licensed as a physician in the state where the facility is located, unless an exception is warranted. The facility may employ or contract directly with the medical director, or may contract with a company or academic program that employs the physician. In multi-facility organizations, arrangements for such services may be made by corporate or regional offices, and policies developed at a corporate level. In these instances, the medical director still must guide the facility to follow appropriate clinical policies and procedures.

It is desirable for the medical director and administrator to jointly develop and update the medical director agreement/contract based on the items discussed herein and adapted to the facility's needs. For example, some facilities want a medical director who primarily provides patient care while others accept a medical director who has little or no patient care responsibilities.

A medical director should consider whether the facility job description is realistic, pertinent, and clearly delineates expectations. The facility should provide the medical director with adequate support and compensation. Surveyor guidance related to F-tag 841 acknowledges that various factors can influence optimal facility patient outcomes, such as resident characteristics and preferences, individual attending physician actions, and facility support. A facility must maintain an environment that supports competent clinical practice. For example, before contacting a practitioner, the staff should be trained to:

• Perform proper assessments and coordinate phone calls.
• Provide accurate information to describe a situation in detail.

- Be prepared to answer the physician's questions about the patient.
- Know what questions to ask the physician.
- Know when to notify the medical director about physician issues and clinical concerns.

The Medical Director's Role in Facility Quality

All health care settings are being required to improve quality. This is being done to improve patient outcomes, improve patient satisfaction and safety, and identify and focus on providing relevant care that uses resources effectively and possibly at lower cost (**Medicare Triple Aim**). In their leadership role to oversee and coordinate medical care, medical directors can help clarify and support the goals and objectives of care, help the organization articulate and strive to meet its goals, show the staff and practitioners how to achieve desired performance, help solve and prevent problems, and help improve employee and patient health, safety, and welfare. Effective problem solving is vital to all aspects of both patient-related and facility-related outcomes. The medical director can improve a facility's problem-solving processes and practices, and ultimately care quality [29].

The medical director should help the facility identify and address potentially remediable issues such as the impact of physician and other licensed health care professional performance and practices. The medical director should guide the facility in determining whether its practices are consistent with accepted clinical standards.

The medical director should learn about regulatory expectations for facilities as well as details about his or her role as medical director by reviewing in the CMS' State Operations Manual (SOM) for surveyors. This review can help the medical director determine whether a facility's care has a clinically sound foundation.

The medical director must also learn about resources that nursing homes can use to improve quality. One example is the CMS "Nursing Home Compare" website (https://www.medicare.gov/nursinghomecompare) that reports quality measures data based on the Minimum Data Set (MDS), as well as staffing and compliance (i.e., survey deficiencies).

The medical director should engage in in-depth case reviews along with other disciplines, looking for care quality and safety issues that may not have been identified by CMS quality measures [30]. The medical director can provide guidance on quality and risk management concerns such as adverse drug events, medication errors, and falls; review accidents and incidents; and advise on infection control policies and practices. The medical director can assist a facility to evaluate the care and performance of medical practitioners (physicians, NPs, etc.) and other licensed health care professionals.

Ultimately, the medical director supports the facility to ensure that its residents and patients receive adequate and appropriate medical care. When needed, the medical director may intervene directly in the care of other physicians' patients by examining the patient and reviewing patient orders. For example, a medical director may intervene if another practitioner does not respond appropriately or in a timely manner to notification of a significant acute change of condition, or is not adequately supervising care provided to a patient by other IDT members.

Pearls for the Practitioner

- Physicians play an important role in long-term care, both in providing direct care and in providing oversight as medical directors.
- Expectations for performance and practice for both practitioners and medical directors come from both regulatory and professional sources, and are generally consistent and widely disseminated.
- Collectively, the physicians and medical director play a vital role in supporting care quality, including facility-wide approaches to clinical reasoning, problem solving, and diagnostic quality.
- A facility's approach to its medical practitioners greatly influences the success of practitioner participation and, in turn, many aspects of the facility's residents/patient outcomes and satisfaction. This includes—but is not limited to—support for the medical director and holding practitioners accountable for resident and patient care.
- Practitioners should view their roles in the context of both the system in which they practice and to medical decision making for individual residents.
- While clinician performance and participation have varied substantially over the years, ranging from excellent to highly problematic, expectations for better practice have grown.
- Changes in the health care system and the increasing provision of post-acute care as well as the initiatives to reduce avoidable hospitalizations from nursing homes has required an increased and more dedicated physician involvement.
- The medical director can have a major impact on a facility's care, influencing both the facility's practices and practitioner performance.
- The medical director is accountable to the facility administrator while licensed health care practitioners and attending physicians should be accountable to the medical director.
- The medical director should inform and educate practitioners on expectations and review and provide feedback on performance.
- Effective medical direction and care given by practitioners can go far toward attaining and sustaining high quality care.

References

1. Levenson SA. Subacute care. In: Capezuti E, Siegler G, Mezey MD, editors. The encyclopedia of elder care. 2nd ed. New York: Springer; 2007.
2. Dimant J. Roles and responsibilities of attending physicians in skilled nursing facilities. J Am Med Dir Assoc. 2003;4:231.
3. Levenson SA. The impact of laws and regulations in improving physician performance and care processes in long-term care. J Am Med Dir Assoc. 2004;5:268.

4. Boyce BF, Bob H, Levenson SA. The preliminary impact of Maryland's medical director and attending physician regulations. J Am Med Dir Assoc. 2003;4:157.
5. Centers for Medicare and Medicaid Services (CMS). State operations manual: Appendix PP—guidance to surveyors for long term care facilities, Revision 52. Physician Services (F483.40). http://www.cms.hhs.gov/manuals/downloads/som107ap_pp_guidelines_ltcf.pdf.
6. Mitchell JB, Hewes HT. Why won't physicians make nursing facility visits? Gerontologist. 1986;26:650.
7. Levenson SA. Medical director and attending physicians policy and procedure manual for long-term care. Dayton: Med-Pass; 2017.
8. American College of Physicians. Teaching clinical reasoning (Teaching Medicine Series). Kindle Edition. 2015.
9. http://www.cms.hhs.gov/manuals/downloads/som107ap_pp_guidelines_ltcf.pdf.
10. Zimmer JG, Watson NM, Levenson SA. Nursing facility medical directors: ideals and realities. J Am Geriatr Soc. 1993;41:127.
11. Department of Health and Human Services, Office of Inspector General. Nursing facility medical directors survey. http://oig.hhs.gov/oei/reports/oei-06-99-00300.pdf.
12. Resnick HE, Manard B, Stone RI, Castle NG. Tenure, certification, and education of nursing facility administrators, medical directors, and directors of nursing in for-profit and not-for-profit nursing facilities: United States 2004. J Am Med Dir Assoc. 2009;10:423.
13. Gladue JR. Evolution of the Medical Director concept. J Am Geriatr Soc. 1974;22:43.
14. Reichel W. Role of the medical director in the skilled nursing facility: historical perspectives. In: Reichel W, editor. Clinical aspects of aging, vol. 570. 2nd ed. Baltimore: Williams and Wilkins; 1983.
15. Gruber HW. The medical director in the nursing facility—a catalyst for quality care. J Am Geriatr Soc. 1977;25:497.
16. HEW guidelines and survey procedures—medical director. J Am Health Care Assoc. 1975;1:29.
17. Levenson SA. Medical direction in long-term care. a guidebook for the future. 2nd ed. Durham: Carolina Academic Press; 1993.
18. Pattee JJ, Otteson O. Medical direction in the nursing facility. Minneapolis: Northridge Press; 1991.
19. Pattee JJ, Altemeier TM. Results of a consensus conference on the role of the nursing facility medical director. Annu Med Direct. 1991;1(1):5.
20. Institute of Medicine. Improving the quality of long-term care. Washington, DC: National Academy Press; 2001.
21. Levenson SA. The Maryland regulations: rethinking physician and medical director accountability in nursing facilities. J Am Med Dir Assoc. 2002;3:79.
22. Centers for Medicare and Medicaid Services (CMS). State operations manual: Appendix PP—guidance to surveyors for long term care facilities, F841- Medical Director (F483.70). https://www.cms.gov/Regulations-and-Guidance/Guidance/Manuals/downloads/som107ap_pp_guidelines_ltcf.pdf.
23. American Medical Directors Association. Roles and responsibilities of the medical director in the nursing facility: position statement A03. J Am Med Dir Assoc. 2005;6:411.
24. Ouslander JG. Medical care in the nursing home. JAMA. 1989;262:2582.
25. Panagioti M, Khan K, Keers RN, Abuzour A, Phipps D, Kontopantelis E, et al. Prevalence, severity, and nature of preventable patient harm across medical care settings: systematic review and meta-analysis. BMJ. 2019;366:l4185. https://doi.org/10.1136/bmj.l4185.
26. Newman Toker DE, Pronovost PJ. Diagnostic errors: the next frontier for patient safety. JAMA. 2009;301:1060–2.
27. Balogh EP, Miller BT, Ball JR. Improving diagnosis in health care. National Academies Press (US). 2015.
28. Henriksen K, Brady J. The pursuit of better diagnostic performance: a human factors perspective. BMJ Qual Saf. 2013;22:ii1–5.

29. Zarowitz BJ, Resnick B, Ouslander JG. Quality clinical care in nursing facilities. J Am Med Dir Assoc. 2018;19(10):833–9. https://doi.org/10.1016/j.jamda.2018.08.008. PMID: 30268289.
30. Levenson SA. Smart case review: a model for successful remote medical direction and enhanced nursing home quality improvement. J Am Med Dir Assoc. 2021;22(10):2212–2215. e6. S1525-8610(21)00564-8. https://doi.org/10.1016/j.jamda.2021.05.043.

Team-Based Care: Nurse Practitioners, Clinical Nurse Specialists, and Physician Assistants

Robert C. Salinas and Peter Winn

Introduction

More than ever before, there is an ongoing national effort to assist older adults attain and maintain their highest functional status and to successfully age in place. With the expansion of telemedicine, remote patient monitoring systems, extended home health care coverage, and emerging home-based primary care models of care, older adults have the possibility to delay nursing home placement [1]. Residents in nursing facilities and assisted living are often the most vulnerable due to multimorbidities, neurocognitive disorders, and psychosocial issues. The complexity of resident healthcare and social needs coupled with the increased burden on physicians to provide care in long-term care has increased the need for collaboration between physicians, the advance nurse practitioners, and physician assistants to provide interdisciplinary/interprofessional team-based care.

Nurse practitioners (NP) are Registered Nurses who have obtained a Master's degree of nursing (MSN) or a clinical doctoral degree as a Doctor of Nursing Practice (DNP). The DNP was established to acknowledge their professional parity with pharmacists and physical therapists who have received a clinical doctorate.

R. C. Salinas (✉) · P. Winn
Department of Family and Preventive Medicine, The University of Oklahoma, College of Medicine, Oklahoma City, OK, USA

© The Author(s), under exclusive license to Springer Nature
Switzerland AG 2023
P. Winn et al. (eds.), *Post-Acute and Long-Term Care Medicine*, Current Clinical Practice, https://doi.org/10.1007/978-3-031-28628-5_7

Nurse practitioners with a DNP have had additional education and clinical training in quality improvement, leadership, and health policy. Nurse practitioners who practice in nursing facilities are usually designated as a gerontological, adult, adult-gerontological, or family NP. Recently the Clinical Nurse Specialist (CNS) education in psychiatric mental health *has been changed to that of a* psychiatric mental health *nurse practitioner.* Nurse practitioners have had greater than 6 years of academic and clinical training [2].

Advanced practice nurses, both nurse practitioners (NP) and clinical nurse specialists (CNS) have shown improvement in several measures of health and the behavior of residents in long-term care as well as better family satisfaction [3–5]. The NP and CNS are autonomous and collaborative members of the interdisciplinary team who enhance the accessibility and quality of care in nursing facilities, and serve as a resource to the assisted living and nursing facility staff who are challenged by the increasingly complex needs of residents [6].

Currently there are over 355,000 NPs licensed in the USA and an increase in "full-time" NPs from 14% in 2008 to 36% in 2018. NPs now represent 60% of full-time primary care practitioners in the LTC sector [7]. Nurse practitioners are trained to perform patient histories and physical exams, to diagnose and treat acute illness, and to manage chronic conditions; can order and interpret laboratory tests, diagnostic reports such as X-rays, Doppler and cardiac studies; are skilled in primary, secondary, and tertiary prevention; may prescribe medication including controlled substances dependent on state regulations; and can provide health teaching, anticipatory guidance, and supportive counseling to patients. As of 2022, there were 24 *full practice states* with practice and licensure law allowing NPs to evaluate patients, diagnose, order, and interpret diagnostic tests, to initiate and manage treatment, including prescribing medication (under the licensure authority of the state boards of nursing). This full practice model has been recommended by the Institute of Medicine and the National Council of State Boards of Nursing. There are 16 states with *reduced practice*, meaning the state practice and licensure law reduces the ability of NPs to engage independently in at least one element of NP practice. These reduced practice States require a *collaborative agreement* with another health discipline (usually a physician) in order for the NP to provide patient care. The remaining 11 states have *restricted practice* (with state practice and licensure laws) that restrict the ability of a NP to engage in at least one element of NP practice. Some States require supervision, delegation or team-management by an outside health entity/practitioner in order for the NP to provide patient care. Information on which states has which NP category can be found at https://www.aanp.org/advocacy/state/state-practice-environment.

It is essential when collaborating with a NP or CNS to have a thorough understanding of their *scope of practice*. The Institute of Medicine report ***The Future of Nursing***: ***Leading Change***, ***Advancing Health*** acknowledges that nurses should practice to the full extent of their education, training and scope of practice in order to meet our nation's health care needs and that nurses be full practice partners with physicians [8].

Partnering with a Nurse Practitioner Nurse or Physician Assistant

Nurse practitioners can achieve better resident health care goals without an increase in the cost of care. NPs and physician assistants (PAs) who practice in LTC can reduce hospital admissions and costs [6]. The Evercare (program) has shown that nursing facilities having a NP manage a resident's care, had half the number of hospitalizations than nursing facilities that did *not* have NP managing the resident's care. NPs can improve the quality and accessibility of primary health care services to this ever-increasing complex resident population through being approachable and respectful of patient, family, and staff. The nursing staff develops trust with NPs and value their knowledge. Meta-analysis studies and systematic reviews have demonstrated *positive results of NP practice in long-term care*:

- High patient satisfaction, decreased hospitalizations, and decreased all-cause mortality compared to physician alone practice.
- Reduced transfers to the emergency department.
- Lower rates of depression, urinary incontinence, pressure ulcers, use of restraints, and less aggressive behavior in residents.
- Practice with a high degree of collaboration with the interprofessional team.
- Provide leadership activities that include education of the interdisciplinary staff in quality improvement, evidence-based practice and practice innovation.

Clinical Nurse Specialists

Clinical Nurse Specialists (CNS) have a Master's degree in nursing and often have further specialized training in a particular area of clinical nursing. Though most frequently employed in Magnet hospitals, they can have a significant positive impact when working in post-acute and long-term care. According to recent statistics, there are 89,000 practicing CNS in the United States [9]. These advanced practice nurses are experts in the diagnosis and treatment of illness, health promotion, and the implementation of evidence-based practice. Through education and consultation with staff, CNS have also been shown to reduce urinary incontinence, pressure ulcers, aggressive behavior, the use of restraints (both physical and pharmacological), to decrease fall-related injuries, and to improve the effect of cognitively impaired residents. Adult and gerontological CNSs are expanding practice in wound care, quality improvement, and education and leadership roles within long-term care. As noted, psychiatric mental health CNS and NPs are trained in the behavioral management of persons afflicted with dementia and others with serious mental illness.

Physician Assistants

There are over 132,940 physician assistants (PAs) currently working in the USA and their number is expected to continue to increase [10]. In 2013, a national survey by the American Academy of Physician Assistants, reported that 0.9 % of PAs were directly *employed* by a nursing facility or other long-term care facility. PA training programs are commonly based at medical schools, hospitals, and other health care facilities. Didactic sessions and clinical rotations are often taken alongside medical students, which helps to cultivate a future collaborative relationship between these two professions. The first year of the 26-month PA program covers the basic medical sciences followed by clinical rotations in all major medical specialties. With over 2000 h of clinical and skill training, PAs are well suited to perform patient histories and physical exams, diagnose, order, interpret test results and manage both acute and chronic conditions, *in collaboration with physicians*. To be able to practice a PA must pass the Physician Assistant National Certifying Exam (PANCE) and require subsequent continuing education in order to recertify every 10 years.

A *PA's scope of practice is defined by four domains: education and experience, state law, facility policy, and the needs of patients.* Each is necessary in order to provide effective patient-centered care. PAs are expected to perform patient care tasks at a similar skill level and competency as a physician. However, State boards do not require a PA to be proficient in any specific tasks.

Collaboration does not necessarily require the constant presence of a physician. In fact, in some rural areas a PA can be a patient's primary care provider with the supervising physician "checking-in" once or twice a week. The PA's scope of practice continues to grow, adapting to changes within the medical profession and state legislatures. *It is imperative that the supervising physicians and the long-term care facility employers be cognizant of changing State regulation.*

Prescribing Privileges of PAs and NPs

A significant difference in prescribing privileges exists between NPs and PAs. Currently all States allow **PAs** to prescribe as long as a physician is either directly involved or available. Most commonly this association is through *delegation* (19 states) and *authorization* (18 states) with other (13 states) specifying that a physician be directly involved in a *supervisory role*. Only Arizona has *specified collaboration. In contrast, 24 states allow **NPs** to have prescriptive authority* where these States have regulations that allow NPs to diagnose and *treat patients independently.* The remaining states require varying levels of collaboration, delegation, and supervision. Prescribing of scheduled drugs is regulated and enforced by individual States through the Drug Enforcement Agency (DEA) [2].

DEA classification of scheduled drugs

Schedule	Medical use/effects	Abuse potential	Examples
I	• No medical use • Research use only	Highest	Heroin, Marihuana, LSD, MDMA
II/IIN	• Severe psychic or physical dependence liability • Narcotic, stimulant, depressant drugs	High	*Narcotic*: Opium, Codeine, Hydromorphone, Methadone, Hydrocodone *Non-narcotic*: Amphetamine, Methamphetamine, Nabilone
III/IIIN	• Moderate or low psychical or physical dependency	High	Narcotic: Acetaminophen with Codeine, Buprenorphine Non-narcotic: Ketamine, Anabolic steroids
IV	• Limited psychological or physical dependency	Low	Chlordiazepoxide, Diazepam, Barbital, Phenobarbital, Clorazepate, Alprazolam
V	• Over the counter or prescription drugs with limited amounts of narcotics • Used for analgesic, antitussive, antidiarrheal	Lowest	Buprenorphine, Propylhexedrine

Controlled (scheduled) drug prescribing is allowed for **PAs** in the majority of states through their collaborative practice with physicians. However, 15 states restrict this privilege to schedule III–V drugs. Florida and Kentucky do not allow for any controlled drugs to be prescribed by a **PA**. All states (except for Florida) allow **NPs** to prescribe controlled substances: the majority of states allow Schedule II through V; however, eight states restrict this to Schedule III through V.

*The registration procedure with the DEA is the same for all Advanced Practitioners and designated as "**mid-level practitioners.**"* Only after successfully completing all requirements imposed by the State in which they will practice and successfully receive a state license are they then able to apply for a DEA registration. Once approved, they will receive a DEA number beginning with "M."

There is a significant lack of PAs who practice in long-term care despite 20% work in primary care. PA programs have shown a propensity for PAs to prefer practice in orthopedics, urgent care, and in-patient care. However, data has shown that PAs have a favorable attitude toward the elderly and would welcome inclusion of a rotation in long-term care during their training.

Collaborative Practice

How and when to develop *Collaborative Practice Agreements* is beyond the scope of this chapter; however, some general comments are noteworthy. *Interprofessional team care has become the gold standard in post-acute and long-term care.* Within this model of care, team members include physicians, Advanced Practice Nurses (NPs and CNS), and PAs. Currently NP and CNS can work independently (depending upon state regulations), whereas PAs must work in collaboration with a physician. There are *six models of care* in collaborative NP/ physician practice at nursing facilities: collaborator, clinician, care coordinator/manager, coach/educator, counselor, and communicator/cheerleader. Combining these models of care can create synergy that positively affects residents, resident families, facilities, and staff. *There are at least seven different forms of collaboration* in practice (1) NP hired by a physician; (2) NP and physician both employed by the long-term care setting; (3) NP contracted (self-employed) or employed by an NP practice; (4) NP employed directly by the nursing facility; (5) NP employed by the payer (e.g., Optum); (6) NP in a specialty collaborative practice that includes consulting; and (7) NP in independent practice employs a physician.

It is encouraging to see the progress that has been made in acknowledging the crucial role that advanced practitioners play in the realm of long-term care and geriatric practice. In 2014, AMDA—The Society for Post-Acute and Long-Term Care Medicine, House of Delegates, voted to permit full membership to NPs and PAs. This resolution allows NPs and PAs to be elected to Board positions and the House of Delegates and thus contribute their expertise to improving patient care [2, 11–13].

Resources for developing collaborative practice agreements can be found through professional organizations including AMDA—The Society of Post-Acute and Long-Term Care Medicine (www.amda.paltc.org), the Gerontological Advanced Practice Nurses Association (www.gapna.org), the American Association of Nurse Practitioners (www.aanp.org), and American Academy of Physician Assistants (www.aapa.org).

Pearls for the Practitioner
- Nurse practitioners and clinical nurse specialists are autonomous and collaborative members of the interprofessional team in both post-acute and long-term care settings.
- Nurse practitioners' scope of practice ranges from state to state: full practice, reduced practice, and restricted practice.
- Physician assistants' scope of practice is determined by education/training, experience, state law, and facility policy.
- Prescribing privileges differ between NPs and PAs and from State to State.
- The DEA designates NPs and PAs as "mid-level practitioners."
- Collaborative practice agreements are often necessary for NPs, CNSs, and PAs.

References

1. Cacchione ZC, Shah R Nurse practitioners, clinical nurse specialists, and physician assistants. In: Fenstemacher P, Winn P, editiors. Post-acute and long-term medicine: a pocket guide. 2nd ed. Humana Press. 2016.
2. American Association of Nurse Practitioners. 2022 nurse practitioner state practice environment. 2022. https://www.aanp.org/advocacy/advocacy-resource/position-statements/scope-of-practice-for-nurse-practitioners. Accessed 26 July 2022.

3. Bakerjian D. Care of nursing home residents by advanced practice nurses. A review of the literature. Res Gerontol Nurs. 2008;1(3):177–85. https://doi.org/10.3928/00220124-20091301-01.
4. Bergman-Evans B. Out of the shadows: nurse practitioner leadership in skilled and long-term care facilities. J Gerontol Nurs. 2021;47(8):3–6. https://doi.org/10.3928/00989134-20210707-01.
5. Rantz MJ, Birtley NM, Flesner M, et al. Call to action: APRNs in U.S. nursing homes to improve care and reduce costs. Nurs Outlook. 2017;65(6):689–96. https://doi.org/10.1016/j.outlook.2017.08.011.
6. Katz PR, Ryskina D, Saliba D, et al. Medical care delivery in U.S. nursing homes: current and future practice. Gerontologist. 2021;61(4):595–604. https://doi.org/10.1093/geront/gnaa141.
7. McGilton KS, Bowers BJ, Resnick B. The future includes nurse practitioner models of care in the long-term care sector. J Am Med Dir Assoc. 2022;23(2):197–200. https://doi.org/10.1016/j.jamda.2021.12.003.
8. The future of nursing: leading change, advancing health. Institute of Medicine (US) Committee on the Robert Wood Johnson Foundation Initiative on the Future of Nursing, at the Institute of Medicine. Washington, DC: National Academies Press (US). 2011. Accessed 26 July 2022.
9. Reed SM, Arbet J, Staubli L. Clinical nurse specialists in the United States registered with a national provider identifier. Clin Nurse Spec. 2021;35(3):119–28.
10. American Medical Association—Advocacy Resource Center. Physician assistant scope of practice. 2018. https://www.ama-assn.org/sites/ama-assn.org/files/corp/media-browser/public/arc-public/state-law-physician-assistant-scope-practice.pdf. Accessed 26 July 2022.
11. Pakizegee, M and Stefanacci R. The ever-expanding role of nurse practitioners in LTC. Ann Long-Term Care. 2019. Accessed 10 Aug 2022.
12. The future of nursing: leading change, advancing health. 2019. National Academies Sciences Engineering Medicine. Accessed 10 Aug 2022.
13. Stucky CH, Brown WJ, Stucky MG. COVID 19: an unprecedented opportunity for nurse practitioners to reform healthcare and advocate for permanent full practice authority. Nurs Forum. 2021;56:222–7.

Common Clinical Conditions in Post-Acute and Long-Term Care

Naushira Pandya

Introduction

The management of medical conditions in the frail elderly who reside in post-acute and long-term care facilities (PALTC) can be challenging due to multimorbidity, progressive functional decline, psychosocial issues, and reduced life expectancy. This chapter will review some of the common clinical conditions that frequently occur in patients in the post-acute and LTC continuum. The treatments prescribed and treatment goals often differ from those of patients in other settings, and thus require an approach that balances the risks/benefits of treatment guided by clinician discussions with the patient and/or surrogate decision-maker. These conditions will be reviewed in the following order:

- Hypertension
- Heart failure
- COPD
- Diabetes
- Anemia
- Thyroid disorders
- B_{12} deficiency
- *Clostridioides difficile infections*
- Scabies
- Herpes Zoster
- Acute kidney injury

N. Pandya (✉)
Department of Geriatrics, Nova Southeastern University, Kiran C Patel College of Osteopathic Medicine, Fort Lauderdale, FL, USA

© The Author(s), under exclusive license to Springer Nature Switzerland AG 2023
P. Winn et al. (eds.), *Post-Acute and Long-Term Care Medicine*, Current Clinical Practice, https://doi.org/10.1007/978-3-031-28628-5_8

Hypertension

The ACC/AHA 2017 [1] guidelines categorize normal BP as <120/<80 and hypertension defined as a blood pressure ≥130/80 mmHg (see Table 1). Hypertension is the most prevalent and modifiable risk factor for cardiovascular disease and death. The National Health and Nutritional Examination Survey (NHANES), reported the prevalence of HTN in those ≥65 years to be 63.6% in women and 65.8% in men. In those ≥75 years, the prevalence is 73.4% in women and 81.2% in men. The age-adjusted prevalence is highest in non-Hispanic black men and women. Up to two-thirds of nursing home patients have HTN. In addition to the well-ascribed risk factors for stroke and cardiovascular disease, persons with HTN are also at increased risk for atrial fibrillation, congestive heart failure (CHF), peripheral arterial disease (PAD), chronic kidney disease (CKD), and cognitive impairment. In older adults, cardiovascular morbidity and mortality have been shown to progressively increase as the systolic blood pressure increases.

Although hypertension (HTN) is not a normal part of aging, its prevalence increases steadily with advancing age. Physiologic changes of aging that contribute to elevated blood pressure include increased arterial stiffness, increased activity of the sympathetic nervous system, increased peripheral resistance, and reduced vascular compliance and vasodilation. In addition, changes in the renin-angiotensin system and kidney function lead to increased salt sensitivity. Obesity and insulin resistance are also contributing factors. Systolic HTN is highly prevalent, more common than diastolic HTN and more closely related to cardiovascular risk than diastolic HTN.

Table 1 HTN definitions and treatment targets – JNC-8 and 2017 ACC/AHA guidelines [1]

	JNC-8	2017 AHA/ACC
Definition of HTN (mmHg) Elevated	Normal <120/<80 Pre-hypertension:120–139/80–89 Stage 1: 140–159/90–99 Stage 2: >160/>100	Normal: <120/80 Increased: SBP 120–129 Stage 1: 130–139/80–89 Stage 2: ≥140/≥90
BP treatment thresholds (mmHg)	≥60 years old: >150/90 <60 years old with diabetes or CKD: >140/90	Adults with history of CVD or ASCVD risk >10%: >130/80 Adults without history of CVD and ASCVD risk <10%: >140/90
BP targets (mmHg)	>60 years old: 150/90 <60 years old: 140/90	<130/80 for all
Therapy selection	Non-Black adults, including with DM: first-line therapy includes ACE inhibitor/ARB, CCB, thiazides (alone or in combination) Black adults, including with DM: first-line therapy includes thiazides or CCB Adults with CKD: first-line therapy includes ACE inhibitor/ARB (alone or in combination)	Non-Black adults: first-line therapy includes thiazides, ACE inhibitor/ARB, CCB Black adults: first-line therapy includes thiazides or CCB

In the PALTC setting, blood pressure measurements may not be accurate and may vary with higher readings in the morning before breakfast and drops after meals. Post-prandial hypotension occurs in one-third of patients and is a risk factor for falls, syncope, stroke, and overall mortality.

Benefits and Risks of Treatment

The benefits of treating HTN in the elderly to reduce cardiovascular and cerebrovascular morbidity and mortality is well established, even in those >80 years old. However, there is insufficient evidence regarding what is the safest and most beneficial treatment strategy for frail older adults.

The Cochrane Review on the treatment of essential HTN in elderly patients (15 trials with 24,055 subjects ≥60 years) reported a reduction in total mortality (RR 0.90) and a reduction in total cardiovascular morbidity and mortality (RR 0.72). *In very elderly patients ≥80 years, the reduction in total cardiovascular mortality and morbidity* was similar (RR 0.75). However, there was no reduction in total mortality, (RR 1.01) [2]. The benefit of antihypertensive treatment in patients age 80 years and older has also been demonstrated by the Hypertension in the Very Elderly (HYVET) trial in which 3845 healthy community individuals over age 80 years with a sustained SBP of ≥160 mmHg were randomized to indapamide or placebo with the addition of perindopril or placebo to achieve a SBP goal of 150 mmHg. However, individuals with immobility, cognitive impairment, and nursing facility residents were excluded from this study. The benefits of treatment were apparent at 1 year, and further increased at 2 years, with a 30% reduction in the incidence of fatal or nonfatal stroke, a 39% reduction in fatal stroke, and a 21% reduction in all-cause mortality [3].

Recently, guidelines for HTN treatment in the elderly have been informed by the Systolic Blood Pressure Intervention Trial (SPRINT), which studied 9361 ambulatory subjects, mean age 68 years with a baseline SBP >130 mmHg. Nursing facility residents, and those with Type 2 diabetes, heart failure, and dementia were excluded. Treatment goal of <120 mmHg was compared to a goal of 140 mmHg and showed a significant decrease in outcomes for cardiovascular events (HR 0.77), and all-cause mortality (HR 0.73) in the intensive treatment group. Subgroup analysis for those classified as frail or having a slow gait speed, showed similar results. Self-reported syncope was more frequent in the intensive treatment group, but falls and falls with injuries were similar in both groups, even in those >75 years. All participants studied in SPRINT-MIND showed a 19% reduction in mild cognitive impairment (MCI), but not in probable dementia [4]. However, the PARTAGE [5] study of 1127 nursing home subjects >80 years in Europe showed a significant relation between SBP <130 mmHg and 2 or more BP-lowering medications and a higher risk of mortality (adjusted HR 1.78; 95% CI 1.34–2.37, both $p < 0.001$).

Other prior randomized trials of HTN treatment in the elderly (SHEP: Systolic Hypertension in the Elderly Program; STOP: Swedish Trial in Old Patients; Sys-Eur:

European Systolic Hypertension in the Elderly; Syst-China: Chinese Trial on Isolated Systolic Hypertension in Elderly) have shown a 32–47% reduction in stroke, a 13–30% reduction in coronary disease, and a 29–58% reduction in heart failure.

Evaluation

The diagnosis of hypertension should be carefully determined. In addition to using an appropriate cuff size and measuring blood pressure in a seated position at rest, it is important that blood pressure be measured as the average of two readings and obtained on at least two occasions. This is especially important in older adults due to blood pressure variability. In the long-term care setting, BP may be highest in the morning and low after meals. Over 90% of elderly with an elevated BP will have essential hypertension, and the majority with *new onset HTN* will have systolic hypertension. As many drugs can increase blood pressure, a careful medication review should be performed. The pulse pressure (defined as SBP minus DBP) increases with age as does white coat hypertension. Nonsteroidal anti-inflammatory drugs (NSAIDs) including COX-2 inhibitors, erythropoietin, alcohol, corticosteroids, and uncontrolled pain are often implicated in elevating BP.

A resident with HTN should be evaluated for the presence of comorbid conditions such as diabetes mellitus, chronic kidney disease (CKD), and sleep apnea that can contribute to HTN. If clinically appropriate, those who present with diastolic HTN or treatment-resistant HTN should be evaluated for a renovascular cause. Patients with unexplained hypokalemia accompanied by metabolic alkalosis may have hyperaldosteronism as a cause of HTN. Although the incidence of pheochromocytoma is low, it may warrant consideration if a resident's BP is unusually labile and weight loss present [6].

Treatment Goals

- For non-institutionalized, mobile, community-dwelling older adults ≥65 years, the ACC/AHA [1] recommends a SBP goal of less than 130 mmHg.
- For older adults ≥65 years with a high disease burden and limited life expectancy and who are unable to live independently, the goals of therapy may differ and need to be determined within the context of patient preference and one's overall clinical status (especially functional and cognitive status, and risk for frequent falls). Consider a discussion with family on the risks vs. benefits of lowering the blood pressure.

Cardiac risk factors should be modified to the extent possible. The elderly should be encouraged to increase physical activity if possible and to stop smoking. The treatment plan should include screening for diabetes and hyperlipidemia, and salt restriction if appropriate. The clinician should be aware that even a relatively simple intervention such as dietary sodium restriction could adversely affect nutritional status and contribute to weight loss. Clinical factors to consider when treating HTN in PALTC patients are reviewed in Table 2. General management guidelines include:

Table 2 Advantages and disadvantages of class of antihypertensive medication

Antihypertensive class	Advantages	Disadvantages	Recommended indications	Cautions
Thiazide diuretics Loop diuretics	Reduction in mortality, stroke, coronary events Daily use Daily use	Hypokalemia Urinary frequency Headaches, ototoxicity, electrolyte disturbances	Systolic hypertension Effective in HTN in HF and CKD	Hyponatremia Gout Urinary frequency Use in am
ACE inhibitors Angiotensin receptor blockers (ARB)	No CNS side effects Preserve renal function Reduce proteinuria Alternative agent if intolerant to ACE inhibitors	Cough Hyperkalemia Hyperkalemia	HF Diabetes ACEi ARBs Microalbuminuria	Renal insufficiency Renal artery stenosis Cough, altered taste, angioedema
Calcium channel antagonists (CCA)	Effective in reducing stroke No CNS side effects No metabolic effects	Constipation Ankle edema Heart block (Non-dihydropyridine CCAs) HF with amlodipine	Systolic hypertension Angina	Left ventricular dysfunction Avoid short-acting CCAs for HTN
Beta adrenergic receptor blockers	None (not recommended as monotherapy)	CNS (Central Nervous System) side effects Increased glucose and lipids with cardio selective	Prior MI Stable angina, ACS HF Atrial fibrillation with rapid rate (*Beneficial in essential tremor, hyperthyroidism*)	COPD PAD Heart block Depression Hyperlipidemia Type 2 DM
Alpha adrenergic receptor blockers	Improved urinary symptoms in prostatic hypertrophy (BPH)	Increased CHF hospitalization	Prostatism	Left ventricular dysfunction Not approved as first-line treatment for HTN
Renin inhibitors	Effective without dose-related adverse effects	No outcome data in the elderly Expensive	Systolic hypertension	Diarrhea

Adapted from Geriatric Medicine and Gerontology, 7th edition. McGraw-Hill [7]

- Initiate treatment with lower doses (half the usual dose) to minimize the risk of side effects.
- A once daily regimen with a long-acting medication is preferred.
- In the absence of a hypertensive emergency or urgency, lower BP gradually over weeks to months as the elderly have impaired baroreceptor and sympathetic neural responses, and impaired cerebral autoregulation.
- Measure supine and standing BP (if possible) prior to initiating treatment for systolic HTN as 20% have orthostatic and/or postprandial hypotension, which increase the risk of falls and hip fracture.
- The degree of blood pressure reduction is the major determinant of cardiovascular risk reduction, not the choice of antihypertensive drug.
- Diuretic therapy is effective in lowering systolic BP and decreases the prevalence of orthostatic hypotension; monitor potassium levels.
- An alternative drug may be selected as the initial agent based on comorbid conditions (DM, HF, CKD).
- If systolic blood pressure goals are not met, addition of a second drug from another class depending on comorbidities is usually necessary
- In Stage 2 hypertension, usually two drugs are required, such as a thiazide diuretic combined with an angiotensin converting enzyme (ACE) inhibitor.
- Combining an ACE inhibitor and an ARB increases the risk of hypotension, syncope, hyperkalemia, and renal dysfunction without improving cardiovascular outcomes [6].
- When control is poor, or deteriorating, consider evaluation for secondary causes.

Resistant Hypertension

Resistant hypertension is defined as poor control despite treatment with 3 antihypertensives that have complementary mechanisms of action (that includes a diuretic), or when control requires ≥4 or more medications. In addition to the contributing factors in Table 3, renal artery stenosis is present in 25% of people with a serum

Table 3 Treatment approach resistant hypertension (ACC/AHA 2017 [1])

• Exclude pseudoresistance (inaccurate BP measurement or poor medication adherence)
• Identify and address contributing lifestyle factors (physical inactivity, uncontrolled pain, excessive alcohol, high salt intake)
• Discontinue or minimize potentially contributing medications (sympathomimetic agents, NSAIDs, erythropoietin, corticosteroids)
• Screen for secondary causes (CKD, primary hyperaldosteronism, obstructive sleep apnea, pheochromocytoma); screening for renal artery stenosis in PALTC with existing renal insufficiency is not recommended
• Modify pharmacological treatment (increase diuretic therapy; addition of a mineralocorticoid receptor antagonist; adding other agents with a different mechanism of action; use a loop diuretic in patients with CKD)

creatinine of >2 mg/dL, and can contribute to heart failure, cardiac ischemia, and "flash" pulmonary edema, especially if bilateral renal stenosis is present. Despite the availability of diagnostic Doppler Ultrasonography, CT or MR angiography, two large studies in subjects >69 years, failed to show benefit of renal artery stenting on either cardiovascular or renal outcomes.

Implications for Long-Term Care

The benefit of lowering blood pressure in the LTC population who are >85 years, frail, or have multiple comorbidities is not clearly established as this population has not been included in clinical studies. Because this population often have a limited life expectancy and are prone to developing orthostatic and post-prandial hypotension, syncope, and falls, the risks of lowering blood pressure are increased and its potential benefit reduced. Data is lacking to help practitioners determine how best to treat hypertension in residents with high-risk conditions such as recent stroke, functional impairment, and aortic aneurysm.

Anemia

Aging predisposes persons to decreased hematopoietic reserve (reduced ability of the pluripotent hematopoietic stem cells to replicate), reduced absorption of essential nutrients, decline in glomerular filtration (GFR) and erythropoietin (EPO) secretion, and increased concentrations of cytokines. The normal pattern of myeloid-lymphoid precursor differentiation is also affected with aging, with a decline in lymphopoiesis and an increase in the differentiation of myeloid clones, which can mutate and cause myeloid neoplasms. However, *anemia is **not** considered a normal part of aging*. Anemia may have an insidious onset with nonspecific symptoms until it is becomes severe. Mild anemia is often assumed as being benign or attributed to the presence of chronic comorbidities. However, studies in community dwelling elders show that anemia may be an independent risk factor for adverse outcomes when DM, CKD, or cardiovascular disease is present. Anemia has been associated with significant physiologic impairments and adverse clinical outcomes (Table 4).

Table 4 Clinical impact of anemia

Physiological impairments	Clinical outcomes
Reduced exercise tolerance	Frailty
Left ventricular hypertrophy	Falls
Decline in renal function	Decline in physical function
Dizziness, autonomic dysfunction	Cognitive dysfunction
Weakness, sarcopenia	Hospitalizations, increased health care costs
Osteoporosis	Mortality

Definition and Prevalence of Anemia

There is no uniform definition of anemia. The World Health Organization defines anemia as a hemoglobin (Hb) level less than 12 g/dL in adult women and less than 13 g/dL in adult men. These cutoffs are based on population data that did not include people >65 years of age, and do not take into account the effect of race and ethnicity. The prevalence of anemia from the NHANES III study in US community-dwelling adults >65 years was 11% in men and 10.2% in women. Anemia increases with each decade of age and is higher in black patients. In acute care, clinics for older adults, and in PALTC the prevalence of anemia is even higher.

From the NHANES III and the Scripps-Kaiser database, new lower limits of normal for men >59 years and women >49 years have been proposed that exclude confounding factors. These normal values were slightly higher for older white men and women (Hb 13.2 and 12.2 g/dL, respectively) and slightly lower for older black men and women (Hb 12.7 and 11.5, respectively). However, these levels may not be optimal with regard to morbidity and mortality. For example, in the Women's Health and Aging Study, a risk gradient for adverse outcomes (mortality, frailty, disability) was present with Hb in the "normal range" as was a rise in the erythropoietin level [8]. In nursing home studies in the USA and Turkey, 56% of residents were anemic, the risk even higher in those who were malnourished [9].

Signs and Symptoms

Signs and symptoms of anemia in long-term care residents may be nonspecific (Table 5). Facility staff need to be aware of their significance and, if present, to report them.

Table 5 Symptoms and signs of anemia

Anorexia, nausea
Chest pain, dyspnea, palpitations, tachycardia
Cold intolerance
Decreased activity level or endurance
Depressive symptoms
Ecchymoses
Gingival bleeding, petechiae
Increase in falls
Increased confusion, headache
Jaundice
Pallor (skin, conjunctivae)

Causes of Anemia

Anemia is generally due to an underlying clinical disorder and warrants an evaluation unless the resident has a reduced life expectancy, is receiving palliative care, or declines further evaluation. A systematic evaluation can help the practitioner make rational treatment decisions. However, using empiric iron replacement, for example, can potentially overlook a significant underlying treatable condition. In community-dwelling adults >65 years, about one-third of anemias are associated with *nutrient deficiencies*, one-third related to *disease* without nutrient deficiencies, and one-third are *unexplained* without nutrient deficiencies. The causes of anemia may be classified by etiology, bearing in mind that more than one cause (such as blood loss, malnutrition or hemolysis) may be present in a given person.

A systematic approach to aide clinical decision-making can be useful in most clinical situations. This includes assessing the resident's medical history, comorbidities, renal function, current and recent medication use, physical findings, and review of laboratory tests. Anemia can then be classified as to whether there is **decreased production** due to a hypoproliferative state or ineffective erythropoiesis, **increased destruction** due to hemolysis, or **blood loss, and** by red cell morphology (see Table 6). It is essential that the evaluation be directed by the most likely and clinically relevant cause, and by involving the patient and/or their health care surrogate in discussions especially if endoscopic studies or bone marrow biopsy would be indicated. Table 7 lists suggested noninvasive diagnostic tests for the evaluation of anemia [10, 11].

Sometimes it can be difficult to differentiate iron deficiency anemia from anemia of chronic inflammation since the typical hematologic abnormalities of advanced iron deficiency occur at a later stage and both types of anemia can coexist. Measurement of the soluble transferrin receptor in conjunction with iron studies and ferritin, may help in differentiating iron deficiency anemia from anemia of chronic inflammation.

Several additional tests are available but are usually not part of the routine evaluation of anemia. These include:

- **Serum erythropoietin:** Increases with severity of anemia but its response may be blunted.
- **Proinflammatory markers:** High sensitivity C-reactive protein, TNF, and IL-6 are established markers and may play a role in the future.
- **Hepcidin:** Increased in inflammation and leads to dysregulation of iron metabolism and systemic iron deficiency or availability; standardized measurement assay not available.
- **Bone marrow biopsy:** Indicated if morphological and laboratory evaluation of anemia is not diagnostic and if multiple cell lines are abnormal (e.g., pancytopenia).

Table 6 Causes of anemia and typical laboratory findings [11]

Classification of anemia	Causes	Typical laboratory findings	Peripheral smear findings
Hypoproliferative	Iron deficiency Possible iron deficiency	MCV decreased Serum ferritin <30 ng/mL and/or TSAT <20% Serum ferritin 30–100 ng/mL and/or TSAT <20%	Microcytosis, hypochromia, anisopoikilocytosis
	Erythropoietin deficiency (CKD, endocrine causes)	eGFR <60	No abnormal cells
	Stem cell dysfunction		
	Aplastic anemia	MCV increased RDW normal	
Ineffective Erythropoiesis	B12 deficiency Folate deficiency	MCV increased RDW increased Low B12, increased homocysteine and methylmalonic acid Low folate, increased homocysteine	Oval macrocytes, spherocytes, hypersegmented neutrophils
	Myelodysplastic syndrome (refractory anemia)	MCV increased Normal RDW B12 and folate normal	Normocytic or macrocytic red cells, dysplastic neutrophils
	Thalassemia Sideroblastic anemia	MCV low	Hypochromic, microcytic cells with target cells and basophilic stippling
Hemolytic	Immunologic (idiopathic or secondary)	Increased reticulocyte count Increased LDH Increased bilirubin Decreased haptoglobin	Schistocytes
	Intrinsic (abnormal hemoglobin, metabolic)		
	Extrinsic (mechanical)		

Anemia of CKD

As renal function declines in people with CKD, the Hb will also decline. This drop in Hb is especially noticeable as the GFR trends below 60 mL/min per 1.73 m^2. The anemia of CKD is typically normochromic and normocytic primarily due to a deficiency of erythropoietin production. These usually is no deficiency of iron, B12, or folate, when the GFR is below 30 mL/min per 1.73 m^2. About 50% of nursing facility residents have a GFR below 60 mL/min per 1.73 m^2 and in one recent study, *60% of residents with Stage III CKD were anemic*.

Table 7 Noninvasive diagnostic tests [10, 11]

• Complete blood count (initial low Hb/Hct may not be evident in volume depletion)
– Absolute reticulocyte count (confirms if appropriate marrow response)
• Peripheral blood smear (if reticulocytes are deficient and if toxic, hormonal, or infectious causes have been excluded)
• Serum iron, ferritin, total iron-binding capacity, transferrin saturation (serum soluble transferring receptor)
• Serum folate and RBC folate
• Vitamin B_{12} (methylmalonic acid, and homocysteine more sensitive)
• Renal function (eGFR)
• Liver function
• Sedimentation rate
• Tests for hemolysis (serum LDH, bilirubin, and haptoglobin)
• Serum protein electrophoresis; and immunofixation
• Stool for occult blood (endoscopy if appropriate)
• Thyroid-stimulating hormone and free T4
• Total testosterone (if hypogonadism is suspected)

Acute or Chronic Immune Activation (ACI)

Acute or chronic immune activation can cause a disturbance of iron homeostasis that limits the availability of iron for erythropoiesis due to the impaired release of iron from macrophages. Ferritin may be increased, while the other iron studies are low. This disturbance in iron homeostasis is mediated by proinflammatory cytokines and the increased production of hepcidin in the liver. Hepcidin decreases duodenal absorption of iron. In addition, erythropoietic cell survival and erythropoietic cell response to EPO is decreased [12]. Some patients may respond to erythropoietin. Persons with chronic disease and hemoglobin levels below 10 g/dL should be evaluated for additional causes of anemia such as blood loss, malnutrition, and hemolysis.

Blood Loss

This is a major concern in older adults with anemia. Loss of blood from the gastrointestinal or genitourinary tract should be investigated. In addition, malignancies, gastritis, angiodysplasia, and benign tumors may be responsible.

Treatment

Treatment of coexistent nutritional deficiencies and hypothyroidism should be initiated. If anemia is related to medication, chronic bleeding, CKD, chronic inflammation, malignancy, or hemolysis, then the underlying condition should be stabilized to the extent possible and any potentially offending drugs discontinued. Treatment options for specific types of anemia and cautions to consider are reviewed in Table 8.

Table 8 Treatment options for anemia based on etiology [11, 12]

Cause of anemia	Treatment options	Cautions
Iron deficiency	• Ferrous sulfate 325 mg daily (65 mg elemental iron) • Ferrous gluconate 300 mg daily (36 mg elemental iron) • Parenteral iron (in cancer, CKD, or intolerance of oral)	• Constipation • GI distress • Consider blood loss • Vit C source if achlorhydria present
Vitamin B_{12} deficiency	• Vitamin B_{12} 1000 μg IM weekly × 1 month, then monthly if malabsorption or neurological complications • Oral B_{12} 1000 μg daily	• Check for concurrent folate deficiency
Folate deficiency	• Folate 1 mg orally, daily or 5 mg daily if severe malabsorption	• Check for concurrent B_{12} deficiency
Anemia of chronic inflammation	• Treat or stabilize the underlying disease	• Anemia may persist • Erythropoietin use is not approved
Anemia of chronic kidney disease	• Epoetin alfa or darbepoetin alfa SC • Control diabetes and HTN	• Maintain Hb 10–11 g/dL • Weekly Hb till stable then monthly • Monitor BP
Hemolytic anemia	• Identify underlying cause • Discontinue any contributing medications	

Blood transfusions are generally given for acute blood loss associated with hypotension and cardiovascular compromise. For chronic anemia, blood transfusion is recommended if the Hb drops below 7 g/dL, the hematocrit decreases to 21%, or in the presence of angina, heart failure, dyspnea, tachycardia, or hypotension.

Heart Failure

Cardiovascular disease is often the primary diagnosis when persons are admitted to nursing facilities. Heart failure (HF) affects 20% of residents. Reduced cardiac function presents with signs and symptoms of reduced cardiac output that occur with exertion or at rest. Heart failure is responsible for significant morbidity and mortality that includes acute care visits and hospital readmissions. The care of HF is complicated by frailty, multimorbidity, cognitive, and functional impairment. Hypertension is a major risk factor for the development of HF, especially HF with preserved ejection fraction (HFpEF). In one study HFpEF was present in 50% of nursing facility residents diagnosed with HF. Moreover, the incidence of HFpEF increases significantly in older adults with diabetes, obesity, female gender, HTN, dyslipidemia, and atrial arrhythmias. Elderly with HF with a markedly high or low BP have a worse prognosis as do those with an abnormal LVEF [13]. SNF rehospitalization rates for HF range from 27 to 43%. Overall, 1-year mortality in LTC residents with HF exceeds 50%, and hospitalization exceeds 50% annually, although there are regional differences [14].

Causes of Heart Failure

Causes of heart failure can be classified as *intrinsic* and *extrinsic*. Be aware that more than one cause may be present in an individual.

- **Intrinsic causes:** Myocardial infection, myocarditis, valvular heart disease, congenital heart disease, nonischemic dilated cardiomyopathy (due to viral disease, alcohol excess, medication-related adverse effects, tachycardia -mediated thyroid disease), cardiac arrhythmias, hypertrophic cardiomyopathy, restrictive cardiomyopathy (from amyloidosis), pericarditis, or cardiac tamponade
- **Extrinsic causes:** Systemic hypertension, chronic obstructive pulmonary disease, pulmonary embolism, anemia, thyrotoxicosis, drug toxicity, excess blood volume/polycythemia

It is important to clarify ejection fraction terminology, and most of the recommendations in this section refer to HF with reduced EF (HFrEF). Three EF categories are currently defined as follows:

- HF with preserved ejection fraction (HFpEF): LV ejection fraction (LVEF) >50%
- HF with mid-range ejection fraction (HFmEF): LVEF 41–49%
- HF with reduced ejection fraction (HFrEF): LVEF <40%

Evaluation

The American College of Cardiology/American Heart Association (ACC/AHA) guidelines for the evaluation and management of HF have classified this condition in four stages (A–D) [15]. The first two stages (A, B) are not symptomatic stages of heart failure but defined to help practitioners identify those at risk for developing HF.

Stage A: At risk for HF but without structural heart disease or symptoms of HF

Stage B: Structural heart disease but without signs or symptoms of HF

Stage C: Structural heart disease with prior or current symptoms of HF

Stage D: Refractory HF requiring specialized interventions

The NYHA functional classification can be used to clarify symptom severity (Table 9).

The clinical differentiation between HF with preserved or reduced EF, although challenging, is helpful in decision-making. A complete history and physical

Table 9 New York Heart Association functional classification of heart failure

Class	Patient symptoms
Class I	No limitation of physical activity. Ordinary physical activity does not cause symptoms of HF
Class II	Slight limitation of physical activity. Comfortable at rest, but ordinary physical activity results in symptoms of HF; can walk two blocks or climb two flights of stairs
Class III	Marked limitation of physical activity. Comfortable at rest, but less than ordinary activity causes symptoms of HF; e.g., walking two blocks
Class IV	Unable to perform any physical activity (including ADLs) without symptoms of HF; or symptoms of HF at rest

examination should be performed in residents with shortness of breath, reduced exercise tolerance, edema, or other symptoms suggestive of HF. Review of prior records, current medications, use of alcohol, and/or illicit drugs and alternative therapies, as well as chemotherapy agents should be considered as contributing factors to HF.

The manifestations of heart failure may be atypical in long-term care residents with frailty, cognitive impairment, and multimorbidity. They may present with fatigue, malaise, lethargy, declining function, neurological symptoms such as confusion, restlessness, sleep disturbance, orthopnea, dyspnea with exertion, cough, and edema. Gastrointestinal manifestations of HF can include anorexia, nausea, abdominal discomfort, and altered bowel function. Remember that exertional symptoms may be less prominent in older adults due to a more sedentary lifestyle.

Patients who have HFpEF are more often female, have a fourth heart sound, sustained PMI, absence of jugular venous distension, absence of peripheral edema, normal heart size on chest -ray, and left ventricular hypertrophy (LVH) on the electrocardiogram (EKG). By contrast, patients with HFrEF are more often male, have a third heart sound, displaced PMI, jugular venous distension, pitting edema, and Q waves on the EKG. There can be up to 8 lbs. of fluid weight gain before a patient may develop peripheral edema.

Remember that peripheral edema may also be caused by venous insufficiency, hepatic or renal failure, hypoalbuminemia, or medication such as calcium channel blockers, and should not be attributed to HF without a more detailed review of comorbidities and the medication regimen. The clinical and laboratory evaluation of HF is summarized in Table 10.

Electrolytes and renal function should be measured regularly. Hypokalemia is a common adverse effect of diuretics and may increase the risk of fatal arrhythmias. Many residents with *hypokalemia* also have *hypomagnesemia*, which can result in an inadequate response to potassium supplementation. Hyperkalemia can be associated with ACE inhibitors, angiotensin II receptor blockers, angiotensin receptor-neprilysin inhibitor (ARNI), and worsening renal function. The development of *hyponatremia* may be an indication of disease progression and is associated with

Table 10 Initial evaluation of heart failure

Test	Purpose
Physical examination; essential	Assess weight, edema, jugular venous distension, cardiac rhythm, third heart sound, hepatojugular reflux, crackles at lung bases, or diminished breath sounds due to pleural effusion
CBC, CMP, magnesium, calcium	Evaluate underlying causes of HF, and suitability for treatment with certain medications
Lipid profile	Evaluate for comorbidities
TSH, free T4	Exclude hypothyroidism or hyperthyroidism
Hemoglobin A1C	Evaluate for presence of diabetes
NT-proBNP or BNP	Assist in the diagnosis of HF if cause of dyspnea is unclear (increase with age, in women, with renal impairment). For age >75 years, NT-proBNP >1800 pg/mL consistent with HF. If BNP <100 pg/mL, HF is unlikely, but likely if BNP >500 pg/mL. Serial measurements are not recommended
Urine microalbumin	Indicates risk for developing HF
Chest X-ray	Pulmonary congestion (may be absent in HF), effusion, exclude pneumonia or chronic lung disease; serial studies not recommended
EKG	Evaluate LVH, ischemia, prior MI, atrial fibrillation (does not diagnose HF)
Echocardiogram with doppler	Determine EF, ventricular size and function, evaluate pericardium, and valvular or other structural heart disease; may be repeated in 3–6 months
Additional tests for selected patients	
Ferritin, TIBC, transferring saturation	Evaluate existing anemia, and exclude hemochromatosis
HIV	Evaluate suitability for particular treatments and detect reversible/treatable causes of HF
Cardiac MRI-ordered by cardiologist	Evaluate for myocardial infiltration (e.g., amyloid), or scar tissue from previous cardiac event
Stress test (echo or nuclear)	If patient has suspected CAD and is willing to undergo cardiac catheterization and surgery for revascularization

reduced survival in the elderly with HF. The resident's functional status should be monitored in addition to the physical examination to include the sitting and standing BP when possible.

Common Precipitants of Heart Failure

In addition to identifying the cause of heart failure, it is also important to assess for conditions that may precipitate an exacerbation of heart failure. Evidence-based medication management and the treatment of coexistent medical conditions can optimize treatment of HF (see Table 11). Cardiologist consultation may be required in some instances.

Table 11 Common factors that precipitate HF

Cardiac
Myocardial infarction or ischemia
Poorly controlled hypertension
Excess of dietary sodium
Medication nonadherence
Excess fluid intake (oral or IV)
Arrhythmias—supraventricular (especially atrial fibrillation with rapid rate), bradycardia, sick sinus syndrome
Associated medical conditions—pulmonary embolism, hypoxia due to chronic lung disease, infection (pneumonia, viral illness, sepsis), anemia, hyperthyroidism, chronic kidney disease (eGFR <30 mL/min)
Medications—alcohol, -β adrenergic blockers (including ophthalmic agents), calcium channel-blockers, NSAIDS, glucocorticosteroids, mineralocorticoids, antiarrhythmic drugs
Provider/system problems (e.g., medication reconciliation errors)

Disease Management and Care Considerations in HF

Close observation and early detection of symptoms and signs which may precede an acute HF episode by several days. Close follow-up may be required for days or months, with the risk of rehospitalization high. The following suggestions can improve patient outcomes of HF:

- Education of first-line caregivers, and nurses to improve recognition, assessment, and monitoring of HF patients.
- Timely intervention by the practitioner (with evaluation of weights, chest X-ray, laboratory tests (see Table 10), determine type of HF, initiation and adjustment of therapy, determination of target weight.
- Determine a regular schedule of clinical follow-up (in person or virtual), weights (3/week, before breakfast, on the same scale), and laboratory testing.
- Engage the interprofessional team (e.g., pharmacists, dietitians, physical therapists) and nurse aides who are essential for care delivery.
- Establish an individualized care plan: Assess patient's self-care ability, cognition, health literacy, and support system in order to plan for appropriate discharge planning and subsequent follow-up.
- Consult a cardiologist or HF nurse specialist for patients who are responding poorly, or experiencing repeated exacerbations and/or hospitalizations.
- Evaluate *facility performance* by developing team-based *quality improvement programs* to track hospitalizations, rehospitalizations, symptom relief, physical function, and strategies to improve outcomes
- Patients with both *frailty and HF* are likely to have higher morbidity so optimize nutrition and rehabilitation.

Management

The following are guidelines and recommendations for the management of HF applicable to NH residents [13, 15]. The choice of pharmacologic and nonpharmacologic therapy will depend on the patient's clinical status, goals of care, comorbid conditions, and frailty. Current treatment recommendations are designed to optimize outcomes, reduce morbidity and mortality, and to break the vicious cycle of hospitalization, hospital discharge, and rehospitalization. Mortality significantly increases with a cardiac ejection fraction ≤30–35%.

Nonpharmacologic therapy is essential:

- Promote smoking cessation.
- Moderate sodium restriction <3 g/day (unless hyponatremic; worse outcome associated with low sodium diets.)
- Avoid excessive fluid intake, but restriction is not usually necessary.
- Record daily weights especially in short stay patients in whom home discharge is anticipated.
- Regular physical activity to the extent tolerated (combine strengthening and gait training if possible).
- Evaluate for anemia and thyroid dysfunction.

In the last 4 years, significant evidence has emerged from large clinical trials on the use of angiotensin receptor-neprilysin inhibitors (ARNIs), sodium-glucose cotransporter-2 inhibitors (SGLT2 inhibitors), and ivabradine (an I_f calcium channel blocker highly specific for the sinoatrial pacemaker current), to improve HF symptoms, reduce hospitalizations, and prolong survival. The SGLT2 inhibitors are beneficial in patients *with and without diabetes*. There is no new data on the use of loop diuretics and digoxin. Figure 1 illustrates a pharmacological approach to HFrEF. The indications, caveats for using medication classes, monitoring, and potential adverse effects in older adults are summarized in Table 12. After the initial diagnosis of HFrEF, it is recommended that medications be adjusted every 2 weeks when indicated, in order to achieve *guideline directed medical therapy*.

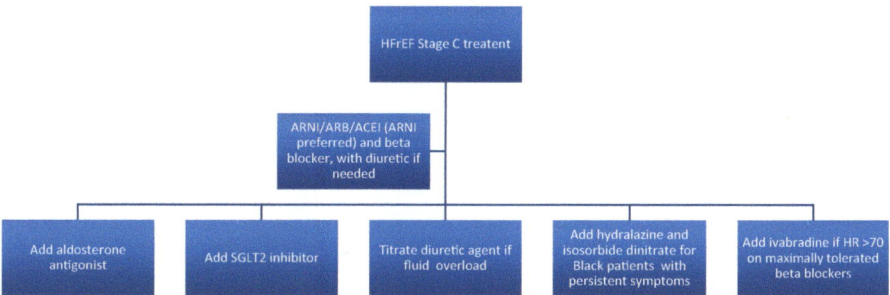

Fig. 1 Pharmacological approach to the management of HFrEF (adapted from the ACC Expert Consensus Decision Pathway for Optimization of Heart Failure Treatment, 2021 [15])

Table 12 Pharmacotherapeutic strategies and selection of treatments for older adults with HFrEF [13, 15, 16]

Medication class	Indication	Outcomes in HF	Contraindications	Adverse events in older adults	Caveats
ACE inhibitors	Consider in patients in whom use of ARNI is not possible	Improved outcomes, reduced mortality	Hyperkalemia (K >5.5 mEq/L), hypotension (syst BP < 80 mm, estimated Cr clearance <30 mL/min	Cough, mild renal function impairment, hypotension, hyperkalemia, angioedema (rare)	Check BP, renal function, and K level weekly when starting and titrating to maximum tolerated dose
Aldosterone antagonists (MRA)	NYHA class III-IV and low EF ≤35%	Reduced mortality and hospitalizations	Serum creatinine ≥2.5 mg/dL, or K ≥5.0 mEq/L	Mild renal function impairment, hyperkalemia	Eplerenone beneficial in HF following MI. Check renal function and K level 2–3 day after initiation, at 7th day, then monthly for 3 months
Angiotensin-receptor blockers (ARBs)	Alternative to ACEI in HF, consider in patients in whom ARNI is not possible	Improved outcomes, reduced mortality	Hyperkalemia (K >5.5 mEq/L), hypotension (syst BP <80 mm, estimated Cr clearance <30 mL/min	Mild renal function impairment, hypotension, hyperkalemia Hyperkalemia may be managed by low potassium diet or scheduled use of potassium binders	Check BP, renal function, and K level weekly when starting and titrating to maximum tolerated dose Combining ACEI and ARB not beneficial and increases adverse events
Beta-Blockers	Newly diagnosed HFrEF, Stage C	Improved ventricular function, reduced cardiac deaths	Severe decompensated HF, marked bradycardia (HR <45–50/min), active bronchospastic lung disease, significant heart block, relative hypotension (SBP <90–100 mmHg)	Worsening of HF (usually transient)	Benefit only demonstrated with carvedilol, metoprolol succinate and bisoprolol. Greatest impact when resting HR <70/min, and patients are "dry"

ARB/ Neprilysin inhibitors	Newly diagnosed HFrEF, Stage C, and NYHA class II + III symptoms	Reduced mortality and HF admissions	Hypotension before treatment, history of angioedema	Mild renal function impairment, hypotension, hyperkalemia, angioedema (rare)	Valsartan plus sacubitril is the first in this class Can be used instead of ACEI, avoid starting within 36 h of last ACEI dose
Digoxin	Persistent limiting HF symptoms or recurrent hospitalizations	Reduced HF hospitalizations, but not mortality		Nausea, visual disturbances, cardiac arrhythmias (bradycardia and SVT or VT) "Therapeutic concentrations" may be associated with toxicity and mortality	Serum levels of 0.5–0.9 ng/ mL are optimal. Lower doses 0.125 mg/day recommended QOD dosing in patients with renal impairment 50% dose reduction if on verapamil, amiodarone, or quinidine
Diuretics	HF with congestion and edema			Hypotension, orthostatic hypotension, hypokalemia	Check BP, renal function, and K. If furosemide dose exceeds 80 md BID, consider a different loop diuretic (e.g., bumetanide) or add a thiazide diuretic (e.g., metolazone)
Hydralazine and nitrates	For Black patients with persistent symptoms despite use of ACEi/ ARBs and beta-blockers, and in HF patients who are unable to take ACEi and ARBs	Improved survival		Headaches with nitrates (resolves with continued use); palpitations, nausea, and dizziness with hydralazine	

(continued)

Table 12 (continued)

Medication class	Indication	Outcomes in HF	Contraindications	Adverse events in older adults	Caveats
Ivabradine	NYHA class II–III HFrEF in sinus rhythm with persistent HR >70/min on maximally tolerated beta-blocker doses	Reduced hospitalizations for HF in patients with NYHA class II–III HFrEF		Transient brightness in some areas of the visual fields	Initiate and titrate beta-blockers to target doses when possible Monitor for bradycardia
SGLT2 inhibitors	Consider in patients with HFrEF, NHHA class II–IV	Improved hospitalization and CV mortality in patients with and without diabetes. Reduced decline in kidney function in HFrEF and CKD		Uncommon but potentially serious genital infections, Fournier gangrene, lower extremity, and acute kidney injury	Dapagliflozin is the current FDA-approved SGLT2 inhibitor for HFrEF
Antiplatelet or Anticoagulant therapy	Routine anticoagulation in HF patients *without atrial fibrillation is not recommended*	Long-term anticoagulation in patients with HF and comorbid atrial fibrillation is indicated in most patients			For anticoagulation, warfarin or one of the newer oral anticoagulants may be used

ACEi angiotensin-converting enzyme inhibitor, *ARB* angiotensin receptor blocker, *ARNI* angiotensin receptor neprilysin inhibitor, *SGLT2i* sodium glucose transporter 2 inhibitor

Rehospitalization for HF

Studies have shown that 20% of patients admitted to the SNF/NF with HF are readmitted to the hospital within 30 days, and up to 50% within 6 months. Not all these rehospitalizations are due to HF; COPD, pneumonia, sepsis, other cardiac events and arrhythmias are contributing causes [17]. The percentage of short stay and long stay patients who are rehospitalized after nursing home admission are CMS nursing home quality measures. Contributing factors for rehospitalization due to HF include:

- Severity of HF and presence of comorbidities.
- Quality of care issues, and suboptimal use of evidence-based therapies for chronic HF.
- Inconsistent availability of practitioners especially during night-time exacerbations.
- Problems with medication administration and weight monitoring, use of NSAIDS.
- Nonadherence to sodium restriction and lack of food choices.
- Problems with care delivery, miscommunication, and with discharge procedures (optimally should include medication reconciliation, transfer of information to community providers, and follow-up appointments).

Refractory HF

HF can have an unpredictable course and a high incidence of sudden death despite intensive medical management. Older adults with HF who are discharged to skilled nursing facilities are known to have high mortality rates (14.4% within 30 days and 53.5% within 1 year). Referral to an advanced heart failure specialist should be considered in patients who have required IV inotropes, had two or more emergency room visits or hospitalizations in the past 12 months for HF exacerbations, persistent fatigue, edema with rising BNP or NT-proBNP, renal failure (creatinine ≥ 1.8 mg/dL or BUN ≥ 43 mg/dL), inability to tolerate appropriately dosed beta blockers, and/or ARB/ACEI/ARNI and/or aldosterone antagonists, development of atrial fibrillation, ventricular arrhythmias or repeated ICD shocks.

Palliative care and end-of-life care should be discussed and considered for those with refractory HF, recurrent hospitalization, and persistence of severe disabling symptoms such as dyspnea, fatigue, pain, sleep disturbance, and functional decline. Palliative care for HF patients has been shown to improve physical, psychosocial, and spiritual well-being. Palliative care consultation is appropriate before placement of an ICD or left ventricular assist device (LVAD) is considered. In addition, an ICD should be inactivated upon admission to hospice if it is consistent with the goals of care [15, 18].

Chronic Obstructive Pulmonary Disease

Chronic obstructive pulmonary disease (COPD) is an insidious, progressive lung disease characterized by airflow obstruction that is not fully reversible. It is the third leading cause of death in older adults. COPD can be difficult to diagnose because persons gradually modify their lifestyle to compensate for progressive fatigue and dyspnea. The main symptoms are dyspnea, cough, and sputum production. COPD continues to be underdiagnosed and undertreated, and often difficult to differentiate from asthma, HF, and other conditions that limit physical activities. One in six patients admitted to a nursing facility may have COPD or emphysema. COPD is responsible for high utilization of acute health care and 34% probability of death in 180 days post hospital discharge to nursing facilities [18, 19].

Identification of COPD

Smoking (90% of cases), advanced age, repeated pulmonary infections, prior tuberculosis, exposure to biomass fuel, air pollution, and alpha-1 antitrypsin deficiency are risk factors for COPD. Early identification of COPD is important since 50% of lung function is lost by the time mild exertional dyspnea occurs and only 30% of lung function remains when there is dyspnea at rest. Residents with dyspnea and other recurrent pulmonary symptoms should be screened for COPD utilizing the clinical indicators listed in Table 13 [18, 19]. A screening tool that uses caregivers to rate residents' symptoms was validated by Zarrowitz et al. who reported that a history of asthma, shortness of breath at rest and shortness of breath on exertion, and smoking are likely to be consistent with a diagnosis of COPD [20].

Table 13 Clinical indicators of COPD in long-term care [18]

Dyspnea (progressive over time, worse with exertion)
Abnormal pulse oximetry
Cough (may be intermittent and unproductive)
Chronic sputum production (any pattern)
Wheezing and chest tightness
Avoidance of activities that lead to dyspnea or impaired performance of ADLs
History of smoking
Recurrent pulmonary infections
Occupational or environmental exposure to occupational dust and chemicals
Weight loss, fatigue, anxiety, cognitive impairment, or sleep disorders

Diagnosis of COPD

On examination, residents with advanced disease may be barrel-chested, have prolonged expiration, use accessory muscles for inspiration, and have wheezing, rhonchi, or distant heart sounds. The signs of *cor pulmonale,* i.e., right-sided HF, include jugular venous distension, hepatic congestion, and pedal edema.

The clinical indicators of COPD and the review of past medical records may help in the diagnose of COPD. Although the definitive method of diagnosis is spirometry, which usually measures FEV_1 (volume of air exhaled in 1 s) to FVC (forced vital capacity or total volume of air able to be exhaled), this is usually not practical in the PALTC setting. The FEV_1 to FVC ratio decreases with aging and hence can lead to overdiagnosis of COPD. Spirometry should be performed in symptomatic individuals when feasible. However, its use in frail or cognitively impaired residents is usually not feasible.

- Normal: $FEV_1/FVC \geq 70\%$ or $FEV_1 \geq 80\%$ of predicted
- COPD: $FEV_1/FVC \leq 70\%$
- Restrictive lung disease: $FEV_1/FVC \geq 90\%$ (pulmonary fibrosis, severe kyphosis)

Other tests may provide useful information when evaluating for the presence of COPD or other conditions with similar signs and symptoms.

- The CBC may have an abnormally high Hb level due to hypoxia
- The chemistry panel may show a high bicarbonate level (metabolic alkalosis) due to hypercapnia
- Chest X-rays are not diagnostic, but may show HF, bullae, pneumonia, pulmonary scarring, hyperinflation, and increased retrosternal airspace, to suggest COPD
- An EKG may show atrial arrhythmias or right heart strain

Pulmonary consultation may be helpful if the cause of dyspnea is not clear or the resident exhibits a poor response to treatment. Clinical judgment is important since the differential diagnosis of COPD can include asthma, heart failure, bronchiectasis, recurrent aspiration, ACE-inhibitor induced cough, vocal cord dysfunction, pulmonary emboli, and respiratory tract tumors. The GOLD criteria classify the severity of COPD (Table 14) [21].

The GOLD ABCD staging [20], may be clinically useful and guide referral to a pulmonologist.

- GOLD A—Fewer symptoms and <2 exacerbations a year
- GOLD B—More symptoms and <2 exacerbations a year
- GOLD C—Fewer symptoms and ≥2 exacerbations a year
- GOLD D—More symptoms and ≥2 exacerbations a year

Table 14 GOLD spirometry classification of airflow obstruction in COPD [21, 22]

Post-bronchodilator FEV$_1$/FVC <70% applies to all categories	
GOLD 1:Mild	FEV$_1$ ≥80% predicted
GOLD 2: Moderate	50% ≤ FEV$_1$ <80% predicted
GOLD 3: Severe	30% ≤ FEV$_1$ <50% predicted
GOLD 4: Very severe	FEV$_1$ <30% predicted
Chronic respiratory failure	

[a]Defined as partial pressure of oxygen less than 60 mmHg with or without partial pressure of carbon dioxide than 50 mmHg while breathing air at sea level

Table 15 Management of COPD [18, 19, 21]

Spirometry	Begin pharmacotherapy if symptomatic
Group A Group B Group C Group D	• A bronchodilator (short or long acting) • A long-acting bronchodilator (LABA or LAMA) • LAMA • LAMA or • LAMA + LABA[a] or • ICS + LABA[b]
Severe progressive disease	• Supplemental oxygen • Theophylline
Other interventions	• Smoking cessation – Physical activity – Improve nutrition • Influenza, pneumococcal, pertussis, and Covid-19 vaccination • Osteopenia/osteoporosis evaluation • Pulmonary rehabilitation • Evaluate for lung-volume reduction surgery
Plan of care	• Identification of care goals and advance care planning • Reinforce proper inhaler technique • Depression and anxiety screening

LABA long-acting bronchodilator, *LAMA* long-acting muscarinic agonist, *ICS* inhaled corticosteroids
Adapted from Ref. [18, 19, 21]
[a]If highly symptomatic
[b]If eosinophils >300/μL

Management of COPD

The main classes of medication therapy include inhaled β–agonists, inhaled or nebulized anticholinergic or antimuscarinic agents, and inhaled corticosteroids. Since staging of COPD by spirometry criteria is not usually possible or practical in PA/LTC, clinical presentation and judgment must be utilized to guide treatment [19, 20] as outlined in Table 15.

Encouraging smoking cessation is important at any stage of this disease; as are measures to improve nutrition, encourage physical activity, and immunizations. Pharmacological treatment should be stepwise and cumulative. Medication can reduce symptoms, increase exercise capacity, and reduce the number and severity of exacerbations; but *no treatment has been shown to modify the progressive decline in lung function*. Complications such as polycythemia, hypoxia, and HF should be treated, and goals of care should be discussed with the resident and family. The following are evidence-based recommendations regarding the use of bronchodilators in stable COPD.

- Long-acting bronchodilators are underutilized, but they are more effective than short-acting bronchodilators or anticholinergics.
- A combination of short-acting agent β–agonists and muscarinic agonists produces a greater change in FEV_1 than either agent alone
- LAMAs and LABAs are effective in improving lung function, dyspnea, and overall health status
- Combination treatment with LAMAs and LABAs improve lung function, symptoms, and reduce exacerbations, compared to monotherapy
- LAMAs are more effective than LABAs in reducing rates of COPD exacerbations and hospitalizations
- Theophylline use may be of modest benefit and have a small effect on bronchodilation

Pharmacologic treatments for COPD are summarized in Table 16.

The routine use of antibiotics is not recommended other than for acute exacerbations. Mucolytics are not recommended, but may be considered for patients with viscous mucous. Although cough is troublesome, the regular use of antitussives is only recommended if it impairs daily activities. *The prolonged use of oral glucocorticoids should be avoided*. Statins and vasodilators do not show any benefit.

Table 16 Commonly used pharmacologic agents: benefits and cautions

Drug class	Drug example	Dosage	Cautions
Short-acting β agonists	Albuterol	2 puffs q6h 2.5–5 mg nebulized q 4–6h	All four drugs may be used for acute bronchospasm
	Levalbuterol	0.63–1.25 mg nebulized q6–8h	
Long-acting β agonists	Formoterol	20 mcg nebulized q12 h	Not for acute bronchospasm. Palpitations, tremor, bronchospasm
	Salmeterol	1 puff q12 h	
	Arformoterol Indacaterol Olodaterol	15 mcg nebulized q12h 1 puff q24h 2 puffs q24h	

(continued)

Table 16 (continued)

Drug class	Drug example	Dosage	Cautions
Anticholinergics Antimuscarinic	Ipratropium bromide	2 puffs q6h 0.5 mg nebulized q6–8h	May be used for acute exacerbation
	Tiotropium MDI&DPI	2 puff q24h or 1 inhalation q24h	For maintenance treatment. Not for acute bronchospasm Caution with BPH and glaucoma
	Umeclidinium DPI	1 inhalation q24h	
	Aclidinium MDA & DPI Glycopyrronium bromide	1 puff or 1 inhalation q12h 1 inhalation q12h	
Inhaled corticosteroids (MDI or DPI)	Beclomethasone	1–2 puffs q 12–24h	For severe COPD with repeated exacerbations; added to routine bronchodilator therapy
	Fluticasone Budesonide Mometasone	1–2 puffs q12h 2 puffs q12h 2 mg nebulized q6h 1–2 puffs q24h	
Oral corticosteroids	Prednisone 5 mg	30–40 mg/day for 5 days	Monitor glucose in patients with DM Osteoporosis, myopathy and cataracts
	Prednisolone 4 mg	24–32 mg/day for 5 days	
Methylxanthines Phosphodiesterase-4 inhibitors Long-term oxygen therapy	Theophylline ER Roflumilast	400 mg/day 500 mcg q24h	*Toxicity and multiple drug interactions.* Caution with liver and cardiac disease. Check levels Adjuvant therapy for severe COPD with exacerbations If resting PaO_2 is $\leq$55 mmHg; use for $\geq$15 h a day improves survival, exercise tolerance and cognition

Acute Exacerbations

Acute exacerbations are often characterized by an increase in dyspnea, wheezing, cough, chest tightness, fever, and a change in sputum color, volume, or consistency. The majority of acute exacerbations may be due to tracheobronchitis, while *one-third of exacerbations may be noninfectious* in origin. However, an exacerbation may be difficult to distinguish from pneumonia, HF, or thromboembolic disease. The following is a protocol for managing a COPD exacerbation [19, 21].

- Increase dosage and/or frequency of β agonists
- Implement use of spacers or nebulizers for better delivery of inhaled medication
- Add oral steroids (e.g., prednisolone 30–40 mg/day) for 5 days
- Antibiotics, if increased sputum volume or purulence (for 5 days; check local resistance patterns)
- Oxygen supplementation (aim for saturation levels of 88–92%)
- CBC, chest X-ray, EKG (sputum culture often difficult to obtain)
- Consider hospitalization if response to treatment is poor and respirations are >28/min

The decision as to whether to hospitalize a resident should be individualized and based on the LTC setting and its ability to treat the resident. In general, *hospitalization should be considered for any patient who fails to respond to treatment, develops tachypnea (respirations >28 breaths/min), remains hypoxic, develops delirium, has high fever, has significant difficulty sleeping or eating, or has serious comorbidities* (HF, DM, CKD, liver disease) [21]. COPD is another major cause of 30-day readmissions to the hospital.

Non-pulmonary complications of COPD increase morbidity and can reduce functional status. Cardiovascular and skeletal muscle changes contribute to reduced lung and exercise capacity. Residents frequently have a reduced BMI, frailty (which increase mortality), and sarcopenia. In addition, male hypogonadism, vitamin D deficiency, glucocorticoid use, and sedentary lifestyle lead to the development of osteoporosis. Residents often experience anxiety, depression, malnutrition, weight loss, sleep disturbance, decreased awareness of hypoxia and hypercapnia, and cognitive dysfunction. A 6-min walk distance of less than 350 m is predictive of future exacerbations and death. In residents with advanced disease, it is important to have an ongoing discussion with the resident and/or family about realistic expectations and treatment goals [18, 21].

Diabetes

Diabetes is one of the most common chronic conditions in older adults and affects over 30% of long-term care residents [23]. It is associated with reduced life expectancy, multiple complications and comorbidities, higher risk of geriatric syndromes, and is an independent predictor of placement into a LTC facility (Table 17). The clinical and economic burden of diabetes in the PALTC setting is high with annual nursing home expenditures estimated to be $18.6 billion. Residents with diabetes are a heterogeneous group characterized by a higher prevalence of cardiovascular disease, infections, lower extremity complications, pain, pressure ulcers, urinary incontinence, injurious falls, poor dentition, cognitive dysfunction, functional dependency. Practitioners face challenges in the management of diabetes due to patient's advanced age, staff and practitioners' issues, site of care capabilities, as well as an evolving therapeutic landscape (see Table 18). There is a paucity of data

Table 17 Problems and complications of diabetes in older adults

- Atherosclerosis with vascular complications (myocardial infarction, stroke)
- Changes in weight (gain or loss)
- Confusion, cognitive impairment
- Dehydration
- Depression
- Excessive skin problems (infections, ulcers, delayed wound healing)
- Visual impairment
- Falls
- Foot ulcers, deformities, gangrene, other foot problems
- Frequent infections
- Impaired pain perception, neuropathy
- Nonketotic hyperosmolar coma
- Oral health problems (caries, periodontal disease, tooth loss, dry mouth, burning mouth)
- Polypharmacy
- Urinary frequency, nocturia, urinary incontinence

Adapted with permission from the AMDA Clinical Practice Guideline; Diabetes Management in the Post-Acute and Long-Term Care, 2015

in PALTC to guide the practitioner in terms of goals of reasonable glycemic control and its impact on clinical outcomes. Many older adults with diabetes have multiple problem and complications that are summarized in Table 17. These need to be evaluated at the time of admission or readmission [23].

Effective diabetes management is multifaceted and requires a protocol-driven, team-based, individualized approach to care. Goals of treatment are affected by life expectancy, patient preferences and values, expected clinical benefit, risks of treatment side effects, particularly hypoglycemia. National organizations have written clinical guidelines in order to improve metabolic control and to reduce debilitating complications of DM. The challenges of managing diabetes in LTC is attributed to multiple factors related to aging, disease burden, institutional, staff, practitioner, and socioeconomic factors (Table 18) [24].

Patients with *prediabetes* may not be recognized nor diligently followed. Intercurrent medical stressors, obesity, pancreatic insufficiency, hyperthyroidism, and medications can cause hyperglycemia, and the development of overt diabetes,

Table 18 Challenges to managing diabetes in PA/LTC [24]

Age and disease	Institution	Staff and practitioner	Socioeconomic factors
Altered glucose metabolism Decline in renal function Variable food intake	Staff turnover and lack of familiarity with residents Varying clinical capacity in ALF and other facilities	Variance in knowledge and treatment preferences Inadequate review of glucose logs Reliance on sliding scale insulin protocols	Limited social support Difficulties in access to care (limited income, health insurance, prescription expense)
Increased risk of hypoglycemia	Restricted dietary practices	Hypoglycemia management (delayed recognition or overcorrection)	Health literacy
Functional impairment (impaired mobility, frailty, sarcopenia) Impaired vision and manual dexterity Multiple comorbidities Polypharmacy and medication side effects Cognitive dysfunction and depression Type 1 diabetes erroneously assumed to be Type 2 Multiple and changing treatment approaches	Lack of facility—specific diabetes treatment algorithms Lack of established blood glucose parameters for physician notification Lack of administrative buy-in	Failure to individualize care Failure of timely and stepwise advances in therapy Therapeutic pessimism Lack of familiarity with diabetes technology (insulin pumps, CGMs)	Complex regimens and delivery systems Transitions of care

even diabetic ketoacidosis. Medications that cause hyperglycemia include glucocorticoids, atypical antipsychotics, β adrenergic agonists, thiazides, and megesterol acetate [23]. Older adults with *undiagnosed* diabetes are at risk of MI, HF, stroke, and complications of diabetes.

Diabetes may present with nonspecific symptoms or geriatrics syndromes in older adults. The latter include failure to thrive, confusion, new onset or worsening urinary incontinence, recurrent infections, dehydration, falls, heart attacks, and stroke. Unique syndromes associated with diabetes include diabetic neuropathic cachexia, diabetic neuropathy (focal or symmetric), renal papillary necrosis with pyelonephritis or UTI, diabetic amyotrophy, diabetic bullae on the palms or soles of the feet, shoulder pain, and diabetic ketoacidosis, the latter possibly caused by antipsychotics or SGLT2-inhibitors.

Type 1 Diabetes in PALTC

Care of patients with Type 1 insulin dependent diabetes can pose challenges to practitioners. The diagnosis of Type 1 diabetes may not be recognized due to incomplete medical records, care transitions, cognitive impairment and lack of social support all of which put the patient at risk of hyperglycemia and hypoglycemia. Practitioners may be unfamiliar with the use of insulin pumps or continuous glucose monitoring devices. Diabetic ketoacidosis can be mistaken for sepsis, organ failure, or metabolic acidosis due to other causes. Hence intensive diabetes education of first-line caregivers, nursing staff, and clinicians is paramount [24, 25].

Key Recommendations for Managing Diabetes in PALTC Settings

A comprehensive position paper published by the American Diabetes Association (ADA) [26] on the management of diabetes in long-term care and skilled nursing facilities had the following recommendations.

- Hypoglycemia risk is an important factor in determining goals of glucose control
- Simplified treatment plan is better tolerated and preferred by patients (and staff)
- The use of a sliding scale insulin regimen as a sole treatment should be avoided
- Use liberal diets to promote adequate intake of food and fluids; less risk than restrictive diets to avoid weight loss and dehydration
- Physical activity and exercise are important and should depend on current functional abilities (Fig. 2).

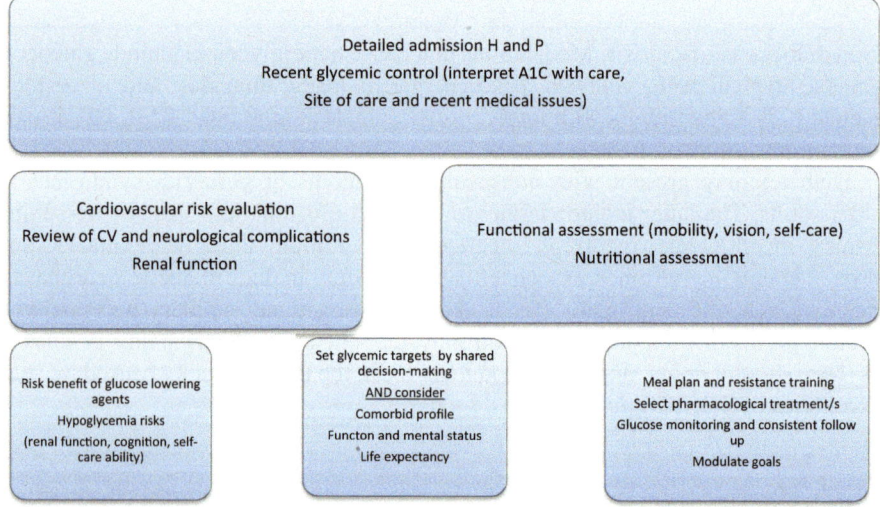

Fig. 2 An approach to individualized diabetic care

Treatment Selection

The general principles for treating diabetes in PA/LTC are similar to those used to treat diabetes in the community. While lifestyle changes are effective, dietary restriction is not recommended in LTC since food enjoyment, quality of life, and prevention of weight loss take precedence. Ambulation, seated exercise and any physical activity (and resistance training) should be encouraged. Type 2 diabetes is a progressive disease and combination treatment with oral agents (to take advantage of their different modes of action) is often required. A stepwise approach to selecting glucose-lowering medication is reviewed in Table 19.

Important considerations in the selection of therapy include the resident's age, functional status, treatment goals (both short and long term), renal impairment, hepatic impairment, and weight loss. The algorithm in Table 19, by the American Diabetes Association represents a feasible approach [26, 27]. Management of blood pressure, lipids, nutritional status, pain control, neuropathic symptoms, lower extremity infections, ulcers, and limb loss must all be considered in the overall care of the resident.

When selecting pharmacological therapies to treat diabetes it is important to be aware of not only specific benefits, but also the potential side effects and cautions within each medication class. These are summarized in Table 20 [28].

Table 19 Stepwise approach to selection of glucose-lowering medication [25–27]

---

1.   Use Metformin as first-line therapy and lifestyle changes to the extent possible
2.   Assess for indicators of high CV risk or established ASCVD, CKD, or HF. **If PRESENT**;
  –   Add a GLP1-RA or a SGLT-2I with proven cardiovascular benefit (can be used in addition if A1C goal is not reached, or instead if one agent is not tolerated)
  –   SGLT-2L with proven cardiovascular benefit if HF with reduced LVEF <45%
  –   SGLT-2L with primary evidence of reducing CKD progression if diabetic kidney disease and albuminuria present
  –   Either GLP1-RA or a SGLT-2I with proven cardiovascular benefit if NO diabetic kidney disease and albuminuria, BUT patients have DM and CKD (eGFR <60 mL/min/1.73 m^2 are at risk of increased CV events)
4.   **If NO** indicators of high CV risk or established ASCVD, CKD or HF, and A1C above individualized target:
  –   treat with any of the following: DPP-4I, GLPI-RA, SGLT2I, TZD (add another agent from this group if A1C goal is not met, or one agent is not tolerated)
  –   DPP-4I and GLP1-RA cannot be used simultaneously
  –   GLPI-RA or SGLT2I if glucose targets not met, or weight loss is desired (based on evidence)
  –   SU or TZD if

DPP-4I dipeptyl peptidase 4inhibitor, GLP-1 RA glucagon-like peptide-1 receptor agonist, SU sulfonylurea, TZD thiazolidinedione, SGLT2I sodium-glucose co-transporter 2 inhibitor

---

Table 20 Commonly used pharmacological therapies in older adults [28]

Medication class	Benefits	Cautions	Caveats and considerations
Biguanides	• Safe if no contraindications • Low risk of hypoglycemia • Low cost	• May cause GI disturbances • Weight loss • Vitamin B12 deficiency • Renal dosing required (safe if eGFR >30 mL/min)	• First-line treatment if no contraindications • Metformin ER may reduce GI disturbances
Sulfonylureas	• Low cost	• Hypoglycemia risk • Drug interactions (e.g., warfarin, allopurinol)	• Short-acting glipizide to reduce hypoglycemia • Avoid glyburide (renal elimination)
Meglitinides	• Skip dose if skipped meal • Useful if variable eating habits	• Increased pill burden • High cost	• Useful with one large meal—controls post-prandial hyperglycemia
Thiazolidinediones	• Low hypoglycemia risk • Can be used in CKD patients	• Edema and HF • Increased bone loss and fracture risk • Bladder cancer concerns	• Contraindications in elderly • Well tolerated, reduces insulin resistance
Glucagon-like peptide 1 receptor agonists	• Consider if overweight or glucose targets not met • Low risk of hypoglycemia • Can use in CKD • Convenience of weekly dosing, reduced nursing time (one oral agent available)	• Nausea, vomiting, diarrhea, satiety • High cost • Usually injectable	• Unintended weight loss • Limited safety profile in elderly
Sodium-glucose transporter 2 inhibitors	• Low risk of hypoglycemia • ASCVD or HF benefit • Decrease renal disease progression	• Genital yeast infections, UTI • Dehydration, increase potassium and LDL	• Limited safety profile in older adults • Avoid if frail, and hydration issues

Insulin

Prolonged severe hyperglycemia leads to glucotoxicity that increases insulin resistance and impairs insulin secretion. Older adults with Type 2 diabetes are known to be more insulinopenic. Timely use of insulin beginning with basal insulin analogs (10 units daily or 0.1–0.2 units/kg/day) with weekly increases of 2–3 units *until desired levels of fasting glucose levels are obtained*, is simple and effective, especially in the elderly over age 80 with liver or chronic kidney disease.

Insulin **should** be used acutely in the following situations [23, 27]:.

- Marked or symptomatic hyperglycemia despite maximal use of oral agents, or increased insulin requirements resulting from infection, stress, surgery, or injury.
- Evidence of catabolism (significant weight loss, ketosis, diabetic ketoacidosis).
- A1C >10% on current treatment regimen
- BG persistently >300 mg/dL

Sulfonylureas may be discontinued and the dose of thiazolidinediones reduced once the fasting glucose levels have been stabilized. If the fasting blood glucose levels are adequately controlled, but the A1C remains elevated despite maximal tolerated treatment with oral agents or a GLP1-RA, prandial insulin (usually a rapid acting insulin analog (4 units or 0.1 units/kg) can be added to the main meal. *Basal analog insulins (U 100 glargine or detemir), or Longer-acting basal analogs (U300 glargine and degludec) may have a lower risk of hypoglycemia and* nocturnal hypoglycemia. Rapid acting analogs can allow flexibility for inconsistent mealtimes and erratic food intake that is not uncommon in PA/LTC. *It is important to be aware that rapid acting insulin analogs should be administered 10–15 min before a meal, while insulin glulisine should be administered 15 min before to up to 20 min after a meal, and insulin lispro can be given 15 min before, or immediately after the meal.*

Sliding-Scale Insulin

Sliding-scale insulin (SSI) as a method of glucose control has many disadvantages. Although widely used alone or as an adjunct to oral agents and/or basal insulin, it is a reactive rather than a proactive approach. Its use is not recommended by any guideline as a primary or sole method of treatment, and is on the Beers criteria for potentially "inappropriate medication use" in older adults. SSI uses hyperglycemia as a threshold (e.g., >200) and often involves "one-size-fits-all" dosing with glucose variability not being assessed (e.g., the practitioner only being contacted if glucose is <60 or >300 mg/dL.) On a practical level, SSI results in an increased number of insulin injections, as many as 60% unnecessary fingersticks, medication errors, increased patient discomfort and increased nursing time [29]. SSI may be more useful as a *correctional scale* to be added to scheduled oral and/or insulin therapy when blood glucose levels are highly variable and the patient medically unstable.

Suggestions for Adjusting Insulin Therapy Based on Glucose Patterns

Maintaining adequate glucose control with insulin requires frequent evaluation of targeted glucose levels and adjusting the insulin dose accordingly. Tables 21 and 22 can be used as guides as to which insulin dose to increase or decrease based on the resident's average glucose levels at various time of the day [23].

Table 21 Standard human insulin therapy: regular and NPH insulin given twice a day

Average blood glucose	Regular AM	Regular PM	NPH AM	NPH PM
Fasting				
LOW				↓
HIGH[a]				↑
Pre lunch				
LOW			↓	
HIGH	↑			
Pre supper				
LOW[b]			↓	
HIGH			↑	
Bedtime				
LOW		↓		↓
HIGH		↑		

Pre-lunch glucose levels are influenced by both the R and NPH given in the AM
Bedtime glucose levels are influenced by both the R and NPH given at the evening meal
[a]Evaluate 3 a.m. blood glucose level to eliminate possible nocturnal hypoglycemia leading to rebound hyperglycemia
[b]Evaluate 3 p.m. BG readings for necessity of afternoon snack

Table 22 Analog insulin therapy: basal insulin with rapid acting insulin at each meal

Average blood glucose	Basal	Rapid[a] Breakfast	Lunch	Supper
Fasting				
LOW	↓			
HIGH[b]	↑			
Pre lunch				
LOW		↓		
HIGH		↑		
Pre supper				
LOW			↓	
HIGH[c]			↑	
Bedtime				
LOW				↓
HIGH				↑

Giving rapid acting insulin up to 15 min after eating may be more appropriate if a patient's eating is unpredictable. This allows for not giving the insulin if the patient does not eat
[a]If a correction dose (sliding scale) is routinely being added to the patient's usual rapid insulin dose at meals due to hyperglycemia, the *average correction* dose used for any particular meal can be used as the number of units to increase the rapid acting insulin dose at the *preceding* meal
[b]Evaluate 3 a.m. BG readings to eliminate possible nocturnal hypoglycemia leading to rebound hyperglycemia
[c]Evaluate 3 p.m. BG readings for necessity of afternoon snack

Goals of Treatment

Treatment goals for diabetes should be individualized and take into account the extent of microvascular and macrovascular disease, life expectancy, resident preferences, functional and cognitive status, presence of any psychiatric disorder, and risk of hypoglycemia. In one study, facility physicians were noted to have managed diabetes less aggressively in residents who were both cognitively and functionally impaired [28]. Less stringent A1C goals (7.5–8.5%) may be appropriate for LTC residents who have a history of hypoglycemia, limited life expectancy, or multimorbidities. Table 23 reviews treatment goals for glycemic control in different PALTC settings proposed by the American Diabetes Association and AMDA [26, 30].

Table 23 Framework for diabetes management goals

Patient characteristics and care status	Reasonable A1C goal[a]	Fasting/premeal glucose targets (mg/dL)	Rationale	Glucose monitoring
Skilled rehabilitation[b]	– A1C unreliable due to recent acute illness – Follow glucose trends	100–200	– Optimize glucose control after recent acute illness	– Monitoring frequency depends on complexity of treatment
Long-term resident	– Avoid relying in A1C; avoid symptomatic hyperglycemia and hypoglycemia – If used, interpret A1C with caution due to conditions that interfere with A1C levels	100–200	– Intensive glycemic control of limited benefit – Focus needs to be on quality of life and reducing glucose excursions	– Monitoring frequency depends on complexity of treatment and hypoglycemia risk
Resident at the end of life[d]	– No role of A1C[a]	– Avoid symptomatic hyperglycemia and hypoglycemia	– No benefit of glycemic control – Avoid symptomatic hypo- and hyperglycemia	– Monitor periodically to avoid symptomatic hypo- and hyperglycemia

Source: Adapted from [26, 27]

[a]Lower goals may be set for individuals if achievable without recurrent or severe hypoglycemia or undue treatment burden

[b]Community-dwelling resident receiving skilled care for short-term rehabilitation and potential discharge to home

[c]Long-term care resident with limited life expectancy and frequent changes in health condition and potential hospitalization, affecting glucose levels

[d]Resident at the end of life; avoiding symptomatic hypoglycemia and hyperglycemia as well as invasive diagnostic or therapeutic procedures is the priority

Medication Management: Focus on Safety and Simplification

As multimorbidities and diabetes-related complications also require pharmacological treatment in addition to glucose-lowering agents, patients are at risk of polypharmacy. Practitioners may have different prescribing preferences and on-call practitioners may alter the regimen without reviewing glucose *trends*. Comparative data on the effectiveness of diabetes treatments is limited in the PALTC setting. The following treatment regimens are suggested to *reduce hypoglycemia risk*, *simplify treatment*, be cautious *in those with renal insufficiency* and to *improve cardiovascular outcomes* [24, 26, 27, 30].

- Administer basal insulin in the morning instead of at night
- The use of oral agents has been shown to achieve comparable glycemic control as to basal insulin; e.g., linagliptin compared to basal insulin showed similar glycemic control with lower rates of hypoglycemia and not require renal dose adjustment
- If a sulfonylurea is used, avoid glyburide; use glimepiride or glipizide, which are primarily eliminated by the liver and monitor for hypoglycemia
- The meglitinides (nateglinide and repaglinide) are useful if meal intake is variable as they can be given when a meal is taken, and help can control postprandial hyperglycemia
- Consider linagliptin as an add-on to oral hypoglyemics and basal insulin, especially in renal insufficiency.
- Consider an SGLT2 inhibitor (e.g., canagliflozin or dapagliflozin) as add-on if heart failure, CKD or albuminuria is present, and the patient has adequate fluid intake, and does not have recurrent UTIs (with eGFR is >45 mL/min/1.73 m^2 or > 60 mL/min/1.73 m^2, respectively).
- Consider adding a GLP1-RA if control is not achieved with oral agents, especially in those with, or at high risk for cardiovascular complications.
- If the patient is stable replace sliding scale insulin with basal insulin or a GLP1-RA.
- Simplify the insulin regimen: titrate basal insulin dose to a BG goal of 90–150 mg/dL (5–8.3mmol/L); if mealtime dose is <10 U consider, discontinuing and add non-insulin agent; if mealtime dose is >10 U, consider decreasing dose by 50% and add non-insulin agent. If GFR is >45 ml/min/1.73m2, start metformin 500 mg/day.
- Consider use of second-generation basal insulins (degludec 200 U/mL, or glargine 300 U/mL) in those requiring a high dose of basal insulin or who have wide fluctuation in glucose levels. These provide similar glycemic control and lower rates of severe hypoglycemia.

Hypoglycemia

Hypoglycemia is defined by its symptoms and confirmed by a low blood glucose. Hypoglycemia is classified into three levels.

Level 1—Glucose <70 mg/dL (3.9 mmol/L) and ≥54 mg/dL (3.0 mmol/L)
Level 2—Glucose <54 mg/dL (3.0 mmol/L)
Level 3—A severe event characterized by altered mental or physical status requiring treatment of hypoglycemia

Recognition of hypoglycemia can be problematic. Symptoms may be atypical: disorientation, lethargy, weakness, falls, aggression, or altered behavior. Neuropsychologic symptoms can be mistakenly attributed to dementia or delirium. Older adults have a lower glucose threshold at which they develop symptoms. Hypoglycemia can increase neuropathic pain. Repeated episodes of hypoglycemia can lead to worsening of dementia (Table 24).

Insulin-induced hypoglycemia can result from delayed insulin clearance as in renal failure, erratic absorption, and increased insulin sensitivity due to weight loss or increased physical activity. Frequent use of SSI, improper timing of insulin relative to food intake, poor meal consumption, inappropriate tight blood glucose control, injection of the wrong type of insulin (e.g., rapid acting instead of long acting), and unawareness of hypoglycemia can all-cause insulin-induced hypoglycemia.

Hypoglycemia may be corrected with ingestion of 15 g of glucose or carbohydrate: equivalent to 1/2 cup juice or soda, 1/2 cup apple sauce, 1 cup milk, 1 tablespoon sugar or honey, 1 mini candy bar, 1 tube of glucose 15 g gel, or 4 glucose tablets. Caregivers should wait *15 min to recheck* blood glucose and if still below the target, give another *15 g* of glucose or carbohydrate. Elderly who are obtunded may be treated with s.c. or i.m. glucagon (1 mg or 1 unit) or 50% dextrose IV (usually 50 mL, or less if hypoglycemia is not severe). Glucagon is now also available as a nasal spray in a prefilled syringe, which does not require mixing. Non-medical personnel and caregivers should be trained in the administration of glucagon.

Table 24 Risk factors for severe hypoglycemia in older adults [31]

- Age
- Black race
- Poor nutrition or variable oral intake
- Cognitive or functional impairment
- Loss of normal counter-regulation
- Unawareness of, or previous severe hypoglycemia
- High doses of insulin or sulfonylureas
- Recent hospitalization or intercurrent illness
- Chronic liver, renal, or cardiovascular disease
- Endocrine deficiency (thyroid, adrenal, or pituitary)
- Alcohol use

Monitoring

Assessment of Glycemic Control

There is no consensus recommendation regarding the frequency of glucose checks in LTC. The practice of routinely checking pre-meal and bedtime glucose should only be used for those receiving multiple insulin injections or insulin pump therapy and for whom this information will be used to adjust insulin dosing. In residents who are on simpler insulin regimen (1–2 doses a day), then twice daily glucose monitoring for at least 3–4 days a week is suggested. For residents receiving oral agents or less frequent insulin injections, a reasonable approach to glucose monitoring would be twice per day for 1–2 weeks after admission, then once or twice per week, and as indicated. Postprandial monitoring may be helpful in situations where the fasting glucose is at goal but the A1C remains elevated [23, 26].

It is recommended that A1C should be monitored every 6 months in patients who are achieving their goals and every 3 months in those who are suboptimally controlled. It is important to carefully interpret A1C results as it can be affected by several factors.

A1C may be <u>increased</u> by: age, race (African American or Hispanic), hypothyroidism, splenectomy, aplastic anemia, polycythemia, hemoglobin variants, iron deficiency anemia, metabolic acidosis/uremia.

A1C may be <u>decreased</u> by: hemolytic anemia, blood loss, transfusions, hemodialysis and hematocrit <30%, liver disease, erythropoietin therapy.

Improving Interprofessional Communication and Facility Care Processes

Successful implementation of a facility-wide diabetes protocols requires buy-in from the administration, and effective education and communication with practitioners, nursing staff, and medical assistants. In an assisted living facility this may be more difficult to accomplish due to variable clinical capabilities. In such situations, the resident may be eligible to receive home health services to complement the care provided by the facility staff. A "diabetes nurse" or champion can help ensure implementation of diabetic protocols. The following are suggestions to improve the care of patients with diabetes [24].

- Thorough evaluation on admission: Type of diabetes, its complications, function, cognition, preferences, goals of care.
- Use a facility protocol for glucose monitoring and parameters for practitioner notification.

- Hypoglycemia: Staff education on recognition, management, and modification of the medication regimen.
- Medication simplification and de-intensification if appropriate.
- Avoid changing the medication regimen based on an isolated hyperglycemic episode.
- Avoid or replace SSI when possible.
- Optimize frequency of glucose monitoring: Avoid routine checks four times a day.
- Frequent foot and skin inspections with prompt intervention for new concerns.
- Prompt evaluation of acute change of condition.
- Facility QI approach: e.g., review hypoglycemia episodes, SSI use, emergency room visits.

Optimizing Transitions of Care

Transitions from hospital or home to LTC, between health care settings, upon discharge to the community, or with a change in practitioners are high risk for patients with diabetes. Poor coordination and continuity of care without a feasible care plan can lead to unnecessary rehospitalizations, duplicate tests, medication errors, delays in diagnosis, and lack of follow-up on referrals. Risk factors for rehospitalization include poor patient health literacy, inadequate social support, black race, age >75 years, male gender, difficulty managing medications, and high comorbidity burden. The following checklist can facilitate a transition in care (Table 25).

Table 25 Suggested checklist for care transitions

From hospital to LTC	From LTC to ALF or home
• History and physical exam, progress notes, consultation reports • Accurate diagnosis list • Laboratory tests and imaging study reports • Current medication list (reconciled) • Time of last basal insulin dose • Hypoglycemia episodes • Approximate meal consumption	• Treatment goals and suggested BG range • Medication reconciliation with written reason for each medication • How and when to take oral agents, insulin, or GLP1-RA • How often to monitor BG • How to treat hypoglycemia (training caregivers on use of glucagon) • When to call the LTC facility and PCP (give numbers) • Home health services requested (agency contacts) • Follow-up appointment details with PCP or specialist

Thyroid Disorders

Though thyroid disorders are common in the elderly, its presentation is often subtle and varied and can range from subclinical disease to overt hypothyroidism or hyperthyroidism. Because of its nonspecific presentation, thyroid disease requires screening and interpretation of thyroid function tests in the context of patient signs and symptoms, clinical scenario, comorbidities, and medication regimen. Subclinical disease requires diligent follow-up and an evidence-based approach to its management. Nodular thyroid disease requires evaluation of thyroid function, imaging, and, if indicated, biopsy, and be consistent with goals of care.

Pathophysiology and Epidemiology of Thyroid Disorders in Older Adults

Normal aging is associated with progressive fibrosis and atrophy of the thyroid gland. However, the hypothalamic-pituitary-thyroid (HPT) axis, remains intact. There is a decline in TSH levels leading to reduced thyroxine (T4) and triiodothyronine (T3) secretion, but due to reduced renal clearance, T4 levels remain normal. T3 declines in advanced old age while the inactive metabolite, reverse T3 (rT3) increases. Acute or chronic *non-thyroidal illness* can lead to abnormalities of thyroid function, as can several medications. Thyroid disease in older adults may be categorized as *functional (hypothyroidism and hyperthyroidism), inflammatory (thyroiditis), and neoplastic (thyroid nodules and malignancies).* Mean TSH levels increase with age as well as thyroid peroxidase antibodies (TPOAb), the latter associated with hypo- or hyperthyroidism. Thyroid disorders are more prevalent in women, and lower in blacks than in whites. Risk factors for hypothyroidism and hyperthyroidism include:

Hypothyroidism: Female, iodine deficiency, autoimmune conditions, (e.g., rheumatoid arthritis), selenium deficiency, medication, syndromic conditions (e.g., Down's)

Hyperthyroidism: Female, iodine deficiency, autoimmune conditions, smoking, selenium deficiency, medication,

Screening for Thyroid Dysfunction

Recommendations on screening for asymptomatic thyroid dysfunction vary, citing the lack of evidence as to the benefit in treating subclinical disease. However, screening in older adults may be justified. In the Colorado Thyroid Disease Prevalence Study, 16% of women and 21% of men over age 74 years had elevated TSH levels [32]. Adults over age 60 have a 2–10% prevalence of hypothyroidism. Conditions for which screening may be reasonable are listed in Table 26. Serum TSH is highly sensitive and is considered the first-line test. In *euthyroid* persons the

Table 26 Conditions associated with thyroid disease

- Biological agents (e.g., interferon, tyrosine kinase inhibitors)
- Chronic kidney disease
- Cognitive impairment/psychiatric illness
- Down's/Turner's syndrome
- Drug therapy (e.g., amiodarone, lithium)
- Hyperlipidemia
- Irradiation of head/neck (recent and remote)
- Pituitary surgery, irradiation
- Radical laryngeal/pharyngeal surgery
- Thyroid disease/surgery in the past, goiter
- Thyroid nodule
- Type 1 diabetes
- Severe head injury
- Unexplained depression/weight loss

normal TSH reference range is 0.4–4.1 mU/L. In those over 80 normal TSH levels can be up to 7.9 mU/L. Hence values above the current upper TSH limit of 4.0–5.0 mU/L may be normal and *not* associated with adverse clinical outcomes. Over diagnosis of hypothyroidism can result in inappropriate treatment (i.e., iatrogenic hyperthyroidism) and other potential adverse effects.

Interpretation of Thyroid Function Tests

Measurement of serum TSH by immunoassay is ultrasensitive and able to distinguish between a normal, low, or high value. However, in the elderly with a pituitary or hypothalamic disorder, the TSH may be misleadingly subnormal or low normal. Thyroid dysfunction occurs with acute or chronic illness, hospitalized patients, those with poor adherence to therapy, or treatment with drugs that alter thyroid hormone levels (see Tables 26 and 27). Measurement of free T4 and total T3 can be useful if hyperthyroidism is suspected.

Non-thyroidal illness due to acute or chronic illness or severe malnutrition can cause a low T3 state with normal TSH, FT4, and T4 (due to inhibition of 5′ deiodinase and decreased conversion of T4 to T3). Patients who are severely ill may have both a low T4 and low T3. TSH can decline with severe illness, while *a transient high TSH may be seen during the recovery phase from an acute illness*. Up to 32% of critically ill inpatients diagnosed with low free T3 levels. It is advisable to repeat thyroid function once a patient is medically stable before initiating treatment with thyroid replacement therapy. There is increasing recognition of *partial hypopituitarism* in

Table 27 Drugs affecting thyroid function [34]

Effect	Drugs
May cause hypothyroidism	Lithium, iodine (all forms, including kelp, contrast media, topical povidone iodine), amiodarone, interferon alpha
May cause hyperthyroidism	Amiodarone, iodine, interleukin-2, interferon alpha
Reduce conversion of T4 to T3	Glucocorticoids, iodine, propylthiouracil, propranolol, amiodarone
Suppress TSH	Dopamine, dobutamine, glucocorticoids, phenytoin, bromocriptine, somatostatin analogs, metformin, mitotane
Increase clearance of T4	Carbamazepine, phenytoin, rifampin, phenobarbital
Reduce binding of T4 to thyroid-binding globulin	Phenytoin, carbamazepine, salsalate, NSAIDS, furosemide, heparin
Influence absorption of thyroxine	Proton-pump inhibitors (PPIs), cholestyramine, aluminum hydroxide, calcium carbonate, ferrous sulfate, sucralfate

Table 28 Interpretation of thyroid function tests

	TSH	FT4	TT3	Tg	Anti-Tg AB
Subclinical hypothyroidism	↑	NL	NL		
Hypothyroidism	↑	↓	NL		
Central hypothyroidism		↓	↓		
Subclinical hyperthyroidism	↓	NL	NL		
Hyperthyroidism	↓	↑	↑		
TSH-producing pituitary adenoma	↑	↑	↑		
Intermittent/poor medication adherence	↑ or NL	↑	↑		
Non-thyroidal illness	NL	↓	NL or ↓		
Thyroiditis/thyroid injury	NL or ↓	NL or ↑	NL or ↑	↑	NL or ↑
Persistent thyroid cancer	NL ↓ ↑[a]	NL ↑↓[b]		NL or ↑	NL or ↑

TSH thyrotropin stimulating hormone, *FT4* free thyroid hormone, *TT3* total triiodothyronine, *Tg* thyroglobulin, *Tg-Ab* anti-Tg antibody
[a] TSH depends on degree of TSH suppression
[b] FT4 depends on degree of thyroid supplementation

frail long-term care residents with cardiovascular disease. When evaluating for thyroid dysfunction a TSH and a free T4 level are the most helpful. Table 28 provides a guide for the interpretation of TSH and free T4 (FT4) levels [33, 34].

Hypothyroidism

Hypothyroidism is defined as a state of reduced thyroid hormone available to peripheral tissues. *Overt hypothyroidism* is diagnosed when serum-free T4 levels are *below* the normal range in the presence of hypothyroid symptoms. Mild

Table 29 Causes of hypothyroidism in the elderly	*Primary hypothyroidism*
	Chronic autoimmune hypothyroidism (Hashimoto's thyroiditis)
	Post ^{131}I treatment for hyperthyroidism
	Subtotal or total thyroidectomy
	Radiation therapy for head and neck cancer
	Drugs
	Central (secondary) hypothyroidism
	Hypothalamic tumors or infiltrative lesions
	Pituitary tumors or infiltrative lesions
	Pituitary surgery
	Head injury or cranial surgery
	Cranial radiation
	Stroke, hemorrhagic, or ischemic

thyroid failure or *subclinical hypothyroidism* is a condition in which the TSH level is elevated in the presence of a normal free T4 level. An increasing TSH level needs to be monitored and a decision made as to whether to start thyroid replacement.

Causes of Hypothyroidism

The majority of residents with hypothyroidism have *primary* hypothyroidism due to thyroid gland failure or dysfunction. *Central* or *secondary* hypothyroidism is rare and accounts for less than 1% of cases. The latter may occur due to lesions of the pituitary or hypothalamus or dysfunction of the hypothalamic–pituitary axis (Table 29).

Clinical Evaluation

Clinical signs and symptoms are often nonspecific. Classical signs and symptoms are listed in Table 30. Fatigue has been noted in 68 % and weakness in 53% [35]. Classical symptoms such as weight gain, cold intolerance, paresthesias, and muscle cramps are less frequent in older adults. *Neuropsychiatric symptoms* (e.g., withdrawal, disorientation, delusions, or psychosis) can develop gradually and be challenging given the prevalence of dementia and the propensity for developing delirium.

Table 30 Symptoms and signs of hypothyroidism in older adults

Symptoms	Signs
Fatigue	Alopecia
Cold intolerance	Xerosis
Constipation	Hoarseness
Dysphagia	Weight gain
Exertional dyspnea, atypical chest pain	Bradycardia, diastolic HTN
Lack of concentration	Worsened congestive heart failure
Memory loss, delusions, or psychosis	Anemia
Hearing loss	Hyperlipidemia, elevated CPK
Depression	Myxedema
Generalized weakness or muscle cramps	Neuropathy, slowed reflexes

Treatment of Clinical Hypothyroidism

The goal of treatment is to normalize the thyroid function test (TSH) to achieve an euthyroid state. The dose of thyroid hormone replacement depends on the age and weight of the resident. Synthetic thyroid hormone preparations (rather than thyroid extracts) are preferred due to a longer half-life and a more constant serum level. The initial replacement dose of levothyroxine is usually 25–50 µg/day, but older adults with significant cardiac comorbidities should be started on 12.5–25 µg/day and the dose adjusted by a similar amount every 3–6 weeks until the TSH has normalized, after which, it is recommended the TSH be checked every 6–12 months. In primary hypothyroidism, the TSH alone can be used to monitor treatment, while in those with central (secondary) hypothyroidism, a free T4 level should be used. If no residual thyroid function exists the daily replacement dose of levothyroxine is usually 1.6 µg/kg body weight (typically 100–150 µg). Dosage adjustments should take into account any concomitant or worsening condition such as atrial fibrillation, HF, or osteoporosis. Low normal or subnormal TSH levels should be avoided, and if needed, thyroxine can be held for days to weeks and restarted at a lower dose once the patient's condition has become stable. It is important to note that *linear changes in the concentration of T4 correspond to logarithmic changes in serum TSH*. If a resident has had an inadvertent discontinuation or omission of levothyroxine therapy during a care transition, there may be a marked increase in the TSH level. *When resuming levothyroxine it should be at the prior documented dose. Measurement of free T4 may be helpful* [35].

Subclinical Hypothyroidism

This condition may also be referred as "mild thyroid failure" and is defined by an elevated TSH with a normal free T4 level. Anti-TPO antibodies are positive in 67% of nursing facility residents with subclinical hypothyroidism. Most elderly are usually asymptomatic. Prevalence of this condition in 80-year-olds ranges from 14 to 20%. The etiology of subclinical hypothyroidism is usually chronic autoimmune thyroiditis, but poor compliance with levothyroxine therapy, suboptimal treatment, recovery from severe illness, thyroiditis, and medications that affect thyroid function should be considered. Hence TSH should be repeated in 1–3 months to confirm this diagnosis. Subclinical hypothyroidism can progress to overt hypothyroidism in 33–55% of individuals, and be associated with elevation of lipid levels, altered mood and cognition, impaired cardiac function, and increased mortality, especially in those with HF. A TSH level >12 mU/L, presence of autoantibodies, goiter, advanced age, and a history of radiation therapy are risk factors for progression to overt hypothyroidism.

Management of Subclinical Hypothyroidism

Current evidence does **not** support a benefit to treating *subclinical* hypothyroidism in an attempt to improve cardiac function or neuropsychiatric symptoms. The current guidelines for the management of subclinical hypothyroidism are the following [36]:

- If the TSH is 4.5–10 mU/L in the **absence** of symptoms, repeat TSH in 6 months and yearly thereafter if patients remain asymptomatic
- If the TSH is above the upper limit of 4.5–6.9 mU/L, no treatment in those >65–70 since TSH is age appropriate; avoid treatment in those over 80 years
- If the TSH is 7.0–9.9 mU/L, treat those who have symptoms of hypothyroidism; the goal of treatment is to achieve a TSH of 3–6 mU/L
- If the TSH is >10 mU/L, in most circumstances administer thyroid treatment.

Hyperthyroidism

It is important to diagnose hyperthyroidism in older adults. If undiagnosed, there is a potential for significant morbidity, mortality, and poor quality of life. Risks include cardiac arrhythmias, worsening osteoporosis, and increased incidence of fracture. Primary and subclinical hyperthyroidism occur more frequently in older adults, reported up to 2% in persons over the age of 60.

The causes of hyperthyroidism in older adults are:

Endogenous: Thyroid hyperfunction due to toxic multinodular goiter (40%), toxic adenoma (30%), Graves' disease (15%), and thyroiditis (5%)

Exogenous: Suppressive dosing of levothyroxine in the treatment of thyroid carcinoma (10%) and excessive dosing of levothyroxine in treating hypothyroidism (5%).

T3 toxicosis can occur where the TSH is low with an *isolated* elevation of T3. It is usually due to excess T3 secretion from a thyroid nodule or goiter. **"T4 toxicosis"** is seen in patients with pre-existing primary hyperthyroidism or concurrent non-thyroidal illness, leading to low or normal T3. **Amiodarone-related thyrotoxicosis** occur more frequently in older adults with atrial fibrillation than younger patients. Prompt identification of clinical signs and diagnostic workup is essential. Amiodarone more often causes hypothyroidism.

Signs and Symptoms of Hyperthyroidism in the Elderly

- Atrial fibrillation (up to 20% of patients)/palpitations
- Unintentional weight loss
- Depression and cognitive decline, delirium, mania
- Lethargy and fatigue
- Heat intolerance
- Sweating
- Tremor
- Diarrhea, vomiting, or constipation
- Exophthalmia
- Alopecia or coarse or thinning hair
- Pretibial myxedema
- Severe osteoporosis and increased fracture risk

Signs and symptoms of hyperthyroidism such as heat intolerance, anxiety, tachycardia, and tremor may be lacking in older adults. Atypical signs or symptoms include vomiting, constipation, depression, and fatigue. *Thyroid storm* is less common and presents with a severe hypermetabolic state, fever, neurocognitive changes, and possibly heart failure. The most common cause of thyroid storm in older adults is infection, rather than due to unprepared thyroid surgery or radioiodine therapy seen in younger patients.

Diagnosis of Hyperthyroidism

Overt, primary hyperthyroidism is diagnosed by low TSH and elevated total and free T4 levels. *Subclinical hyperthyroidism* is diagnosed by the presence of low TSH and normal levels of total or Free T4. The latter may also indicate T3 toxicosis. Positive thyroid-stimulating immunoglobulin (TSI) or other thyroid antibodies can help confirm a diagnosis of Graves' disease. Review medications regimen to evaluate iatrogenic causes of hyperthyroidism.

Management of hyperthyroidism in older adults depends on its underlying etiology, comorbidities, and the patient's goals of care. Management is summarized in Table 31 [33, 37].

Table 31 Causes and management of hyperthyroidism

Causes of hyperthyroidism	Management	Caveats
Subacute thyroiditis	• Beta blockers for hyperadrenergic symptoms • Glucocorticoids if refractory thyroiditis • NSAIDS for inflammatory pain (low dose)	• Avoid in decompensated HF, asthma, and Raynaud's disease
Grave's disease	• Antithyroid medications; methimazole, propylthiouracil (PTU) • Radioiodine therapy	• Elevated risk of agranulocytosis, during the first 90 days with PTU • Monitor LFT regularly • Short course before radiodine therapy • Favored over long-term medications or surgery; reduction of mortality
Toxic multinodular goiter or toxic adenoma	• Antithyroid medications; methimazole, propylthiouracil (PTU) • Radioiodine therapy • Surgery for large obstructive goiters	• Elevated risk of agranulocytosis, during the first 90 days with PTU • Monitor LFT regularly • Short course before radiodine therapy • Favored over long-term medications or surgery; reduction of mortality
Amiodarone-induced thyrotoxicosis type 1 Amiodarone-induced thyrotoxicosis type 2	• Antithyroid medications; methimazole, propylthiouracil (PTU) • Long course of glucocorticoids	• High doses of methimazole [40–60 mg/day] or PTU [600–800 mg/day]) to block thyroid hormone synthesis • Glucocorticoids for relapse
Thyroid storm	• Fluid and electrolyte stabilization • High doses of methimazole (40–80 mg/day) or PTU (200 mg q 6 h) • Beta blocking agent • Stress dose glucocorticoids • Potassium iodide 1 h after antithyroid medication	• Other agents may be used to lower thyroid hormone levels; sodium iodate, potassium perchlorate, and cholestyramine
Subclinical hyperthyroidism	• Same treatment as for overt hyperthyroidism when TSH levels are <0.1 mIU per L	

LFT liver function tests

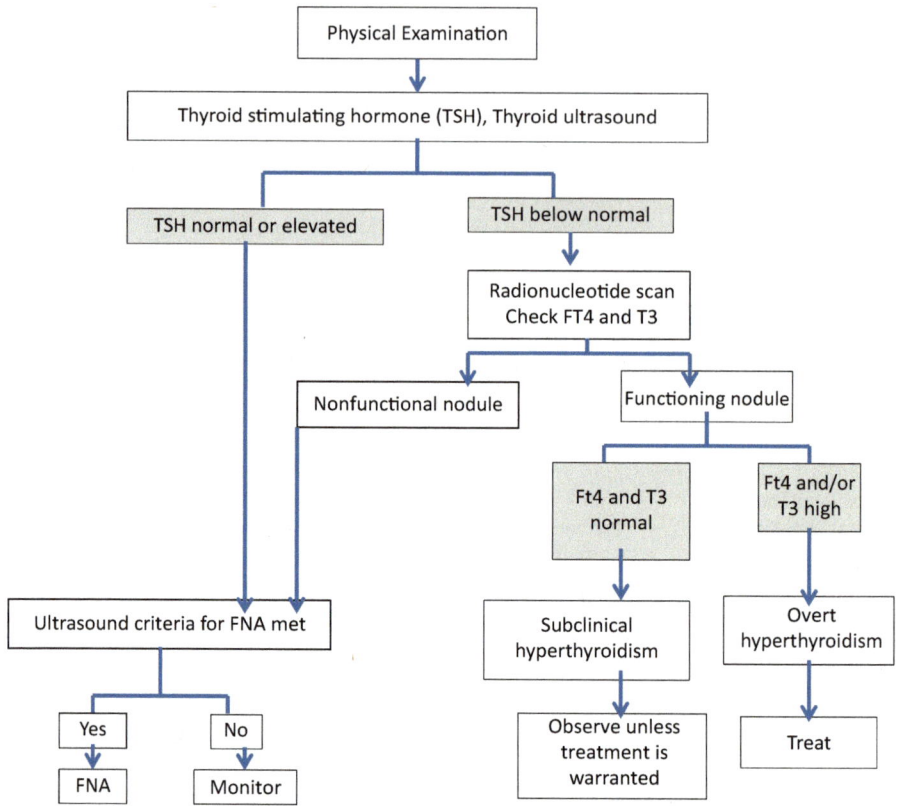

Fig. 3 Initial approach to a patient with a thyroid nodule (adapted from American Thyroid Association) [38]

Thyroid Nodules and Thyroid Cancer

Thyroid nodules become more prevalent with age. Over age 65, 50% have thyroid nodules detected by ultrasound and 5% of thyroid nodules may be malignant. The prevalence of thyroid cancer is higher in those over 60–65 years of age, history of head and neck irradiation, family history of thyroid cancer, history of total body irradiation for bone marrow transplantation, multiple endocrine neoplasia type 2 (MEN2), and familial adenomatous polyposis, or Cowden syndrome. The following algorithm provides an initial approach to patients with a thyroid nodule [38] (Fig. 3).

Follow-Up of Patients with a History of Thyroid Cancer

It is not uncommon to assume the care a of newly established patient who has had a history thyroid cancer. The history is usually unclear, and thus it is important to question why patients are on thyroid supplementation, to palpate the neck for thyroid nodules, goiter, and lymphadenopathy, and to look for neck incisional scars. Unexplained hypocalcemia, may be due to hypoparathyroidism related to partial parathyroidectomy during previous thyroid surgery. The presence of exophthalmos in persons on thyroid supplementation suggests prior treatment of Grave's disease with radioiodine ablation or thyroidectomy. Patients who have been treated with thyroidectomy followed by radioiodine ablation or had treatment for thyroid cancer, should be referred to an endocrinologist or oncologist [39]. Pre-referral studies to consider:

- **TSH**: Identify appropriate TSH goal: TSH suppression with levothyroxine may not be necessary if the cancer was low risk and without recurrence, or the patient has cardiac arrhythmias or a low bone density.
- **Thyroglobulin**: Should be undetectable with TSH stimulation.
- **Anti-Tg antibodies:** If present, the serum Tg level alone cannot be used as a marker for recurrent or persistent thyroid cancer and further imaging will be necessary.
- **Neck ultrasound:** Identifies malignant cervical lymph nodes (common site for recurrence of papillary thyroid cancer)

Vitamin B$_{12}$ Deficiency

- B$_{12}$ deficiency is common in older adults and can lead to hematological abnormalities *(though often there is no associated anemia or macrocytosis)* as well as potentially serious and irreversible neurological consequences. Population studies show a prevalence of B$_{12}$ deficiency of 10–15% in older adults, with one study of hospitalized elderly from the community and nursing facilities reporting a prevalence of 5% with low B$_{12}$ (<200 pg/mL or 150 pmol/L), and 20% with marginal B$_{12}$ (200–349 pg/mL or 150–260 pmol/L). The signs and symptoms of B$_{12}$ deficiency are nonspecific and varied and can be misattributed to other disorders or the neurological changes of normal aging. The elderly may have "subtle B$_{12}$ deficiency" with only a biochemical deficiency. In a population in which the prevalence of dementia and other neurological and neuropsychiatric abnormalities are high, early recognition and treatment of B$_{12}$ deficiency can be beneficial [40]. Older age and more established symptoms of B$_{12}$ deficiency are associated with lower likelihood of neurologic improvement when treatment is delayed. Vitamin B$_{12}$ deficiency has also been associated with low bone mineral density and been implicated in pre-frailty.

Risk factors and causes of B$_{12}$ deficiency are listed Table 32. Dietary cobalamin deficiency is responsible for about 40–50% of B$_{12}$ deficiency, and pernicious anemia (due to decreased gastric intrinsic factor production) for about 10%. Hypochlorhydria and atrophic gastritis are important contributing factors. Stomach acid is necessary for the release of vitamin B-12 from food, which then binds to haptocorrin, undergoes degradation by pancreatic enzymes, then binds to intrinsic factor, and finally is absorbed in the terminal ileum. The B-12 intrinsic factor complex then binds to transcobalamin for transport in the blood.

Table 32 Causes of B_{12} deficiency [40]

• Atrophic gastritis and hypochlorhydria
• Chronic antacid use (histamine-2 blockers, proton pump inhibitors)
• Gastrectomy (total or partial), gastric by-pass surgery
• Ileal resection
• Small intestine and terminal ileum disorders (Crohn's disease, sprue, malabsorption)
• Pancreatic insufficiency
• *Helicobacter pylori* infection
• Bacterial overgrowth syndromes
• Strict vegetarian diet
• Pernicious anemia (positive anti-intrinsic factor antibodies)
• AIDS and AIDS treatment (zidovudine)
• Metformin

Table 33 Signs and symptoms of B_{12} deficiency [40]

Hematologic: Macrocytosis, anemia, neutrophil hypersegmentation, pancytopenia
Neurologic: Peripheral neuropathy, paresthesias, spinal column lesions (loss of vibration, position sense, ataxia), extensor plantars, orthostasic hypotension, limb weakness
Neuropsychiatric: Delirium, slow thinking, depression, confusion, memory loss
Other: Glossitis, pallor

B_{12} deficiency should be suspected in residents with unexplained anemia or neurological symptoms, glossitis, anorexia, diarrhea, or other gastrointestinal disorders as well as the presence of autoimmune diseases such as thyroiditis and vitiligo. Signs and symptoms of vitamin B_{12} deficiency are listed in Table 33.

Diagnosis

- Measure vitamin B_{12} levels in frail older adults, those with macrocytic anemia, hypersegmented neutrophils, gait disorders, peripheral neuropathy, or neuropsychiatric symptoms without obvious cause.
- Serum B12 levels less than 200 pg/mL (150 pmol/L) are consistent with a diagnosis of B_{12} deficiency.

    - *Falsely low levels of B_{12} may be seen* in AIDS, multiple myeloma, folate deficiency, and excessive vitamin C intake.
    - *Falsely normal or high levels of B_{12}* may be seen in transcobalamin II deficiency, certain myeloproliferative disorders (chronic myelogenous leukemia), liver disease, and intestinal bacterial overgrowth.

- Serum B_{12} levels between 200 and 350 pg/mL (150–260 pmol/L) indicate a borderline B_{12} deficiency that can be treated by supplementation.
- Methylmalonic acid (MMA) by serum or urine testing is specific for B_{12} deficiency, and should be considered in patients with borderline B12 levels if neces-

sary to confirm clinically significant B_{12} deficiency. MMA levels will normalize with treatment. Falsely elevated levels of MMA may be seen in hypovolemia and renal insufficiency.

- *Consider Helicobacter pylori* testing when evaluating patients with B_{12} deficiency.
- Folate deficiency can coexist, and it is prudent to check folate levels when B_{12} deficiency is diagnosed. Failure to treat folate deficiency prior to starting B12 replacement can result in spinal cord demyelination.
- No further evaluation is usually required once the diagnosis of B12 deficiency is made by a low blood B_{12} level. The Shilling test or other tests of gastric function are rarely of added benefit to a workup. Bone marrow biopsy is rarely needed but should be considered in cases of pancytopenia [40, 41].

Treatment

In *symptomatic* patients a common treatment is to replace B_{12} in the form of 1000 µg cyanocobalamin by intramuscular injection weekly for 3 weeks, then monthly, or every other month. For residents in whom B_{12} was discovered incidentally it may be replaced orally. Crystalline B_{12} administered orally is well absorbed and at least 500–1000 µg/day is required to reverse the biochemical disorder of B_{12} deficiency. Patients with impaired absorption of B_{12} may respond to higher oral doses (1000–2000 mcg daily) if there is a lack of intrinsic factor or pathology of the terminal ileum. Sublingual, transdermal, and intranasal forms of B_{12} are more costly and have been less rigorously tested. There is no evidence for the use of supplemental B_{12} as a tonic to improve well-being.

Monitoring recommendations vary and depend on the manifestation and severity of B_{12} deficiency. Elderly with anemia due to B_{12} deficiency should have a reticulocyte count checked in 1 week after starting treatment and hemoglobin level in 1–2 months. Treatment of B_{12} deficiency may unmask underlying folate and iron deficiency. Thus, as red cell production increases, folate and iron supplementation may be required.

Skin Disorders

Scabies

Scabies is a contagious parasitic infestation of the skin caused by the human itch mite *Sarcoptes scabiei var hominis*. It can cause extensive outbreaks among residents and staff unless timely treated and system-wide infection control protocols followed. The severity of a scabies infection depends on the number of mites infesting the skin. *Norwegian scabies* is a severe atypical infection characterized by extremely pruritic crusty skin lesions with thousands to millions of live mites. Mental retardation, dementia, immunodeficiency states, renal failure, malnutrition, HIV, insulin-treated diabetes, and administration of topical and systemic corticosteroids can increase the severity of scabies.

Transmission and Diagnosis

The incubation period of scabies is 2–6 weeks. Healthy individuals without prior infestation may be asymptomatic during this period. Those with previous infestation are sensitized and often develop pruritis within 48 h of reinfection as the itching originates from an allergic reaction to the mite. This itching is often severe, particularly at night. Skin areas typically affect the web spaces between the digits, breast folds, buttocks, genitalia, and flexor surfaces of the wrists, elbows, and axillae. Skin lesions consist of erythematous papules and linear excoriations. The differential diagnosis will include eczema, folliculitis, tinea, psoriasis, insect bites, or dermatitis herpetiformis.

A scabies outbreak is defined as one or more confirmed cases within a finite period of time and in a defined facility location (e.g., a nursing unit or ward). Norwegian scabies causes on extremely high rate of transmission. Transmission of scabies occurs from person to person skin contact or infested clothing. Chair covers and bed linens play a smaller role in transmission.

Skin scrapings of affected areas by microscopic exam for the presence of mites, eggs, or fecal pellets will confirm the diagnosis of scabies. However, in recently exposed persons, skin scrapings can be negative and the Burrows Ink Test may then provide clues to infestation. The Burrows Ink Test is performed by running a black or green felt tip pen over the waxy red raised burrows, and then wiping the skin off with alcohol to reveal a black or green zigzag line under magnification [40]. An eczematous eruption can frequently be seen covering the trunk of elderly who are infected with scabies, but this is usually an allergic reaction to the mite and may show little or no evidence of mite infestation. Skin biopsies are not recommended due to low yield. Hence empiric treatment based on symptoms may be necessary. Dermatology consultation may be needed for an indeterminate rash.

Controlling the Outbreak

Barrier precautions using gowns and gloves should be used until the diagnosis of scabies has been eliminated as a possibility. The medical director should be notified and treatment ordered and other practitioners notified. The infection control professional should track cases and contacts as well as implement barrier precautions. The staff needs to treat all residents in an area if multiple cases are found. Any caregivers, exposed visitors, and volunteers should be treated as well. The local health department or the state regulatory agency should also be notified.

Contact precautions should be used for at least 24 h after initiating treatment. Residents with crusted scabies will require several treatments and may be contagious for several weeks. *In the case of crusted scabies contact isolation in a single room should be continued until three consecutive skin scrapings are negative.* Clothing, pillows, blankets, and wheelchair pads should be washed in hot water, sealed in plastic for 5–7 days, or placed in a hot dryer. Environmental surfaces, beds, assistive devices, diagnostic and therapy equipment should be cleaned with an Environmental Protection Agency (EPA)-registered cleaning product. Furniture with fabric upholstery will need to be removed for 5–7 days, topical creams and lotions discarded, all carpets vacuumed and the vacuum bag disposed of immediately.

Treatment of Scabies [41, 42]

- Gamma-hexachlorocyclohexane (Lindane) *is no longer recommended due to resistance of the mites* and *neurotoxicity* concerns.
- Permethrin 5% (Elimite) cream applied head to toe and left on for 8–14 h is 90% effective after the first application. In some patients, *a second application after 7–10 days may be necessary*
- All symptomatic patients, and close contacts including staff should be treated with permethrin in the same 24–48 h period.
- Health care workers and their household contacts should be treated at the end of the work shift. *Leave permethrin cream on and shower after 8–12 h.*
- Permethrin should be applied on the *entire area of skin from the hairline to the feet*, including the palms and soles, under the fingernails and toenails; the scalp may rarely need treatment unless infested.
- Topical steroid creams or antihistamines to treat pruritis *should not be applied until the scabicide has been removed.*
- *Oral ivermectin* (Stromectol) is an effective and cost-comparable alternative to topical scabicides although it is not FDA approved for use in scabies. It may be particularly useful in patients with dementia, in large outbreaks, and in the treatment of severely crusted scabies in immunocompromised residents or when topical therapy has failed. A single dose of 200 µg/kg is effective or a *standard dose of 6 mg for a 70 kg adult.*
- *A second treatment is needed in 1–2 weeks* after the eggs mature (since therapies are not effective against mite eggs)

Herpes Zoster

Herpes zoster (HZ) is caused by reactivation of the varicella zoster virus (VZV), which is latent in the sensory ganglia. The prevalence of HZ in PALTC residents is unknown, but two-thirds of cases are diagnosed in >50-year olds. Herpes zoster is characterized by a pruritic, maculopapular vesicular rash that evolves into *noninfectious dried crusts* over a 5- to 6-day period. It is triggered by a decline in cell-mediated immunity that facilitates the reactivation of latent varicella virus. Long-term care residents are at greater risk because of age-related decline in cell-medicated immunity, malnutrition, multimorbidity, and frailty. They also have diminished reserves to respond to stress that can trigger an episode of HZ.

Prodromal symptoms can include hyperesthesia, localized pain, or itching. The lesions of HZ are often described as a "dew drops on a rose petal," which are clustered in a dermatomal distribution and not crossing the midline. Most often, HZ is diagnosed clinically, but the laboratory diagnosis can be made by isolation of the varicella virus from a lesion. Rapid varicella virus identification using PCR is preferred if available, but direct fluorescent antibody (DFA) testing can be used to make the diagnosis as well.

About 20% of affected older persons may develop *post-herpetic neuralgia* (PHN). This can be a devastating complication requiring prolonged pharmacotherapy and pain management and lead to depression and a decline in function. Other complications may include involvement of the ophthalmic branch of the trigeminal branch (leading to uveitis, keratitis, blindness), the nasociliary branch (vesicles in the pharynx and tip of the nose), and the Ramsay Hunt syndrome (vesicles in the ear, deafness, facial palsy, vertigo).

General Measures

The nursing leadership and medical staff should educate the resident and direct staff caregivers regarding the nature of the infection and the risk of viral transmission to individuals who have not had chickenpox. HZ is not contagious to those who have a history of chicken pox or adequate titers of IgG to varicella. Skin lesions should be kept clean and dry to *avoid* bacterial superinfection. Antibiotic ointments and adhesive dressings should be avoided since healing and drying of the lesions will be delayed. Shingles in immunocompromised individuals and those with ophthalmic zoster must be treated with antiviral agents

Vaccination

Encourage Zoster vaccination for persons 50 years and older, regardless of prior history of a natural HZ infection unless a contraindication exists. It is not recommended for immunocompromised individuals [42]. *Although zoster vaccine (Zostavax) in general has been associated with 51% fewer episodes of HZ, and 66% less PHN, these figures were only 18% and 26%, respectively, in those 80 and over.* Hence response to the vaccine in LTC residents cannot reliably be predicted and facility immunization programs for herpes zoster are not currently recommended.

The Shingrix vaccine released in 2019 is 97% effective in preventing HZ in those >50 years, and should be given in two doses, 2–6 months apart [42, 43].

Treatment

- *Topical antiviral* treatment is **not** efficacious.
- *Systemic antiviral treatment* is recommended if ≥50 year age, moderate to severe pain or rash; or have non-truncal involvement within 72 h of rash onset. Begin immediately or sooner than 72 h, if neurologic or ocular signs, severe pain, and/ or rash. Monitor renal function in those with renal insufficiency.

    - Acyclovir 800 mg, *five* times daily (every 4–5 h) for 7–10 days (less preferred due to dosing schedule)
    - Famciclovir 500 mg, *three* times daily for 7 days
    - Valacyclovir 1000 mg, *three* times daily 7 days

- Adjuncts to antiviral therapy consider:

    - Analgesics (acetaminophen, opioids, tramadol)
    - Gabapentin (maximum 3600 mg daily), pregabalin (75 mg twice daily), or a low dose tricyclic antidepressant (nortriptyline 25 mg at bedtime, occasionally up to 150 mg daily), if no improvement in pain

- Oral corticosteroid use is common but lacks evidence in improving quality of life or reducing the incidence of PHN.
- Referral to a pain specialist is recommended to evaluate for neural blockade if analgesics, adjunct therapies, and corticosteroids have not been effective in relieving post-herpetic neuralgia.
- Psychosocial evaluation if severe depression
- Attention to both nutrition and maintenance of functional status

Clostridioides difficile Infection

Clostridioides difficile (*C. difficile*) infections (CDI) are a serious cause of morbidity and mortality in the post-acute and long-term care setting. Nationwide 500,000 infections occur annually. One in six patients with CDI experience a recurrence in the subsequent 2–8 weeks, and one in eleven adults over 65 years diagnosed with a healthcare-associated CDI, die within 1 month [CDC website] [43, 44]. *C. difficile* colonizes the gut after the normal gut flora has been altered by antibiotic treatment. More virulent strains are emerging and the NAP1/BI/027 strain has been implicated in CDI outbreaks, and is capable of increased production of toxins A and B. About 8–10% of PA/LTC residents are thought to be carriers. The infection is transmitted in health care facilities from environmental surface contamination, hand carriage by staff members, and infected patients (Table 34).

Table 34 Risk factors for *C. difficile*

• Advanced age
• Frequent need for hospitalization
• Recurrent exposure to antibiotics (especially clindamycin, third-generation cephalosporins, and fluoroquinolones)
• Presence of comorbid medical conditions
• Use of proton-pump inhibitors or histamine 2 receptor antagonists for gastric acid suppression
• Immunosuppression (organ transplant with immunosuppressive therapy, HIV/AIDS, cancer)

Clinical Features

Older adults may be asymptomatic, or symptomatic with watery diarrhea, abdominal cramps, constipation or ileus, and fever, though patients may be afebrile. *Symptoms may begin during antibiotic treatment or up to 8 weeks after completion of antibiotics.* In PA/LTC residents, diarrhea may not be the initial problem, but fever, confusion, abdominal pain, anorexia, nausea, leukocytosis (often >20,000 WBC), and hypoalbuminemia. A distinctive fecal odor is also a manifestation of CDI. The differential diagnosis of CDI includes an acute abdomen (due to ileus, volvulus, ischemia), shock (due to sepsis or cardiogenic), infectious diarrhea (due to antibiotics or *salmonella or clostridium perfringens)*, or noninfectious causes (e.g., celiac disease, Crohn's, ulcerative colitis, collagenous colitis, IBS, fecal impaction).

Diagnosis should be made by testing diarrheal stool. Options are:

- *C. diff* toxin testing by enzyme immunoassay (EIA) for toxins A and B
- PCR testing for toxins A and B is superior and can be available in 1 h. Beware of false positives.
- EIA testing for *C. difficile* glutamate dehydrogenase (GDH), but it cannot distinguish between toxigenic and nontoxigenic strains; results available in 1 h and may be used as a screening test.
- *Repeat testing to confirm cure is not recommended!*
- Discontinue the use of any potentially inciting antibiotics and avoid the use of antiperistaltic agents!
- Consider discontinuing proton pump inhibitors (PPIs).

Management

- *For mild to moderate disease* (diarrhea plus other symptoms not meeting severe or complicated criteria);

  - Metronidazole 500 mg p.o. TID for 10–14 days
  - Discontinue unnecessary antibiotics

- Vancomycin 125 mg p.o. QID if unable to take metronidazole or no improvement in 5–7 days

- *For severe disease* (albumin <3 g/dL **and** one of the following: WBC >15,000, or abdominal tenderness);

  – Vancomycin 125 mg p.o. QID

- *For severe and complicated disease* (ICU admission, hypotension, fever, ileus or abdominal distension, confusion, WBC >35,000 or <2000), lactate >2 mmol/L)

  – Vancomycin 500 mg p.o. QID
  – Vancomycin by enema (500 mg in 500 mL normal saline QID **and** metronidazole 500 mg IV q 8 h if oral therapy is not tolerated

- *For recurrent C. diff infection* (10–20% recur within 8 weeks)

  – Confirm diagnosis
  – Conservative treatment for mild symptoms
  – Same regimen as for the initial episode
  – "Pulsed vancomycin" regimen
  – Fidaxomycin 200 mg BID for 10 days (questionable efficacy) (expensive)
  – Fecal microbiota transplantation may be safe and effective in restoring normal flora

The use of private rooms will reduce transmission. *Antibiotic stewardship* is crucial as is *hand hygiene* and the maintenance of *contact precautions* using gowns and gloves when entering the room of a patient with CDI. Environmental surfaces should be disinfected using an approved sporicidal agent. Proton pump inhibitors should be used judiciously or discontinued. Moreover, there is no conclusive evidence supporting the use of probiotics though commonly prescribed during *C. difficile* treatment or as preventive therapy when antibiotics are prescribed for other infections.

Acute Kidney Injury

Renal function declines in many older adults, and thus are vulnerable to acute kidney injury due to age-related changes in renal functions that include:

- Decrease in glomerular filtration rate (GFR)
- Decrease in urine concentrating ability (leading to nocturia, hypernatremia, poor compensation for hypovolemia)
- Reduced sodium conservation in the face of low sodium intake (risk of volume depletion)
- Reduced sodium excretion in the face of high sodium intake (risk of edema and salt-sensitive HTN)
- Decreased potassium excretion (risk of hyperkalemia)

Acute kidney injury (AKI), is defined as an acute increase in creatinine or a decrease in urine output to <0.5 mL/kg/h for at least 6 h. It is increasingly common in older adults and can result in increased morbidity and even the need for dialysis. Its incidence increases with older age, male gender, black race, chronic inflammation, and those with poor nutritional status [44, 45]. The causes of AKI and its evaluation are reviewed in Table 35 [45]. Due to low muscle mass related to aging and frailty, serum creatinine may be normal or near normal despite severe impairment of renal function. In evaluating for the cause of AKI, it is useful to classify it as prerenal, intrinsic renal (glomerular, tubulointerstitial, and vascular), and postrenal causes.

Table 35 Causes of AKI and evaluation

Category of AKI	Causes	Clinical findings	Treatment
Prerenal azotemia	• Hypoperfusion due to volume depletion (reduced fluid intake, acute illness, GI fluid loss, diuresis) • Low arterial volume (decompensated HF) • Renal hypoperfusion (e.g., bilateral renal artery stenosis) • Medications (e.g., ACEI, ARBs, NSAIDS, diuretics, SGLT2i)	• History • Orthostatic hypotension • Urinalysis: high specific gravity, bland urine sediment	• Stop or reduce offending medications • Restore intravascular circulating volume with oral hydration or intravenous fluids
Obstructive uropathy	• Bladder outlet obstruction (e.g., BPH in men) • Bladder carcinoma • Urethral stricture • Functional outlet obstruction (e.g., anticholinergic medications, spinal cord injury, diabetic autonomic neuropathy) • Ureteral obstruction (stones, strictures, or retroperitoneal malignancy)	• Urinary hesitancy, nocturia, overflow incontinence • GFR maintained if only one kidney affected (unless unilateral kidney present) • Renal ultrasound shows hydronephrosis, stones	• Bladder emptying (may need to be scheduled or indwelling bladder catheter) • Specific treatment depending on the cause and level of obstruction

Table 35 (continued)

Category of AKI	Causes	Clinical findings	Treatment
Intrinsic renal disease (selected types): – Acute tubular necrosis (ATN) – Acute interstitial nephritis – Multiple myeloma and other plasma cell dyscrasias	• Ischemia • Sepsis • Nephrotoxins (cisplatin, vancomycin, aminoglycosides, rhabdomyolysis, iodinated contrast agents) • Allergic response to medication (NSAIDS, PPIs, and antibiotics) • Infections • Rheumatological disorders • Increased prevalence with age • Acute or chronic kidney disease • AKI caused by cast nephropathy	• Urine sediment includes epithelial cells and granular casts • FE_{Na} >2% (usually <1% in prerenal azotemia • Urine sediment shows white cells with or without WBC casts, absence of infection • Eosinophilia on CBC with differential • Low anion gap • High globulin • Hypercalcemia • SPEP and immunofixation	• Complex conditions usually require nephrology consultation • Supportive treatment (may include dialysis) • Optimize volume status • Avoid nephrotoxins • Stop offending medication • Corticosteroids may hasten recovery (after kidney biopsy to confirm diagnosis) • Treat dysproteinemia • Supportive renal care

Hyperkalemia often coexists with AKI and be aware that medications may be a contributing factor. These include ACE inhibitors, angiotensin receptor blockers, renin inhibitors, NSAIDS, spirono-lactone, amiloride, cyclosporine, tacrolimus, trimethoprim-sulfamethoxazole, and pentamidine. *NSAIDS* non-steroidal anti-inflammatory drugs, *FENa* fractional excretion of sodium, *SPEP* serum protein electrophoresis

Conclusion

The management of medical conditions in patients and residents in the long-term care continuum is challenging due to patient complexity, multimorbidities, guarded prognosis, individual advance directives for health care, goals of care, and the health care setting in which care is being provided by an interprofessional team, under the scrutiny of government and survey agencies. It is essential for practitioners to determine the risks and benefits to patients in the identification, assessment, treatment, and monitoring in the management of multiple clinical conditions. Practitioners need not forget *less common conditions* that can afflict residents such as cancer, Parkinson's disease, polymyalgia rheumatica, traumatic brain injury, and abuse and neglect.

Peals for the Practitioner
- Studies have shown that the treatment of HTN in those over age 80 can result in a significant reduction in fatal and nonfatal stroke and all-cause mortality within 1–2 years of starting antihypertensive treatment.
- A systematic evaluation is recommended for residents with anemia, and should be evaluated for comorbid conditions such as loss of physical function, risk for falls, and cognitive impairment.

- Residents with HF have a 74% or 92% 5-year mortality with either a normal or reduced LVEF, respectively. HF is a major cause of hospital admissions and readmissions.
- COPD, the third leading cause of US deaths, is present in one in six people admitted to nursing facilities and yet remains either unrecognized or suboptimally treated.
- Effective management of diabetes requires an approach that is multifaceted, protocol-driven, interdisciplinary, and individualized. If used, sliding-scale insulin is best utilized as a supplement to scheduled oral hypoglycemic agents and/or basal insulin therapy and not as a primary means to control blood glucose.
- Subclinical hypothyroidism is both common and not associated with the classic signs and symptoms of hypothyroidism are often seen in younger adults. It is not uncommon in those already diagnosed with DM or vitamin B_{12} deficiency.
- Vitamin B_{12} deficiency in older adults is commonly *not* associated with anemia or macrocytosis, so a high index of suspicion is warranted as to its possible presence.
- For scabies, permethrin 5% cream has a 90% effective cure rate after its first application. A second application may be necessary 7–10 days.
- Shingrix vaccine is 97% effective in preventing HZ in those 50 years and older. It is given in two doses, 2–6 months apart.

Websites
- AMDA-The Society of Post-Acute and Long-Term Care Medicine. https://paltc.org
- AHA. www.americanheart.org.
- American College of Cardiology. www.acc.org.
- The Global Initiative for Chronic Obstructive Lung Disease. www.goldcopd.com.
- American Diabetes Association. www.diabetes.org.
- American Thyroid Association Professional Guidelines. www.thyroidguidelines.net.
- Center for Disease Control and Prevention. www.cdc.gov.
- www.kidney.org/professionals/KDOQI/gfr_calculator.

References

Hypertension

1. 2017 ACC/AHA/AAPA/ABC/ACPM/AGS/APhA/ASH/ASPC/NMA/PCNA guideline for the prevention, detection, evaluation, and management of high blood pressure in adults: a report of the American College of Cardiology/American Heart Association Task Force on Clinical Practice Guidelines. Hypertension. 2018;71:e13–e115. https://doi.org/10.1161/HYP.0000000000000065.
2. Musini VM, Tejani AM, et al. Pharmacotherapy for hypertension in the elderly. Cochrane Database Syst Rev. 2009;4:CD000028. https://doi.org/10.1002/14651858.CD000028.pub2.

3. Beckett NS, et al. Treatment of hypertension in patients 80 years of age or older. N Engl J Med. 2008;358(18):1887–98.
4. The Sprint Research Group, Wright JT, Williamson JD, Whelton PK, et al. A randomized trial of intensive versus standard blood pressure control. N Engl J Med. 2015;373:2103–16.
5. Benetos A, Labat C, Rossignol P, et al. Treatment with multiple blood pressure medications, achieved blood pressure, and mortality in older nursing home residents: the PARTAGE study. JAMA Intern Med. 2015;175(6):989–95. https://doi.org/10.1001/jamainternmed.2014.8012.
6. Vongpatanasin WL. Resistant hypertension: a review of diagnosis and management. JAMA. 2014;311(21):2216–24.
7. Halter JB, Ouslander JG, Tinetti ME, et al. Chapter 82. Hazzard's geriatric medicine and gerontology, 7th ed. McGraw Hill. 2017.

Anemia

8. Chaves P, Ashar T, Guralnik JM, et al. Looking at the relationship between hemoglobin concentration and previous mobility difficulty in older women: should the criteria used to define anemia in older people be changed? J Am Geriatr Soc. 2002;50:1257–64.
9. Pandya N, et al. Study of anemia in long-term care (SALT): prevalence of anemia and its relationship with the risk of falls in nursing home residents. Curr Med Res Opin. 2008;24(8):2139–49.
10. AMDA, Society for Post-Acute and Long-term Care Medicine. Anemia in the long-term care setting. Clinical practice guideline. Columbia: AMDA. 2007.
11. Halter JB, Ouslander JG, Tinetti ME, Studenski S, High KP, Asthana S. Chapter 103. Hazzard's geriatric medicine and gerontology, 7th ed. McGraw Hill.
12. Weiss G, Goodnough L. Anemia of chronic disease. N Engl J Med. 2005;352:1011–23.

Heart Failure

13. Heckman GA, Shamji AK, et al. Heart failure management in nursing homes: a scoping literature review. Can J Cardiol, 2018 34, 7, 871-880
14. Hutt E, Elder SJ, Fish R, Min S. Regional variation in mortality and subsequent hospitalization of nursing residents with heart failure. J Am Med Dir Assoc. 2003;12(8):595–601.
15. 2021 update to the 2017 ACC expert consensus decision pathway for optimization of heart failure treatment: answers to 10 pivotal issues about heart failure with reduced ejection fraction. J Am Coll Cardiol. 2021;77(6):772–810.
16. Daamen MA, Hamers JP, Gorgels AP, Tan FE, Schols JM, Brunner-la Rocca HP. Treatment of heart failure in nursing home residents. J Geriatr Cardiol. 2016;13(1):44.
17. Hutt E, Frederickson E, Ecord M, Kramer AM. Associations among processes and outcomes of care for Medicare nursing home residents with acute heart failure. J Am Med Dir Assoc. 2003;4(4):195–9.
18. Rogers JG, Patel CB, Mentz RJ, et al. Palliative care in heart failure: the PAL-HF randomized, controlled clinical trial. J Am Coll Cardiol. 2017;70(3):331–41.

COPD

19. AMDA-The Society for Post-Acute and Long-Term Care Medicine. COPD management in the post-acute and long-term care setting. Clinical practice guideline. Columbia: AMDA; 2016.
20. Patel M, Steinberg K, Suarez-Barcelo M, Saffel D, Foley R, Worz C. Chronic obstructive pulmonary disease in post-acute/long-term care settings: seizing opportunities to individualize treatment and device selection. J Am Med Dir Assoc. 2017;18(6):553.e17–22.

21. Zarowitz BJ, O'Shea T. Chronic obstructive pulmonary disease: prevalence, characteristics, and pharmacologic treatment in nursing home residents with cognitive impairment. J Manag Care Pharm. 2012;18(8):598–606.
22. Singh D, Agusti A, Anzueto A, Barnes PJ, Bourbeau J, Celli BR, Criner GJ, Frith P, Halpin DMG, Meilan H, Varela MVL, Martinez F, de Oca MM, Papi A, Pavord ID, Roche N, Sin DD, Stockley R, Vestbo J, Wedzicha JA, Vogelmeier C. Global strategy for the diagnosis, management, and prevention of chronic obstructive lung disease: the GOLD Science Committee report 2019. Eur Respir J. 2019;53(5):1900164. https://doi.org/10.1183/13993003.00164-2019.

Diabetes

23. Dybicz SB, Thompson S, Molotsky S, Stuart B. Prevalence of diabetes and the burden of comorbid conditions among elderly nursing home residents. Am J Geriatr Pharmacother. 2011;9(4):212–23.
24. American Medical Directors Association (AMDA). Diabetes management in the post-acute and long-term care setting. Clinical practice guideline. Columbia: American Medical Directors Association (AMDA); 2015.
25. Pandya N, Hames E, Sandhu S. Challenges and strategies for managing diabetes in the elderly in long-term care settings. Diabetes Spectr. 2020;33:236–45.
26. Pandya N, Patel M. Textbook chapter—Evidence-based geriatrics, a case-based approach. 2022.
27. Munshi MN, Florez H, Huang ES, et al. Management of diabetes in long-term care and skilled nursing facilities: a position statement of the American Diabetes Association. Diabetes Care. 2016;39:308–18.
28. American Diabetes Association. Older adults: standards of medical care in diabetes—2020. Diabetes Care. 2020;43(suppl 1):S152–62.
29. Leung E, Wongrakpanich S, Munshi MN. Diabetes management in the elderly. Diabetes Spectr. 2018;31(3):245–53.
30. Pandya N, Wei W, Meyers JL, et al. Burden of sliding scale insulin use in elderly long-term care residents with type 2 diabetes mellitus. J Am Geriatr Soc. 2013;61:2103–10. https://doi.org/10.1111/jgs.12547.
31. Sloane PD, Pandya N. Individualizing diabetes care in older persons with multimorbidity. J Am Med Dir Assoc. 2021;22(9):1884–8.
32. Chelliah A, Burge MR. Hypoglycaemia in elderly patients with diabetes mellitus: causes and strategies for prevention. Drugs Aging. 2004;21(8):511–30.

Thyroid Disease

33. Canaris GJ, Manowitz NR, Mayor G, Ridgway EC. The Colorado thyroid disease prevalence study. Arch Intern Med. 2000;160:526–34.
34. Ajish TP, Jayakumar RV. Geriatric thyroidology: an update. Indian J Endocrinol Metab. 2012;16(4):542–7.
35. Mitrou P, Raptis S, Dimitriadis G. Thyroid disease in older people. Maturitas. 2011;70:5–9.
36. Garber JR, Cobin RH. Clinical practice guidelines for hypothyroidism in adults: cosponsored by the American Association of Clinical Endocrinologists and the American Thyroid Association. ATA/AACE guidelines. 2012;18(6):988–1028.
37. Hennessey JV, Espaillat R. Diagnosis and management of subclinical hypothyroidism in elderly adults: a review of the literature. J Am Geriatr Soc. 2015;63(8):1663–73.

38. Ross B, et al. 2016 American Thyroid Association guidelines for diagnosis and management of hyperthyroidism and other causes of thyrotoxicosis. Thyroid. 2016;26(10):1343–421.
39. Haugen A, et al. 2015 American Thyroid Association management guidelines for adult patients with thyroid nodules and differentiated thyroid cancer: the American Thyroid Association guidelines task force on thyroid nodules and differentiated thyroid cancer. Thyroid. 2016;26(1):1–133.

Vitamin B$_{12}$ Deficiency

40. Malouf R, Evans GJ. Folic acid with or without vitamin B12 for the prevention and treatment of healthy elderly and demented people [update of Cochrane Database Syst Rev. 2003;(4):CD004514;PMID: 14584018][Review][121 refs]. Cochrane Database Syst Rev. 2008;(4):CD004514.
41. Green R, Allen LH, Bjørke-Monsen AL, Brito A, Guéant JL, Miller JW, et al. Vitamin B12 deficiency. Nat Rev Dis Primers. 2017;3(1):1–20.

Scabies

42. Shimose L, Munoz-Price LS. Diagnosis, prevention, and treatment of scabies. Curr Infect Dis Rep. 2013;15(5):426–31.

Herpes Zoster

43. Heineman TC, Cunningham A, Levin M. Understanding the immunology of Shingrix, a recombinant glycoprotein E adjuvanted herpes zoster vaccine. Curr Opin Immunol. 2019;59:42–4.

Clostridium difficile

44. Lessa FC, et al. Burden of Clostridium Difficile infection in the United States. N Engl J Med. 2015;372:825–32.

Acute Kidney Injury

45. Anderson S, Eldadah B, Halter JB, et al. Acute kidney injury in older adults. JASN. 2011;22(1):28–38. https://doi.org/10.1681/ASN.2010090934.

Preventing Hospital Admissions and Readmissions

R. Scott DeLong

Introduction

Over the past decade, there has been increasing attention directed toward reducing the number of hospital admissions and readmissions from nursing facilities (NF) and skilled nursing facilities (SNF). However, the national average for readmissions stills remains high at approximately 18% for FY 2019 according to the most recent data from the Centers for Medicare and Medicaid Services [1].

The Affordable Care Act established the Hospital Readmissions Reduction Program (HRRP) starting October 1, 2012. The goal of the HRRP is to "encourage hospitals to improve communication and care coordination to better engage patients and caregivers in discharge plans and in turn to reduce avoidable hospital readmissions" [2]. The goal is to motivate hospitals to improve communication and care transitions by *linking payment to the quality of medical care* provided at the time of discharge. CMS continues to monitor these efforts by reviewing the excess readmission ratio (ERR). The ERR is a "ratio of the predicted-to-expected readmissions rates" [2]. Moreover, the ERR measures a hospital's performance compared to regional and national readmission rates. CMS currently evaluates six medical diagnoses based on the ERR:

- Heart failure
- Acute myocardial infarction
- Chronic obstructive pulmonary disease

R. S. DeLong (✉)
Geriatrics at Home Program, Penn Medicine Lancaster General Health/Penn Medicine Geriatric Fellowship, Lancaster, PA, USA

P. Winn et al. (eds.), *Post-Acute and Long-Term Care Medicine*, Current Clinical Practice, https://doi.org/10.1007/978-3-031-28628-5_9

- Pneumonia
- Coronary artery bypass graft surgery
- Elective primary total hip arthroplasty and/or total knee arthroplasty

The HRRP reports a "30-day risk standardized unplanned readmission rate that includes unplanned *readmissions that happen within 30 days of discharge* from the index admission and patients who are readmitted to the same hospital, or another applicable acute care hospital *for any reason*" [2].

The Protecting Access to Medicare Act of 2014 *mandated penalties for NFs and SNFs* starting October 1, 2018 *for excessive readmissions to the hospital* in an effort to transition from a fee-for-service to a *value-based payment model* [3]. *The Patient Drive Payment Model* (PDPM) went into effect in the fiscal year 2020 to replace fee-for-service. CMS provided NFs and SNFs quarterly readmission reports starting October 2016 prior to the payment model change starting fiscal year 2019 when facilities could obtain a 1.6% Medicare Part A *payment bonus* **or** a 2% *payment reduction* based on each facilities *readmission* data [3]. Data shows that 3% of SNFs received the maximum bonus of 1.6% while approximately 20% of SNFs got the maximum cut of 2% with the remaining facilities falling in between the two extremes [3].

Hospitals continue to remain an important and appropriate medical setting to receive intermittent care for residents in NFs/SNFs depending on the goals of care of the resident. However, unintended adverse events can occur during a hospital admission. In a 2016 JAMDA article, Dr. Ouslander and others described many adverse hospital events and admonished patients, families, and NF/SNF providers that the hospital may not be the safest setting for frail elder adults. Adverse hospital outcomes included [4]:

- Distress and discomfort for the resident and family
- Delirium at least partially related to a change in environment
- Polypharmacy and drug errors during transitions between care settings
- Falls/fractures in the hospital setting
- Incontinence and improper catheter use
- Hospital acquired infections (HAI)
- Unintentional weight loss and poor nutrition
- Immobility, de-conditioning, and pressure wounds

There continues to be a growing number of physicians, CNRPs, and PAs providing care in nursing facilities with an increasing number of these providers receiving specialized training in Post-Acute and Long Term Care Medicine (PALTC). These providers in collaboration with other disciplines (i.e., nursing, therapy services, and social services) have made great strides in *reducing the number of avoidable hospitalizations*. This chapter will review strategies and tools in preventing avoidable hospital admissions and readmissions. The topics to be covered include the following:

- Transitions of care
- Accountable Care Organizations (ACOs)

- Acute change in condition
- Physician Orders for Life-Sustaining Treatment (POLST) and goals of care discussions

Transitions of Care

Care transitions primarily involve three systems of care that have the potential to reduce avoidable hospitalizations and improve the quality of care: the NF/SNF, the hospital, and primary care based in the community. Most of these transitions are from *hospital to NF/SNF, NF/SNF to hospital*, and *NF/SNF to the community*. Research has focused on transitions between the hospital and NF/SNF. Recent research has studied transfers between the NF and the community. While each setting is unique and under various state and federal regulations, the key elements needed for successful transfers include the following:

1. Patient-centered and family-oriented care
2. Effective communication between all systems that provide care to patients

An important component of patient-centered and family-oriented care is the involvement of a patient advocate for an older frail adult. There are many tasks required of a *patient advocate* that includes listening, asking questions, and requesting clarification of instructions. Many patients experience various degrees of memory, hearing, and visual loss. Therefore, there is a concern that discharge instructions may not be heard, understood clearly, or later misread by the patient and/or patient advocate. Whenever possible it is imperative to review the plan of care with the health care proxy, power of attorney (POA), and/or family caregivers as well as the patient.

When a patient transitions to the hospital, NF, or back home in the community, it is critical that goals of care are reviewed with the patient, assuming the patient has the capacity to understand and appreciate a goals of care discussion. If the patient has memory loss, future goals should be discussed and clarified with the patient's proxy or surrogate decision maker.

During a care transition important opportunities arise to talk about the "what ifs" that may occur in the future. *"What if"* you are unable to care for yourself? *"What if"* you have a CHF exacerbation for the 4th time in 3 months"? Care transitions are an opportune time to clarify a patient's wishes for future hospitalizations, emergency room visits, and NF/SNF care. Goals of care should include discussions regarding orders on cardiopulmonary resuscitation (CPR), do not resuscitate (DNR), and if appropriate, "do not transfer to the ER" or "do not admit to hospital."

There has been increasing effort by many medical communities and organizations to create an "age-friendly" health care system. In 2017 the Institute for Healthcare Improvement (IHI) and the American Hospital Association (AHA) collaborated to create the Geriatrics 4M model of care. The Geriatrics 4M model includes assessment and management of the following:

- Mind: (e.g., dementia evaluation; delirium evaluation)
- Mobility: (e.g., fall prevention; fall evaluation)
- Medications: (e.g., polypharmacy review; de-prescribing)
- Matters Most: (e.g., advance care planning; serious illness conversation)

These four domains form the foundation for excellence in geriatric care and its implementation can help to reduce avoidable hospitalizations [5, 6]. Some organizations have now *added a 5thM termed multi-morbidity (or multi-complexity)* that reflects the complex medical management of older adults and is an additional key factor in reducing avoidable hospitalizations [7].

Effective Communication

Effective communication with the patient, the POA, and the receiving health care provider should be a gold standard of health care. Written communication is most effective when transferring patients from one system of care to another. Ideally, a discharge summary should be sent with the patient at the time of discharge. Another copy should be sent/emailed/faxed to the primary care physician. A discharge summary should be succinct and include the following information [4]:

- Up-to-date discharge medication list and reasons for any medication changes
- Discharge instructions from the facility's primary provider
- Medical conditions to be monitored (e.g., daily weights for CHF, fall prevention interventions if high fall risk)
- Contact person at the discharging facility for answering any care questions
- Pertinent consultations, emergency room visits, and scheduled follow-up visits with the primary care provider and any consultants
- Copies of any advanced directives and goals of care discussions, including DNR status

Many hospitals and NFs currently have processes in place to call discharged patients or caregivers to ensure the patient has experienced a safe transition back to home or into the NF/SNF. The follow-up phone call should discuss:

- Medication-related issues (e.g., medication reconciliation)
- Planned follow-up visits (primary care physician, consultants)
- Follow-up laboratory work and testing that has been recommended

If NFs/SNFs are to improve transitions of care and to reduce avoidable hospital admissions, there are two very important elements of care:

1. That practitioners must acquire and maintain excellent geriatric competencies in caring for frail older adults.
2. The NF/SNF must ensure patients are seen for follow-up in a timely manner upon admission to the facility or for an acute change in condition.

Practitioners must be knowledgeable on the diagnosis and treatment of complex geriatric syndromes such as dysphagia associated with aspiration pneumonitis, fever, difficult behaviors (not responding to behavioral interventions), and delirium. Many NF/SNF providers have been able to decrease avoidable hospitalizations by focusing on the Geriatric 4Ms (Mind, Mobility, Medications, and what Matters Most). Core geriatric principles can assist practitioners in evaluating patients in a person-centered approach that can reduce avoidable admissions and readmissions.

Below are some practical tips and guidance regarding a PCP Fax as a transitional care summary from SNF to home.

PCP Fax Transitional Care Summary: SNF to Home

Guidance:
- The nursing facility discharge summary (if done!) frequently is not completed by the day of discharge and may not be received by the PCP in a timely manner causing a delay in information transfer.
- Many NF discharge summaries lack complete clinical information that the PCP requires to assume care coordination for the patient.
- The PCP Fax Summary ensures timely communication of critical clinical information to the PCP on the day of discharge from the facility.
- The PCP Fax is a collaborative document that is to be completed prior to discharge from the facility. Elements of the form may be completed by the attending physician, other providers, and the nursing staff.

Instructions for Use:

1. The PCP Fax Summary should be completed and faxed on the day of discharge to the patients PCP—the physician who will be assuming the care of the patient.
2. The Summary should not be faxed prior to the day of transfer as it may be incomplete. It should not be faxed after the day of transfer as the task may be forgotten by the facility staff.
3. The name and contact number of the Attending Physician and SNF staff contact person should be written on the form.
4. The form does not require a signature as this would delay its completion.
5. Additional documents such as the medication list, list of referrals, admission history, and physical exam, should be faxed along with the form for completeness and to avoid redundancy.
6. Do not provide a copy of the form to the patient in lieu of faxing, as it may not be reliably received by the PCP in a timely way, (remembering that the PCP may begin to receive phone calls regarding the patient's care as early as the day of discharge).

Accountable Care Organizations (ACO)

CMS created ACOs in an attempt to emphasize prevention and early treatment of serious medical illness in an effort in reduce avoidable admissions. CMS defines ACOs as "groups of doctors, hospitals, and other health care providers, who come together voluntarily to give coordinated high-quality care to Medicare patients" [8]. Medicare decided to incentivize ACOs by allowing individual ACOs to share with Medicare any cost savings while at the same time placing the ACO at risk for financial losses if quality of care has not meet set standards.

There continues to be growing evidence that NFs will need to work collaboratively and successfully with other organizations in the health care system in order to be successful in the ACO market. If a NF is considering involvement with an ACO there are at least three important questions that should be addressed:

1. Can the NF/SNF promote a culture of timely assessment, diagnosis, and treatment for a patient's change of condition?
2. Is the NF/SNF prepared to develop better educational programs to train staff and providers?
3. Are the practitioners readily available to assess patients when a change in condition occurs?

Medicare data and that from the Agency for Healthcare Research and Quality (AHRQ) demonstrates three diagnoses that consistently are *common reasons for hospitalization: septicemia, congestive heart failure, and pneumonia.* The medical literature reports that 60–75% of the hospital admissions for these three conditions **from** NF/SNFs are potentially avoidable.

ACOs can also impact NFs/SNFs by referring frail adults suffering from an acute illness directly to the NFs/SNFs rather than admitting them to the hospital. Frail adults, who are medically stable but unable to care for themselves during an acute illness, could be referred directly to a NF/SNF from the hospital emergency room. Nursing facilities that are prepared to receive admissions 24/7, including holidays, and which demonstrate improved outcomes at less cost will be role models in defining how future care will be provided for the elderly. Successful nursing facilities will be effective partners for ACOs because they will help to ensure the ACOs success in reducing avoidable hospitalizations.

Acute Changes in Condition

When nursing facilities make a commitment to reduce preventable hospital admissions and readmissions, there needs to be a focus on appropriate training of licensed staff in the early recognition and assessment of patients experiencing an acute change in condition. There are many excellent materials available to assist in this training. One of the best educational tools is the Know-It-All series available at the

PALTC.org web site. It is a detailed assessment tool for many common geriatric syndromes and symptoms. Moreover, it is user-friendly and improves the skills of licensed clinical staff. Dr. Ouslander and colleagues previously developed an excellent tool, INTERACT II, which when implemented in nursing homes has demonstrated improved quality of care and reduction of avoidable hospitalizations [9].

In addition to a well-trained staff, it is equally important to have physicians, nurse practitioners, and physician assistants available to assess patients within 24–48 h when an acute change in condition occurs. While the 48-h guideline may be a hardship, frequent contact with well-trained licensed staff is important. Timely communication needs to continue until the change in condition is promptly assessed, treatment initiated, stabilization obtained, and improvement begins to occur. Moreover, there are various telemedicine models that can assist in the timely assessment of patients.

While the list of acute changes in condition is extensive, some of the more common conditions of which licensed nursing staff should be knowledgeable include the following:

- Change in mental status
- Chest pain
- Congestive heart failure
- Dehydration
- Acute onset of physical or verbal aggressive behavior
- Fever of unknown origin
- Urinary tract infection and asymptomatic bacteriuria
- Pneumonia.

Change in Mental Status

An acute change in mental status commonly occurs among frail older adults. More frequent causes include medication side effects, new-onset infections, progression of cognitive decline, and/or pain. Research suggests that the prevalence of memory loss in NF patients varies between 50% and 80%. Therefore, it is critical to obtain a baseline cognitive assessment within the first few days after a patient's admission to a nursing or assisted living facility. When a recently admitted patient is diagnosed with delirium (encephalopathy) and/or depression, their cognition baseline should be reevaluated after resolution of the acute change in mental status (see Chapter on "Dementia, Delirium, and Depression" for further discussion).

Many clinicians have heard staff report, "the patient seems more confused." When this occurs, it is a good opportunity to educate staff that an increase in confusion is more appropriately called delirium and reinforce the importance of recognizing such a change and urgently notifying the PCP. After recognizing a change in mental status and obtaining vital signs, staff should contact the PCP. The patient's complaints and any significant physical findings on nurse assessment need to be discussed with the PCP. The PCP should then inquire about the patient's medical history, medications, and recent laboratory studies. Vital signs should be monitored each shift for at least 3 days. When reviewing the patient's medications, it is important to look for any problematic medications and recent medication changes (see Chapter on "Medication Management in Long Term Care" for further discussion). Recent laboratory studies should be reviewed for any evidence of disease progression or newly identified conditions. Important lab to be ordered include but are not limited to hematologic, liver, and renal evaluation.

Nursing facilities should have well-established systems of care that facilitate licensed staff in assessing a resident's acute change in condition. Early recognition, diagnosis, and treatment of an acute change of condition is imperative to prevent an avoidable hospitalization or hospital readmissions.

Chest Pain

Chest pain is an emergency in any medical setting. However, calling 911 may not always be the best immediate response depending on a patient's goals of care. Determine if there have been prior convesations with the patient and/or POA regarding the risks and benefits of hospitalization. Many practitioners note that residents prefer treatment in the NF when possible. This is especially true for patients who have established "comfort" as their goal of care. Pain relief is a primary concern when the focus is on *comfort care* rather than immediate transfer to the hospital. Consequently, treating chest pain with aspirin, sublingual nitroglycerin, and sublingual morphine sulfate, when needed, would be appropriate in such a situation (especially if the resident is receiving hospice services).

Congestive Heart Failure (CHF)

Unexpected rapid weight gain (not due to overeating) can be caused by congestive heart failure. CHF is one of the most common diagnoses for which NF residents are transferred to hospital, and in many cases, such hospitalizations are avoidable [10]. During monthly or bimonthly visits, the residents' weights should be reviewed. Except for very rare situations (e.g., ruptured heart valve), PCPs should be able to treat CHF at the facility and avoid hospitalization unless refractory pulmonary edema develops. The management of heart failure is thoroughly reviewed in AMDA's Clinical Practice Guideline on *Heart Failure in the Post-Acute and Long-Term Settings* (see Chapter on "Common Clinical Conditions in Post-Acute and Long-Term Care" for further discussion).

Dehydration

Dehydration is frequently caused by acute onset of protracted vomiting and/or diarrhea without adequate fluid replacement. Early diagnosis and intervention can potentially prevent an avoidable hospitalization or readmission. Early interventions include symptom management (i.e., starting an antiemetic medication), holding or reducing the dose of medication that may cause further adverse effects (such as warfarin, diuretics, insulin, oral diabetic medications, and GI medications), and administering intravenous (IV) fluids or encouraging increase oral fluid intake. Intravenous fluids may not be appropriate in patients who have multi-morbidities associated with progressive unavoidable weight loss (see Chapter on "Weight and Nutrition in Post Acute and Long Term Care" for further discussion) or if the intervention is counter to the patient's goals of care.

The decision to withhold artificial hydration or to not hospitalize is usually less difficult for the patient POA if goals of care were previously addressed. If the problem is acute with a reasonable chance for improvement, some patients and/or POAs may request IV therapy at the nursing facility. Since more than 60% of long-term care facility (LTCF) residents have significant cognitive impairment, it may be appropriate to offer that a family member be present when administering IV therapy. The family member can potentially calm a delirious patient and prevent the accidental removal of the IV line. Replacement of an accidently removed IV line should always be discussed with the POA since many families may not want to replace the IV line if it has led the patient to becoming agitated.

Behavioral Problems

Acute onset of physically or verbally aggressive behavior is common among NF residents, especially in those with cognitive impairment. The PCP should have a conversation with the POA regarding physical or verbal abusive behaviors that are unresponsive to behavioral or non-pharmacological interventions. This is especially important when a resident is attempting to harm self, staff, or other residents or visitors to the facility.

Hospitalizing residents with serious behavioral problems has little benefit other than temporarily removing them from the NF until the staff can successfully de-escalate the behaviors of the remaining patients. Successful memory loss units have experienced staff who can use creative behavioral interventions to de-escalate most physically or verbally aggressive behavior. Maintaining an educated and consistent staff that are familiar with the nuances of the residents is extremely important though sometimes difficult to achieve due to staffing issues and staff turnover.

Due to the lack of psychiatrists trained in geriatrics, many NF PCPs use psychiatrists trained in adult psychiatry to assist with residents who have challenging behaviors. Unfortunately, many of these well-intended psychiatrists often lack adequate training in evaluating and treating behavioral problems in residents with cognitive impairment. There are no psychotropic medications approved by the FDA in treating behavioral and psychological symptoms of dementia. Although there are few medications that have been shown to improve the behaviors of residents with dementia, many facilities have found the advice of psychologists helpful.

As a last resort, medications can be used off-label in an effort to lessen disruptive resident behaviors. Before deciding to prescribe any off-labeled medication, a family member or the resident's POA may be able to assist with de-escalating their family member's behavior either by phone contact or by a visit to the NF. If a PCP is considering the use of an off-label medication, it is important that the PCP or staff member share with the POA the risks and benefits of using these medications (e.g., discussing the "black box warning" of antipsychotics).

Acute Onset of Fever

One of the most commonly overlooked vital signs in a NF population is a slightly elevated temperature. Unfortunately, it is common for fever to be symptomatically treated as if the patients were younger and healthier. NFs should avoid standing orders of anti-pyretics without notifying PCP of a temperature change. Giving medication for a fever without identifying the underlying cause can lead to a poor outcome and possible hospitalization. Castle et al. have reported that repeated oral temperatures greater than 99 °F (37.2 °C) has a sensitivity of 80% and specificity of 89% for fever. In addition, Castle advised that either *a single oral temperature greater than 100 °F (37.8 °C) or,* a single temperature 2 °F (1.1 °C) above a patient's baseline, *or* repeated oral temperatures greater than 99 °F (37.2 °C) are significant for infection and need to be reported to the PCP [11]. CMS has reported that pneumonia and urosepsis are two common diagnoses among NF/SNF residents that lead to hospitalization. Many of these hospitalizations result from poor monitoring of vital signs, lack of licensed staff adequately assessing ill residents, and lack of timely notification of the PCP regarding an acute change [12].

Asymptomatic Bacteriuria and Urinary Tract Infections

Guidelines for Diagnosing Urinary Tract Infection or Urosepsis
Whether to initiate treatment or not for an abnormal urinalysis is a common dilemma in the NF. Moreover, knowing when to order a urinalysis is a diagnostic challenge for the clinician. Often when a cognitively impaired resident demonstrates disruptive behavior or a change in mental status, the nursing home staff or family request a urinalysis. However, over 40% of all urine specimens of frail older adult females residing in nursing facilities will have bacteriuria. If a resident only has a mental status change and no other signs of symptoms to suggest a UTI, it has

been found that only 11% of these residents will have a UTI [13]. *Unless a resident meets the criteria for a UTI/urospesis with or without an indwelling catheter (see criteria below), the clinician should refrain from diagnosing a UTI or urosepsis.*

Criteria have been developed for LTC facility-acquired infections by *the Society for Healthcare Epidemiology of America (SHEA)* [14]. This criterion for urinary tract infections addresses residents with and without a urinary catheter.

1. For residents *without* an indwelling urinary catheter (both criteria 1 and 2 must be present)

   (a) At least one of the following signs or symptom subcriteria.

      (i) Acute dysuria or acute pain, swelling, or tenderness of the testes, epididymis, or prostate.

      (ii) *Fever or leukocytosis* (neutrophilia >14,000 or left shift >6% bands or 1500 or more bands/mm^3) and *at least one of the following localizing urinary tract* subcriteria:

      - Acute costovertebral angle pain or tenderness
      - Suprapubic pain
      - Gross hematuria
      - New or marked increase in urgency
      - New or marked increase in incontinence
      - New or marked increase in frequency

      (iii) *In the absence fever or leukocytosis, then two or more of the following* localizing urinary tract subcriteria

      - Suprapubic pain
      - Gross hematuria
      - New or marked increase in incontinence
      - New or marked increase in urgency
      - New or marked increase in frequency

   (b) One of the following microbiologic subcriteria

      (i) At least 100,000 cfu/mL of *no more than two species* of microorganism in a voided urine sample

      (ii) *At least 100 cfu/mL* if any number of organisms in a specimen collected by in-and-out catheter

2. For residents *with* an indwelling catheter (*both criteria 1 and 2 must be present*)

   (a) At least one of the following sign or symptom subcriteria

      (i) Fever, rigors, or new-onset hypotension, with no alternate site of infection

      (ii) Either acute change in mental status or acute functional decline, with no alternate diagnosis and leukocytosis

(iii) New-onset suprapubic pain or costovertebral angle pain or tenderness

(iv) Purulent discharge from around the catheter or acute pain, swelling, or tenderness of the testes, epididymis, or prostate

(b) Urinary catheter specimen culture with at least 100,000 cfu/mL of any organism(s)

If the resident has an indwelling catheter, the Infectious Disease Society of America (IDSA) *recommends changing the catheter* **before** *collecting a urine specimen for a culture and sensitivity (C&S)*. However, it is common to culture two or three organisms identified even with a catheter change. The clinician must then decide which, if any of these organisms, are responsible for the resident's illness. To help better identify the offending organism(s) in a catheterized resident with urosepsis (fever, shaking chills, hypotension, and/or delirium), it is prudent to obtain blood cultures. While waiting for the results of the blood cultures, aggressive treatment with a broad-spectrum antibiotic is recommended.

Multiple studies have demonstrated that within a month of inserting an indwelling catheter, a resident has a 75–95% chance of developing bacteriuria, with the risk of bacteriuria is 18–40% 1 month after replacement of a suprapubic catheter [15]. Use of a condom catheter reduces the risk of bacteriuria to 12%. Finally, the risk of bacteriuria is lowest with proper hygiene and self-catheterization, 1–3% in 1 month [15].

Nursing Home Acquired Pneumonia

Pneumonia is a common infection in PA/LTC. Some studies have suggested that lower respiratory infections are more common than UTIs, considering that many presumed UTIs are actually treated cases of asymptomatic bacteriuria. The incidence rates of pneumonia in the nursing facility setting range from 0.3 to 2.5 infections/1000 resident care-days [16]. In addition, a number of residents may be inappropriately diagnosed with bacterial pneumonia when in fact the resident has aspiration (chemical) pneumonitis in which antibiotic therapy often is not indicated.

There is a tenfold increase in the incidence of pneumonia in LTC residents compared to age-matched persons living in the community [17]. LTC residents are predisposed to lower respiratory infections because they have a decreased ability to clear mucus from the airways, are more prone to swallowing difficulties due to decreased oral and pharyngeal swallowing and thus more prone to aspiration. Research has demonstrated that the increased bacterial load in the mouth due to poor oral care increases the risk for pneumonia.

The criteria for diagnosing pneumonia in the NF/SNF setting has been revised by SHEA [18]. The following criteria are the most current guidelines for LTCFs:

Pneumonia Criterion (*all three criteria must be met*)

1. Interpretation of a chest radiograph as demonstrating pneumonia or the presence of a new infiltrate
2. **At least one of the following respiratory** subcriteria

   (a) New or increased cough
   (b) New or increased sputum production
   (c) Oxygen saturation <94% on room air or a reduction in oxygen saturation of 3% from baseline
   (d) New or changed lung examination abnormalities
   (e) Pleuritic chest pain
   (f) Respiratory rate of 25 or greater breaths/min

3. **At least one of the constitutional criteria** in residents of LTCFs are included in the following list: (Constitutional Criteria in Residents of LTC Facilities)

   (a) Fever

      (i) Single oral temperature >37.8 °C (>100 F) or
      (ii) Repeated oral temperatures >37.2 °C (99 F) or rectal temp. >37.5 °C (99.4 F) or
      (iii) Single temperature >1.1 °C (2 F) over baseline form any site (Oral, tympanic, axillary)

   (b) Leukocytosis

      (i) Neutrophilia (>14,000 leukocytes/mm^3) or
      (ii) Left shift (6% bands or 1500 or more bands/mm^3)

   (c) Acute change in mental status from baseline (criteria for delirium assessment, Confusion Assessment Method {CAM}, must be present—See chapter "Dementia, Delirium, and Depression" for further discussion of delirium)

      (i) Acute onset
      (ii) Fluctuating course
      (iii) Inattention
            and
      (iv) Either disorganized thinking or altered level of consciousness

   (d) Acute functional decline

      (i) A new 3-point increase in total activities of daily living (ADL) score (range 0–28) from baseline based on the following 6 ADL items. Each scored form 0 (independent) to 4 (total dependence)

      • Bed mobility
      • Transfer
      • Locomotion within LTCF
      • Dressing
      • Toilet use
      • Personal hygiene

Use of diagnostic criteria is critical to prevent a potentially avoidable hospitalization for pneumonia. Rapid diagnosis and early treatment with antibiotics are very important and lead to better clinical outcomes.

Many factors contribute to determining the most appropriate setting for the treatment of pneumonia. If the resident is stable with acceptable oxygen saturations (with or without O_2 therapy) and the staff can closely monitor the resident's condition, then many clinicians are comfortable treating pneumonia in the NF/SNF setting as long as the treatment plan agrees with previously discussed goals of care of the resident. If the resident and/or health care proxy want aggressive treatment including respiratory ventilation if needed, then hospitalization would be appropriate. However, patients and/or health care proxies may request treatment for pneumonia be provided "in place" based on a "comfort care" goal and have no desire to receive artificial respiratory ventilation or cardiopulmonary resuscitation. Furthermore, undesirable risks that commonly occur with hospitalization include:

• Development of pressure ulcers
• Colonization with highly virulent or drug-resistant organisms
• Delirium, especially in residents with dementia
• Difficult-to-manage behaviors from being in a strange physical and people environment, especially among residents with an underlying cognitive disorder

In addition, patients are at an increased risk for hospital readmission and mortality following a hospital admission for pneumonia based on:

• Higher number of comorbidities
• Increased number of medications
• Prior admissions to health care facilities [19]

Physician Order for Life Sustaining Treatment (POLST) and Advance Directives

It is difficult to reduce hospital admissions and readmissions without addressing resident goals of care. Experienced practitioners who take the time to have these discussions with patients and families are less likely to find families expecting aggressive interventions in a frail resident with advanced, life-limiting illness near the end-of-life. Unfortunately, many patients/families have never had a conversation with their PCP regarding goals of care until a medical crisis occurs. A conversation regarding goals of care in the midst of a crisis is not an ideal time for these difficult decisions. During a crisis, there are *three fundamental questions* that are usually asked by the patient [20]. "What is happening to me and why?" "What does this mean for my future?" "What can be done about it and how will it change my future?" Having a conversation regarding goals of care will help the practitioner to build a trusting relationship and to better help answer these fundamental questions.

The Serious Illness Conversation Guide (SICG) is a useful tool developed by Ariadne Labs [21].

- This tool helps clinicians have effective conversations with patients regarding their "values, goals, and preferences."
- This tool was shown in multiple clinical trials to "result in more, better, and earlier serious illness conversations, positive impact on patients, and cost reductions in the last 6 months of life."
- The current guide is based on numerous patient and clinician feedback regarding the effectiveness of the guide for these conversations. The guide is a one-page script that demonstrates the use of "patient-tested language," which helps clinicians when talking about serious illness and avoiding unwanted hospitalizations.

Hospital systems, emergency medical staff, and nursing facilities in many US states have adopted the Physician Orders for Life Sustaining Treatment (POLST). The website "POLST.org" is a great resource to research both national and state efforts in adopting the POLST paradigm. While, this document may have different names in the 50 states and the District of Columbia, the goal of POLST is to have a portable document that communicates wishes for medical care for patients experiencing serious illness.

It is critically important that the PCP have a conversation with the patient/POA upon every admission to the NF/SNF. Most families desire the *highest quality of life possible* for their ill family member and have less interest in maintaining life as long as possible. Accordingly, one can shift the conversation from simply clarification of code status to goals, wishes, expectations of the patient and family if an acute change in condition occurs. When families learn that a NF/SNF can treat frail adults in place rather transferring to the hospital, it is frequently easier for the patient or POA to agree to "NO HOSPITALIZATION" and "NO EMERGENCY ROOM VISIT." In many cases, the resident should only be hospitalized when the NF/SNF is unable to provide sufficient treatment and comfort to meet the resident's needs based on the goals of care.

Summary

Preventing avoidable hospital admissions and readmissions is challenging. If the nursing home is committed to reducing hospitalizations, its culture should reflect the following:

- PCPs must acquire and maintain skills to care for frail adults with complex multi-morbidities (e.g., Geriatric 4Ms model of care).
- Regular educational activities for all NF/SNF staff are a priority.
- The management team should work closely with local hospitals and home health care and hospice agencies to develop transitions of care that are person-centered and have clearly defined expectations.

- GOALS OF CARE should be discussed with all resident/patients (POAs when appropriate) during every care transition (e.g., Serious Illness Conversation Guide).
- The PCP should discuss expectations of care. (e.g., DNR/CPR, ER visits, or hospitalizations) prior to any acute change in condition.
- Newly admitted residents be seen within 2–5 days of admission or within 12–24 h when a significant change in condition occurs.
- The management team and staff should be committed and able to treat residents in place when appropriate and congruent with the wishes of the patient/POA.
- PCPs and licensed nursing staff should provide timely and frequent communication with the patient/POA whenever a significant change in condition occurs.
- Have an effective antibiotic stewardship program that uses the updated LTCF criteria by SHEA in defining LTCF-acquired infections.

Pearls for the Practitioner
- Preventing avoidable hospitalizations requires skilled and timely resident assessment whenever a resident experience a change in condition.
- Preventing avoidable hospital admissions requires a conversation between the patient and/or proxy decision maker and the PCP regarding goals of care.
- When a resident with memory loss demonstrates increase behavioral problems without meeting criteria for a UTI, the medical literature indicates only 11% will have a UTI.
- Avoid standing orders to treat elevated temperatures without notifying the PCP.
- Do not treat residents with urinary catheters for a UTI unless they meet the SHEA criteria for a UTI/urosepsis.
- If a clinician suspects urosepsis, blood cultures should be drawn before initiation of broad-spectrum antibiotics, which will be helpful in determining appropriate antibiotic choice than the results of a urine C & S.
- Aspiration pneumonitis without pneumonia does not require antibiotic treatment.

Suggested Websites
- Centers for Medicare and Medicaid Services (CMS): https://www.CMS.gov
- American Geriatric Society (AGS): https://www.americangeriatrics.org
- AMDA/The Society for Post-Acute and Long-Term Care Medicine: https://www.paltc.org
- Pathway Health/INTERACT: https://www.pathway-interact.com
- National POLST: https://www.polst.org
- Serious Illness conversation: https://www.ariadnelabs.org/areas-of-work/serious-illness-care
- The Society for Healthcare Epidemiology of America (SHEA): https://www.shea-online.org

References

1. Baker B, et al. Skilled nursing facility 30-day all-cause readmission measure (SNFRM) NQF #2510: all-cause risk-standardized readmission measure; April 2019. https://www.cms.gov/ Medicare/Quality-Initiatives-Patient-Assessment-Instruments/Value-Based-Programs/SNF-- VBP/Downloads/SNFRM-TechReportSupp-2019-.pdf
2. Centers for Medicare and Medicaid Services. Hospital Readmissions Reduction Program (HRRP). https://www.cms.gov/Medicare/Medicare-Fee-for-Service Payment/ AcuteInpatientPPS/Readmissions-Reduction-Program. Accessed June 2021.
3. Centers for Medicare and Medicaid Services. SNF PPS payment model research. https://www. cms.gov/Medicare/Medicare-Fee-for-Service-Payment/SNFPPS/therapyresearch. Accessed June 2021.
4. Ouslander J, et al. Root cause analyses of transfers of skilled nursing facility patients to acute hospitals: lessons learned for reducing unnecessary hospitalizations. J Am Med Dir Assoc. 2016;17:256–62.
5. Denson S, et al. Age friendly healthcare delivery: the 4Ms #93. https://www.geriatricfastfacts. com/fast-facts/age-friendly-healthcare-delivery-4ms. Accessed June 2021.
6. Institute for Healthcare Improvement. Age-friendly health systems: guide to using the 4Ms in the care of older adults; July 2020. http://www.ihi.org/Engage/Initiatives/Age-Friendly-- Health-Systems/Documents/IHIAgeFriendlyHealthSystems_GuidetoUsing4MsCare.pdf.
7. Molnar F, et al. The 5Ms of geriatrics. HealthinAging.org. https://www.healthinaging.org/ tools-and-tips/tip-sheet-5ms-geriatrics. Accessed June 2021.
8. Centers for Medicare and Medicaid Services. Shared savings program. https://www.cms.gov/ Medicare/Medicare-Fee-for-Service-Payment/sharedsavingsprogram. Accessed June 2021.
9. Ouslander J. Overview of the INTERACT program and curriculum. https://pathway-interact. com/interact-training/. Accessed June 2021.
10. Weerahandi H, et al. Risk of readmission after discharge from skilled nursing facilities following heart failure hospitalization: a retrospective cohort study. JAMDA. 2019;20:432–7.
11. Castle SC, et al. Lowering the temperature criterion improves detection of infections in nursing home residents. Aging Immunol Infect Dis. 1993;4:67–76.
12. Chandra A, et al. Risk of 30-day hospital readmission among patients discharged to skilled nursing facilities: development and validation of a risk-prediction model. J Am Med Dir Assoc. 2019;20:444–50.
13. Noelle LE, et al. SHEA Long-Term-Care Committee. Urinary tract infections in long-term care facilities. Infect Control Hosp Epidemiol. 2001;22:167–75.
14. Stone, ND et. al. Surveillance definitions of infections in long term care facilities: reviewing the McGeer criteria. Infect Control Hosp Epidemiol 2012; 33(10): 965-977
15. Saint S, Lipsky BA. Preventing catheter-related bacteriuria: should we? Can we? How? Arch Intern Med. 1999;159(8):800–8.
16. Loeb M, Mcgeer A, McArthur M, et al. Risk factors for pneumonia and other lower respiratory tract infections in elderly residents of long-term care facilities. Arch Intern Med. 1999;159:2058–64.
17. Muder RR. Pneumonia in residents of long-term care facilities: epidemiology, etiology, management, and prevention. Am J Med. 1998;105(4):319–30.
18. Smith P, et al. SHEA/APIC Guideline: Infection prevention and control in the long-term care facility. Am J Infect Control 2008; 39(7): 504-535.
19. Graversen, S. et. al. Factors associated with 30-day rehospitalization and mortality in older patients after a pneumonia admission. J Am Med Dir Assoc 2020; 21: 1869-1878.
20. Manish S, et al. DeGowin's diagnostic examination (11th edition electronic). New York: McGraw-Hill Education; 2020.
21. Ariadne Labs. Serious illness care. https://www.ariadnelabs.org/areas-of-work/serious-illness-- care/. Accessed June 2021.

Goals of Care and Prevention

Introduction

A resident of a nursing facility has multimorbidities of diabetes, hypertension, chronic renal insufficiency, and peripheral arterial disease. Interventions such as aspirin to prevent a cardiac event or stroke, meticulous foot care to prevent infection and subsequent amputation, and tightly controlled diabetes and hypertension are to be instituted. But how do these interventions reflect the resident's goals of care? Does the resident have days, months or years to live? What if the resident is a frail 97-year-old female with dementia who frequently refuses her medication and resists care and who now has unavoidable weight loss? Her goals of care need to be considered with every intervention as to benefit vs. risk. How are her goals of care to be determined?

Providing person-centered care is essential to the provision of high quality and excellence in geriatric care. Age-friendly care should respect the goals and wishes of the patient and compels us to put aside enough time to ask what is most important to them. Documenting the practitioner's discussion on goals of care *and* determining whether the patient can make *informed* decisions is vital to diligent and safe practice. Every patient and family situation is unique and presents its own challenges to ensure that care is congruent with the goals of the patient. One of the four components of age-friendly care [1], encouraged by the Institute for Health Care Improvement (IHI), is asking the patient "what matters most" in their day-to-day life. Once we know what matters, we can then institute a better plan of care.

C. Kuttner (✉)
Wilmington VA Medical Center, Wilmington VA Community Living Center, Wilmington, DE, USA

183

P. Winn et al. (eds.), *Post-Acute and Long-Term Care Medicine*, Current Clinical Practice, https://doi.org/10.1007/978-3-031-28628-5_10

This chapter will help practitioners evaluate the needs of patients/residents as to goals of care, fall prevention, immunizations, nutrition, exercise, and the US Preventive Services Task Force recommendations on screening as to benefit and risk.

Goals of Care

Determining a resident's goals of care and understanding their wishes and preferences for care is an entrusted responsibility of all practitioners. Anticipating that goals of care frequently change over an illness trajectory is crucial. These changes need to be acknowledged and incorporated into the plan of care to ensure that all care is patient centered. Currently there is no nationwide or state database for persons to document their wishes and preferences for care. Currently many states use the *POLST* (Physician Orders for Life-Sustaining Treatment) [2] or the *MOLST* (Medical Orders for Life-Sustaining Treatment) [3] to document patient wishes on the use (or not) of CPR, airway intubation, feeding tubes, IV therapy, and antibiotics. Most states also have laws pertaining to the use of advance directives on health care such as a *living will* or a *durable power of attorney* for health care, which can further enable persons to document their wishes and preferences for care (see Chapter "Ethical and Legal Issues in Post-Acute and Long-Term Care" for further discussion). The Veterans Administration uses "life sustaining treatment orders" to document the wishes of veterans in its health system.

Providing quality medical and nursing care is more complex than writing a "do not resuscitate" or "full code" order. Practitioners and the staff of nursing or assisted living facilities should meet with patients and family to review their expectations on admission to a facility or program and to establish overall goals of care. Meetings with family or guardians may be in person, by phone, or by telemedicine services such as a videochat.

Periodic follow-up meetings are often necessary as illness progresses and crises occur that will necessitate modification of the goals of care. For example, if a patient has dysphagia and speech therapy has recommended an altered diet with thickened liquids, a discussion about aspiration and feeding tubes is vital (see Chapter "Weight and Nutrition in Post-Acute and Long-Term Care" for further discussion). The patient or surrogate decision maker may decide that thickened liquids and pureed foods are worsening the patient's quality of life, and may decide instead to liberalize the diet despite the risk of aspiration and pneumonia. For a patient with severe COPD, a discussion on the benefits and burden of CPR, bipap, and respirators is essential. The patient and family may decide that bipap is acceptable, but a respirator is not, and instead prefer to be treated in place at the nursing facility rather than transferred to the hospital.

Most people appreciate the opportunity to discuss end-of-life care and have often had previous experiences with the death of friends or family members that will influence their thoughts and decisions.

Listening to the stories of the resident and family can provide the health care team invaluable information on resident beliefs and values, which can assist the team to provide the intensity of care desired. The COVID-19 pandemic sadly created an urgent need for more of these discussions. The silver lining is that it encouraged practitioners to discuss advance care planning with family members and residents to state what they wanted or did not want if they became ill and unable to make their own decisions. Specifically asking patients what they understand about their illness and what their hopes are for the future can be very revealing. Patients tend to minimize the severity of their illness with hopes that unfortunately may not be realistic. Understanding the level of knowledge and insight of patients can help to better direct education on prognosis and palliative approaches to treatment when a cure is not possible.

Recently a new approach called "age friendly care" has focused on the 4 Ms—Mobility, Mentation, Medication, and "what Matters" to the patient. This simple but sensible strategy can help practitioners and staff to better know patients and to provide the person-centered care that we all strive to achieve [1]. For example, a patient may state hopes to return home to care for a son who has been developmentally disabled since childhood. Or that a patient longs to visit a sister to mend a fractured relationship before either one dies.

Fall Prevention

Falls are an all too common event in long-term care. Falls are potentially life threatening and can result in serious fractures, particularly of the hip or pelvis, or a traumatic brain injury. An increasing number of residents are taking anticoagulants and thus have an increased risk of serious bleeding when a fall occurs. Falls are a frequent reason for admission to a nursing facility due to safety concerns at home, which can overwhelm caregivers. CDC reports that in 2018, 27.5% of people over the age of 65 reported at least one fall in the past year, and 10.2% reported a fall-related injury [4]. Newly admitted patients are at high risk; one study showed that 21% of newly admitted nursing home residents had fallen within 30 days of admission [5]. A fall with injury can result in liability to the nursing facility, poor facility quality measures, and survey citations.

The 2010 AGS Clinical Practice Guideline: "Prevention of Falls in Older Persons" has excellent recommendations on the screening and assessment of patients at increased risk of falls or who have fallen [6]. All patients should be questioned about a history of falls and the circumstances surrounding those falls. A multifactorial fall risk assessment should be completed on nursing home (or assisted living) admission as well as a physical exam that includes a gait and balance evaluation. A *focused history* on falls includes all medications being taken (including OTC medications) and risk factors. The latter include: diabetic neuropathy, urinary urgency, antihypertensive medication, depression, psychotropic medication, foot deformities, orthostasis, muscle weakness, vision impairment, cognitive impairment, delirium, and vestibular dysfunction. Chronic conditions or diseases such as Parkinson's disease, anemia, osteoarthritis, diabetes, cerebrovascular disease, cardiovascular disease, bladder incontinence, dementia, and chronic pain are frequent comorbidities that increase the risk of falls. Patient care plans should reflect the interventions put in place to help prevent falls such as frequent toileting, non-skid footwear, keeping personal items within reach on the bedside table, and having assistive devices close at hand.

According to the AMDA The Society for Post-Acute and Long-Term Medicine clinical practice guideline on falls [7], it is important to document a *fall risk assessment* for each patient, and to discuss those risks at the care plan conference. After a fall, a *huddle* should occur in which the possible factors contributing to the fall are reviewed. The guidelines state that a "multicomponent intervention by a multidisciplinary team may reduce the *number of falls* and the *number of fallers* in the long term care setting."

When performing the *Physical Examination*, it is important to assess gait, balance, mobility, lower extremity joint stability, muscle strength, and overall function. The neurologic exam should include an evaluation of cognition, peripheral proprioception, reflexes, cortical and extrapyramidal and cerebellar function, and muscle strength of the lower extremities. Cardiovascular assessment should include heart rate and rhythm, blood pressure, orthostatic blood pressure, and peripheral pulses. Test visual acuity and check feet and footwear. The *Functional Assessment* should include an assessment of ADLs and adaptive equipment including mobility aids. Query on the fear of falling and any self-imposed limitations due to that fear. An *Environmental Assessment* should be done to check for lighting, obstacles, uneven surfaces, and other hazards, especially in community dwelling older adults. Specific tests that may be useful include the "get up and go" test [8], the "functional reach test" [9], the "Berg balance test" [10], and the "POMA-*performance oriented mobility assessment*" [11]. Carotid sinus massage-induced bradycardia may also be diagnostic in patients with repeated falls of unknown etiology.

Recommendations to decrease fall risk include:

- Exercise programs to maintain strength and mobility and decrease risk of falls. Yoga, Tai Chi, and weight-bearing exercises are most helpful.
- Supplement residents with at least 800 IU of vitamin D daily for those with vitamin D deficiency and/or impaired balance. Patients who have vitamin D levels less than 20 ng/mL may have a decreased fall risk with vitamin D supplementation.
- Consider dose reduction of medications that can cause orthostasis or increase risk of falls (psychotropic medications particularly benzodiazepines, sedatives, and anxiolytics) or use of multiple antihypertensives (see Chapter "Medication Management in Long-Term Care" for further discussion), and opioids.
- Consider treatment of osteoporosis in residents who can tolerate pharmacologic therapy and have a life expectancy of 5–10 years, particularly for those who have had a prior wrist, vertebral or hip fracture(s).
- Residents with cognitive impairment may be impulsive and unable to remember information taught on fall prevention. Frequent monitoring and regular toileting may decrease but not eliminate their risk of falls.

Bed and chair alarms do not prevent falls; they only alert staff to a resident who is trying to stand or get out of bed. Most nursing facilities are now alarm free. Restraints should be avoided at all times (both chemical and physical) because they neither prevent falls nor injury and instead increase falls and injuries! The use of side rails is controversial, with double rails considered a restraint. Many side rail injuries are linked to older beds, which allowed entrapment of the patient between the rails and mattress or the side rail and the wall. There is also a great risk that a patient climbing over the side rail and falling from this higher height to the floor can suffer a more severe impact injury than a fall from bed without a rail in place. The efficacy of hip protectors is controversial [12]. There is limited evidence that they are effective and many patients are reluctant to wear them. Putting them on requires extra effort by the nursing staff. Given the high risk of falls and injuries, if a patient is willing to wear hip protectors, consider a trial.

Nursing facilities may have a "fall teams" or a falls protocol to evaluate each fall and to determine what preventive interventions to initiate such as the use of low bed. Input by the practitioner can be vital due to his/her expertise to take into account *intrinsic* and *extrinsic* risk factors, patient multimorbidities, and to guide the inter-disciplinary term to create an appropriate plan of care to lessen fall risk. *Medication review performed by the practitioner and the facility contract pharmacist can provide critical input to lessen fall risk.*

AHRQ has excellent resources to help identify medication that may increase risk of falls as does the Beers criteria. *Deprescribing* can be helpful in reducing risk [13]. An optimal falls team would include an occupational therapist, physical therapist, pharmacist, nurse/nursing assistant, recreation therapist, and either physician or nurse practitioner. Decreasing falls and avoiding major injury is an excellent quality improvement project (PIP) for the IDT team to undertake under Quality Assurance and Performance Improvement (QA-PI).

Immunizations

Vaccines currently recommended for the elderly include the influenza vaccine, pneumococcal vaccine, herpes zoster vaccine (Shingrix), tetanus (Tdap) booster, and the COVID-19 vaccine.

Influenza

Efficacy of the influenza vaccine varies from year to year, depending upon the strains selected for the vaccine and those strains that infect the population. *It is paramount to vaccinate residents, staff, and visiting family members while discouraging sick visitors from coming into the facility during influenza season.* If unvaccinated staff become ill with influenza, it can result in the widespread dissemination of the flu virus to residents, patients, and other staff, causing absenteeism and increased workload on remaining staff. Influenza can be a life-threatening illness, so practitioners and staff should be vigilant as to the possibility that an influenza outbreak has occurred. Some facilities are now mandating flu vaccine as a condition of employment unless there is a medical or religious contraindication. Staff vaccination rates of 60–70% may decrease the likelihood of an outbreak in the facility among patients and staff.

The facility medical director should be notified when an outbreak of influenza occurs and to decide if and when to provide prophylaxis to all residents in the facility. CDC.gov provides an excellent "Toolkit for Post-Acute and Long-term Care Facilities" that describes all aspects of influenza prophylaxis and treatment [14]. *Vaccination of residents and staff with the trivalent influenza vaccine should start as soon as the vaccine is available* (usually in September or early October). Having *standing orders to vaccinate residents* and vaccinating all staff unless there is a medical contraindication or personal choice not to receive the vaccine can increase compliance. For residents, consent can be obtained from the health care power of attorney or guardian if the resident is unable to give informed consent due to incapacity or lack of decision-making capacity.

An outbreak in a nursing facility is defined when two residents are sick with flu-like symptoms within a 72-h period and one has confirmed Influenza by viral testing. When this occurs, all residents should be treated or prophylaxed with either oseltamivir or zanamivir for 5 days. Transit between facility units by staff and residents should be limited. Standard and droplet precautions should be followed for all residents with suspected or confirmed influenza. To help prevent further spread, dining and activities may need to occur in patient rooms rather than in common areas. Note that *amantadine and rimantadine are no longer considered to be effective* due to the development of resistance and thus should not be used for treatment or prophylaxis. It is essential to have a policy and procedure at the facility on how to manage an influenza outbreak including its isolation protocol. The medical director should collaborate with the infection preventionist in the building to create durable policies and procedures to keep patients, staff, and visitors safe.

Pneumococcus

Currently there are several recommended vaccines to help prevent pneumococcal disease in older adults: the *Prevnar 20*, *Pneumovax 23*, *Prevnar 15* and the *Prevnar 13*. Common presentations of pneumococcal disease in older adults are pneumonia, sepsis, and meningitis [15]. PCV 13, 15 and 20 are conjugate vaccines and the PPS 23 is a pneumococcal polysaccharide vaccine. Current recommendations are on the CDC website and continue to evolve for different age groups. For adults 19–64 years of age, there is a long list of diagnoses such as alcoholism, diabetes, chronic renal failure, that put patients at higher risk for severe pneumococcal disease. These patients should receive the PCV 20 or PCV 15, followed by the PPS 23 in 1 year. All patients over 65 years of age are recommended to receive pneumococcal vaccination. They can either receive a dose of PCV 15 followed by PPS 23 in a year, or a one time dose of PCV20.

Shingles (Herpes Zoster)

The Herpes Zoster vaccine (Shingrix) has been shown to decrease the risk of shingles and post-herpetic neuralgia [17]. *This recombinant vaccine is much more effective than the prior vaccine (Zostavax) and can prevent 90% of herpes zoster and 89% of post-herpetic neuralgia.* Shingrix was approved in 2017, and it is effective in preventing shingles for at least 4 years. This vaccination is a two part series, with the second dose being given 2 months after the first dose [16].

Tdap is preventive for tetanus, which can occur in long-term care patients with wounds. It is given as an IM vaccination every 10 years. In addition to preventing tetanus in wounds, it may also prevent pertussis infection which can be serious in older patients.

COVID-19 Vaccination

In 2020 several vaccines to prevent COVID-19 infection were approved. The science and technology of these vaccines is rapidly evolving; however, they have been very effective in preventing COVID infection in many nursing home and assisted living residents and reducing the severity of illness in the few patients who do become infected after having had a previous COVID-19 vaccination. It has been determined that ongoing boosters will be needed to maintain immunity. Monoclonal antibody treatments are also being utilized to decrease severity and duration of illness and prevent hospitalizations.

Nutrition and Vitamin and Mineral Supplementation

"We are what we eat," continues to be true in the LTC setting. There are consequences to being underweight and overweight. Being *underweight* increases risk for infections, pressure ulcers, physical decline, cognitive decline, and death. Malnutrition and dehydration are common in the NF setting, with a recent article identifying the prevalence of malnutrition at about 20% depending on the patient population [17]. Being *overweight* increases risks of developing metabolic syndrome, hypertension, diabetes, and the personal need for more physical assistance from staff for daily tasks of living (ADLs).

A nutritional and dietary plan is required for all residents in order to ensure that nutrient and calorie needs are being met. Goals of care are paramount. *Resident rights* allow patients to decline a prescribed diet and to eat what they choose, even if it compromises their medical condition. This can complicate the treatment of diabetes, CHF, and renal disease, and raise conflict between health care providers and the resident/patient. However, the nursing or assisted living facility is their "home" and just like community dwelling persons, residents are entitled to make informed decisions on food preferences. Despite this, care planning requires the facility to set goals for residents in order to achieve adequate nutrition. At times this can be challenging. If the dietician has a goal that the resident needs to lose 10 lbs and achieve a hemoglobin A1C of 7% but the patient eats double portions and snacks throughout the day, the listed goals in the care plan may not be realistic. Conversely, if a patient with dysphagia is on a pureed diet with thickened liquids and the patient refuses to eat the prescribed diet, the goal to gain weight may be futile and paradoxically result in weight loss!

Poor dentition can be a barrier to adequate nutrition. Encouraging the nursing staff to provide routine and thorough mouth care is essential. Engaging a dentist with an interest in geriatrics to come to the facility can be invaluable, but also challenging. Some dentists may offer on-site bedside dental care such as cleaning and tooth extractions. Starting a tooth brushing or mouth swabbing program (for patients who are edentulous) will improve oral hygiene and may decrease rates of aspiration pneumonia.

Another common problem is swallowing dysfunction (*dysphagia*) due presbyesophagus or neurologic conditions such as Parkinson's or cerebrovascular disease. Dysphagia can affect the texture of food and liquids that can be tolerated. A visit to the dining room at mealtime to observe how the patient is eating can be very informative. Is staff assistance needed ? How is the food texture and liquid consistency being tolerated? Such a visit can provide insight into why a resident is losing weight and suggest possible therapeutic interventions. If a resident has advanced dementia and the family chooses comfort care, hand feeding to the best of the staff's ability is the best option to offer meal with dignity. Choosing Wisely guidelines from AGS and AMDA strongly advise against insertion of feeding tubes in those with dementia (see Chapter "Weight and Nutrition in Post-Acute and Long-Term Care" for further discussion) [18].

The dietician, the speech language therapist, and the pharmacist can be allies in the management of unintended weight loss. The dietician can offer preferred foods after the speech therapist determines which foods and consistency are safe for the patient to eat. The pharmacist can advise which medications may be affecting taste and appetite and suggest a trial of deprescribing.

A diet balanced with protein, carbohydrates, and fats can help residents maintain good health, muscle strength, and mental vigor. Fresh fruit and vegetables, often absent in dietary plans, should be encouraged in order to provide natural nutrients, hydration, and fiber. The medical director can encourage the facility administration and dietary to supply more fresh fruit and vegetables on the meal plan as well as healthy snacks between meals. Fruit and vegetable smoothies or pureed fruits may be a good choice for those with dysphagia. Frozen fruits and vegetables can also provide excellent nutritional options if fresh products are not available. *If patients eat a healthy diet, a supplemental multivitamin may not be needed.* However, if not eating a balanced diet, a vitamin/mineral supplement may be reasonable.

The most common electrolyte abnormalities in nursing home residents are hypokalemia related to diuretics and abnormalities in sodium (either hypo or hypernatremia) related to fluid balance abnormalities. Avoiding fluid restrictions whenever possible and providing fluids in between meals can help to avert dehydration. Consider a hydration cart with flavored water and other healthy drinks that can be given to residents several times a day. Providing extra fluid at the times of medication administration is another option.

Many residents are deficient in vitamin D deficiency, which has been associated with falls, fractures, musculoskeletal pain, and muscle weakness [19]. Routine testing of 25-hydroxyvitamin D levels is usually not needed when a vitamin D supplement is being given. However, if checked, a level of at least 40–50 is optimal. Different organizations recommend differing doses of vitamin D supplements, ranging from 800 IU to 4000 IU a day. Residents at highest risk of vitamin D deficiency include those with dark pigmented skin, obesity, malabsorption, and who take medications that accelerate the breakdown of vitamin D (such as phenytoin and phenobarbital) or bind oral vitamin D (such as cholestyramine). Consider a calcium supplement of 1000–1200 mg daily *with* vitamin D if dietary intake is poor and supplementation is consistent with goals of care. Calcium supplements enhance the benefit of vitamin D on bone mineral density; however, calcium supplements can be constipating. If the calcium supplements result in a need for additional laxatives, this may cause a *prescribing cascade* where the risks outweigh its benefits.

Magnesium is often deficient, particularly in residents on diuretics or proton pump inhibitors that have been taken for an extended period of time and in those with diabetes mellitus [20]. Oral zinc replacement has been found to be beneficial in patients who have zinc deficiency and a wound; the optimal amount of supplementation and duration of therapy is currently being studied. There seems to be a correlation between adequate zinc levels and cognition and depression [21].

Screening Tests

Screening for Osteoporosis

The US Preventive Services Task Force has *not made a specific recommendation about resident screening for osteoporosis in nursing homes.* However, it does recommend consideration of screening in women over age 65. Currently there is inadequate evidence to recommend screening in men. On the other hand, the National Osteoporosis Foundation recommends screening in women over 65 and men over 70 [22]. Screening options may include *DEXA scanning* of the lumbar spine and hip, quantitative ultrasound of the calcaneum or *FRAX risk calculation* [23]. Some residents may have already sustained an osteoporotic fracture or have an elevated Dexa T-score greater than −2.5. Life expectancy, prognosis, and clinical judgment may determine which residents would be most appropriate for screening. For many, treatment with bisphosphonates or other agents may be appropriate and tolerated; for others, it is burdensome and inconvenient and has potential adverse side effects such as GERD, osteonecrosis, and atypical fractures. The lag effect for benefits needs to be considered; if a patient is at end of life, treatment of osteoporosis should not be prioritized. *Residents in assisted living may be more appropriate for screening than those in a nursing facility.*

Tuberculosis Screening

Recommendations for tuberculosis screening in nursing homes has changed over the past 10 years due to declines in both active and latent tuberculosis in the USA. Tuberculosis screening of residents is recommended on admission to nursing facilities and for a facility tuberculosis risk assessment. The initial testing should be done with a *two-step tuberculin skin test* (TST) or an IGRA (interferon gamma release assay) blood test. Many older people are anergic due to immunosenescence and may not respond to skin testing (manifest as a false negative). Symptoms suggestive of active or reactivated TB should be aggressively pursued. Fortunately, this situation is infrequent in most US NFs. Many NFs (especially those at low risk) use an annual "symptom screen" rather than repeating the TST every year. It is no longer recommended to do a TB skin test or an IGRA test yearly if the incidence of tuberculosis is low in the facility.

Cancer Screening

Cancer screening of residents in NFs and assisted living may be reasonable if consistent with residents' goals of care. Depending on the age, prognosis, and physical/cognitive function of the patient, decisions about whether or not to screen should be made in concert with the patient/family.

Cervical Cancer screening should *rarely if ever be needed* and *Breast Cancer screening* can be considered if the patient is able to participate in mammography; however, many nursing home residents are unable to stand and be properly positioned for a mammogram. Some may be unwilling to undergo surgery and potential radiation and chemotherapy if a cancer is found. Physical exam can detect most significant breast cancers in elderly residents. Workup and treatment of any breast mass should be discussed with the patient/family. Periodic clinical breast exams by the practitioner are prudent and reasonable if the resident provides consent. Consider mammograms for residents in assisted living.

Colon cancer screening is *not recommended over the age of 75 by the USPSTF*, and should only be undertaken if the patient is willing and able to undergo major surgery.

Screening for lung cancer with low dose CT scan is limited to select patient populations who are under the age of 75 and have smoked at least 40 pack years and would be willing/able to undergo treatment if cancer is found. This CT screening recommendation was *intended for otherwise healthy patients in the community; not for frail elderly in a nursing* facility.

Prostate Cancer screening with PSA testing is *NOT recommended* for most male residents, as it has no mortality benefit and it may be associated with increased morbidity and mortality resulting from diagnostic workup and unnecessary treatment.

AMDA discussed cancer screening in its "Choosing Wisely" campaign. It did **not** recommend screening for breast, colorectal, or prostate cancer unless life expectancy is estimated to be over 10 years and stated that for most long-term residents over age 75 the burdens of screening likely outweigh any benefits

Exercise

Exercise is a low risk activity with high benefit to improve function and prevent physical decline in residents. Exercise has shown to have positive effects on mood and to help maintain physical function in patients with Alzheimer's disease [24, 25]. The best benefits involve an exercise program that includes walking, strength training, balance, and flexibility exercise. Unfortunately, not all residents are able to walk, but restorative programs can keep many residents ambulatory for longer than expected. Restorative programs are generally provided by nursing, based on recommendations from rehabilitation therapy and the restorative care coordinator. Exercise programs for people who are wheelchair-dependent or bedbound are also helpful. Yoga, Tai Chi, and stretching programs have been adapted for those chairbound [26]. Exercise for bedbound patients is more challenging, but less intense programs can be given based on individual needs and capabilities. Exercise combined with music has been shown to be effective in patients with Parkinson's disease [27]. Further research on best practices is ongoing to avert increased frailty and sarcopenia. Exercise training, particularly resistance/muscle training and weight-bearing are the most effective [28].

Mental exercise is important as well. Depending on the cognitive reserve of the resident, there are opportunities for mental stimulation. Reminiscence, music, sensory activities, arts, current events, and visits from family and friends are all important in maintaining cognitive vitality.

Peals for the Practitioner
- Discuss, revisit, and then document residents' revised goals of care when a change in condition occurs.
- Preventive health interventions and treatments are guided by residents' multi-morbidities, prognosis, advance directives, and goals of care.

- Fall prevention should always include a medication review and attempts to discontinue medications that potentially increase fall risk.
- Vaccination of residents and staff is vital to maintaining personal health and preventing outbreaks of infectious disease in the facility.
- Good nutrition is key to the maintenance of physical and cognitive health. Observation of residents at mealtime may help determine interventions in those with weight loss.
- Liberal diets are appropriate for most frail older patients. Restrictive diets should be avoided unless medically necessary. And may cause loss of appetite, refusal to eat, and weight loss.
- Screening for cancer in asymptomatic residents should be individualized and generally minimized. But may be more appropriate for residents in assisted living who tend to be younger and independent than those in a nursing facility.
- Mental and physical exercise programs improve quality of life of residents; meeting the exercise needs of individual residents requires thought, teamwork, and creativity.

References

1. Age-friendly health systems. Guide to using the 4Ms in the care of older adults-institute for health care improvement; July 2020.
2. POLST, physician orders for life-sustaining treatment paradigm®. http://www.polst.org. Accessed 1 July 2021.
3. Medical orders for life sustaining treatment; MOLST. https://www.molst.org. Accessed 1 July 2021
4. Trends in non-fatal falls and fall-related injuries among adults greater than 65 years-United States, 2012-2018. https://www.cdc.gov/mmwr/volumes/69/wr/mm6927a5htm. Accessed 1 July 2021.
5. Leland NE, et al. Falls in newly admitted nursing home residents: a national study. JAGS. 2012;60(5):939–45.
6. American Geriatrics Society. AGS/BGS clinical practice guideline: prevention of falls in older persons, summary of recommendations. http://www.americangeriatrics.org/health_care_professionals/clinical_practice/clinical_guidelines_recommendations/prevention_of_falls_summary_of_recommendations.
7. AMDA Clinical Practice Guideline on Falls. Accessed 1 July 2021.
8. Balance in elderly patients: the "get up and go" test. Arch Phys Med Rehabil Jun 1986 67(6):387–9.
9. de Waroquier-Leroy L, et al. The functional reach test: strategies, performance and the influence of age. Ann Phys Rehabil Med. 2014;57(6–7):452–64.
10. Neuls P, et al. Usefulness of the berg balance scale to predict falls in the elderly. J Geriatr Phys Ther. 2011;34(1):3–10.
11. Tinetti ME. Performance-oriented assessment of mobility problems in elderly patients. JAGS. 1986;34:119–26.
12. Santesso N, Carrasco-Labra A, Brignardello-Petersen R. Hip protectors for preventing hip fractures in older people. Cochrane Database Syst Rev. 2014;3:CD001255. https://doi.org/10.1002/14651858.CD001255.pub5.

13. AHRQ "Preventing Falls in Hospitals". Tool 31:Medical Fall Risk Score and Evaluation Tools. Accessed 1 July 2021.
14. Centers for Disease Control and Prevention. Post-acute and long-term-care facility toolkit: Influenza. https://www.cdc.gov/flu/toolkit/long-term-care. Accessed 28 April 2023.
15. ACIP Vaccine Recommendations and Schedules. https://www.cdc.gov/vaccines/acip/recommendations.html. Accessed 28 April 2023.
16. James S. Shingrix: the new adjuvanted recombinant herpes zoster vaccine. Ann Pharmacother. 2018;52(7):673–80.
17. Bell C, et al. Malnutrition in the Nursing Home. Curr Opin Clin Nutr Metab Care. 2015;18(1):17–23.
18. https://www.choosingwisely.org. Accessed 28 April 2023.
19. Yanamadala M, et al. Ensuring Vitamin D supplementation in nursing home patients: a quality improvement project. J Nutr Gerontol Geriatr. 2012;31(2):158–71.
20. Arinzon Z, Peisakh A, Schrire S, Berner YN. Prevalence of hypomagnesemia (HM) in a geriatric long-term care (LTC) setting. Arch Gerontol Geriatr. 2010;51(1):36–40.
21. Markiewicz-Żukowska R, Gutowska A, Borawska MH. Serum zinc concentrations correlate with mental and physical status of nursing home residents. PLoS One. 2015;10(1):e0117257.
22. https://www.nof.org. Accessed 28 April 2023.
23. Welcome to FRAX®. FRAX® WHO fracture risk assessment tool. http://www.shef.ac.uk/FRAX. Accessed 28 April 2023.
24. Rolland Y, Pillard F, Klapouszczak A, et al. Exercise program for nursing home residents with Alzheimer's disease: a 1-year randomized, controlled trial. J Am Geriatr Soc. 2007;55(2):158–65.
25. Williams CL, Tappen RM. Effect of exercise on mood in nursing home residents with Alzheimer's disease. Am J Alzheimers Dis Other Demen. 2007;22(5):389–97.
26. Cordes T, et al. Chair-based exercise interventions for nursing home residents: a systematic review. JAMDA. 22(4):733–40.
27. de Dreu MJ, van der Wilk AS, Poppe E. Rehabilitation, exercise therapy and music in patients with Parkinson's disease: a meta-analysis of the effects of music-based movement therapy on walking ability, balance and quality of life. Parkinsonism Relat Disord. 2012;18(Suppl 1):S114–9.
28. Levinger I, Duque G. Sarcopenia: innovation and challenges. JAMDA. 22(4):728–30.

Integrating Palliative Care into Long-Term Care

Peter Winn

Introduction

Practitioners in post-acute and long-term care (LTC) are challenged in caring for an ever-increasing number of persons who face serious and life-limiting illness due to multiple chronic conditions (multimorbidities) and who reside either at home or in a LTC setting (i.e., nursing facility, SNF, assisted living or residential care). The Center to Advance Palliative Care (CAPC) has reported that up to 80% of residents in nursing facilities could benefit from palliative care. As many facilities lack on-site access to a specialist palliative care consultation service, it is essential that practitioner's acquire competency to integrate palliative care into daily practice. In addition, practitioners must acquire skills (cultural competency) to effectively communicate and interact with *both* patients' families *and* health care workers of different cultures and diversity [1]. A well-referenced editorial by Kristler, Sloane, and Zimmerman [2] stresses that core areas of palliative care that challenge practitioners, patients, and families include: *advance care planning* (prognostication and values clarification, through both family-centered and patient-centered decision making); *symptom management;* and *psychosocial support.*

Irrespective of a patient's non-cancer or cancer prognosis, palliative care can supplement traditional medical care, such that disease-modifying treatments are not necessarily abandoned if congruent with patients' values, preferences, and goals of care and *goals of "life."* Such "total care" must be safe, effective, patient-centered, timely, efficient, and equitable, all consistent with the six aims of the Institute of Medicine 2001 report to improve health care in the United States. The overarching goal of care in nursing facilities is to provide residents with treatment and services

P. Winn (✉)
Department of Family and Preventive Medicine, University of Oklahoma, College of Medicine, Oklahoma City, OK, USA

© The Author(s), under exclusive license to Springer Nature Switzerland AG 2023
P. Winn et al. (eds.), *Post-Acute and Long-Term Care Medicine*, Current Clinical Practice, https://doi.org/10.1007/978-3-031-28628-5_11

to attain and maintain the highest practical physical, mental, and psychosocial well-being and functioning despite the resident's medical condition and normal aging process. As such all residents in PA and LTC can benefit from integration of palliative care into practitioner practice. F-Tags 684, 697, 849, and 744 of the State Operations Manual provides guidance to State surveyors (as well as practitioners!) as to the provision of care to all residents, including those approaching end-of-life or receiving hospice services. This encompasses the recognition and management of pain, non-pain symptoms, and the behavioral and psychologic symptoms of dementia, all essential to provision of effective and holistic palliative care to residents.

- F-Tag 684, Quality of Care: Relates to Hospice Care, Palliative Care, and the Terminally ill
- F-Tag 697, Pain Management
- F-Tag 849, Hospice Services
- F-Tag 744, Care of residents with dementia
- F-Tag 757, Unnecessary Drug Use

The provision of palliative care in Post-Acute and Long-Term Care Medicine aligns with the Centers for Medicare and Medicaid Services (CMS) Quadruple Aim: to *improve the health* of *patient populations,* in this case, the PA and LTC resident population we serve; to enhance patient and patients *family experience* and *satisfaction*; to *reduce health care costs* (for example by reducing ER transfers from LTC to the hospital and hospital admissions); and to *improve job satisfaction* (among LTC health care workers and providers).

This chapter will focus on the following:

- Principles of palliative care in post-acute and long-term care
- Illness trajectories and prognostication for those who have serious and life-limiting illness.
- Pain and non-pain symptom management
- Hospice eligibility guidelines
- Palliative care during the last days and weeks of life

Guiding Principles of Palliative Care

Irrespective of the age of a patient, the clinical setting, place of resident care, or whether a person is suffering from a serious chronic acute or life-limiting illness, the *core principles of palliative care* are to:

- Reduce the symptom burden from pain and other distressful symptoms, to include the relief of suffering.
- Recognize and address the physical, psycho-emotional, social and spiritual/existential needs, and dimensions of pain and other symptoms experienced by *both* the *patient and family*.
- Provide medical treatment that is goal-congruent with the wishes, values, preferences, beliefs, culture, and concerns of the patient and family (advance care planning).

- Promote care that is both interdisciplinary and multidisciplinary.
- Assist the patient, family, facility staff, *and* practitioners with health care ethical and legal issues.

Practitioners must be committed to the highest quality (palliative) care that is both timely and comprehensive. To do so, requires regular clinical assessment, diagnosis, care planning, interventions, and monitoring the patient's response to these interventions while recognizing the natural trajectory of the disease. Practitioners must anticipate and prevent/alleviate distressful symptoms and suffering. Care should be *patient-centered* and *family-focused*. All practitioners and health care providers are challenged on many levels to provide seamless transitions in care between institutional, ER/hospital, and home care settings. Effective communication skills are essential.

For the patient and family, the primary goals of palliative care include:

- To strive for the highest practical quality of life, despite late stage illness.
- To be in control (autonomy) and to maintain one's dignity.
- To relieve distressful symptoms and suffering (social, spiritual, existential).
- To alleviate family burden (can be psycho-emotional, financial, practical).
- And to mend estranged relationships, if possible.

In LTC Medicine, the goals of palliative care are similar whether patients are at end-of-life on hospice or not. Medical care should be delivered in accordance within the ethical principles of heath care, its legal framework (State and Federal), the practitioner's scope of practice, and provided with cultural sensitivity and competency (see Chapters on "Ethical and Legal Issues in Post-Acute and Long-Term Care" and "Working with Families and Person-Centered Care").

Illness Trajectories and Prognostication

Irrespective of a person's place of residence, currently the leading causes of death in the United States are heart disease, cancer, stroke, lung disease, Alzheimer's, influenza and pneumonia, and kidney disease, in addition to unintentional injuries, diabetes, septicemia, and the COVID-19 pandemic of 2020–2021. These diseases commonly afflict patients/residents in the LTC continuum who can benefit from the integration of effective palliative care into their traditional medical treatment, whether it be during the early, middle, late, or terminal phase of their illness trajectory.

For persons who reside in nursing facilities, the common causes of death have been [3, 4]

- 30–60% cardiovascular (includes sudden cardiac death, myocardial infarction, heart failure, and stroke).
- 1–23% pulmonary (COPD, pneumonia, lung cancer).
- 36% Alzheimer's disease and other dementia (10% of all dementia deaths occur in nursing facilities).
- 7–9% cancer.
- 2–3% end stage renal disease.

As of June 2021, CMS had reported 657,457 total resident COVID-19 confirmed cases and 133,210 COVID-19 resident deaths in nursing facilities and 586,899 confirmed cases and 1,949 deaths among the staff of nursing facilities.

Generally, ***Illness trajectories*** that lead to death manifest in one of *four ways* [5]:

- *A **short period of rapid decline*** before death (usually a few weeks or months) often seen in cancer.
- ***Prolonged dwindling over several years***. Often seen in those afflicted with dementia or progressive frailty and debility due to neurologic disease such as Parkinson's, multiple sclerosis, and Lou Gehrig's.
- ***Progressive functional decline over 2–5 years with intermittent serious episodes of acute illness,*** often associated with multiple ER visits and hospitalizations, with only partial recovery of functional status after each episode, leading to eventual death, often seen in advanced cardiac or pulmonary disease.
- ***An acute catastrophic event leading to death within 7–14 days***. Often seen with acute stroke, myocardial infarction, respiratory or renal failure, coma, or severe gastrointestinal bleeding for which blood transfusion may have been deferred.

When patients manifest a given trajectory, practitioners should anticipate the need to "breaking bad news" and take the initiative to engage patients, caregivers, and family members in "advance care planning" that may eventually transition to "terminal care planning" as end-of-life and death approaches.

Though it is challenging to prognosticate in the chronically ill, the Flacker Mortality Score can provide a percentage probability of death in 1 year in newly admitted residents to nursing home aged 65 and older [6] while other patient characteristics (available from the MDS) can also assist in prognostication (e.g., significant weight loss, swallowing problems, BMI <22, age >88, CHF, shortness of breath, male sex). Another prognostic tool is the Palliative Prognostic Score that may predict 30-day survival [7]. Note that the presence of delirium is another significant prognostic factor.

General Indicators and Clinical Parameters of Serious Illness

General indicators and clinical parameters that can forewarn a practitioner that a patient may be at risk of death within the next 6–12 months include the following:

- Repeated ER visits and frequent hospitalizations.
- Recurrent life-threatening infections such as pneumonia, UTI, and sepsis.
- Progressive decline in residential functional status as determined by the Palliative Performance Score [8] of less than 50–70%, (see Table 1) or increasing dependency in 2 or more Basic Activities of Daily Living (i.e., BADLs).

Table 1 Symptom prevalence in advanced illness

Symptom	Cancer	Non-cancer	Cancer, AIDS, COPD, Heart and renal diseases
Fatigue	72–74%	76%	32–90%
Pain	71–74%	67%	34–96%
Lack of energy	69%		
Weakness	60%		
Appetite loss	53–70%	55%	
Breathlessness	36%	36%	60–95%
Anxiety/depression	40%	57%	

- Progressive *unavoidable weight loss*, of 5% body weight in 3 months or 10% in 6 months.
- Serum albumin less than 2.5 gm/dL.
- Presence of one or more stage 3 or 4 pressure ulcers (a.k.a. "injuries").
- *Progressive decline* in Body Mass Index to less than 22, (especially <20).
- Advanced age greater than 88.
- Severe refractory symptoms such as fatigue, shortness of breath, peripheral edema, or bowel obstruction.

A resident's emotional demeanor, and their acknowledgment and acceptance of serious illness can be an opportunity to review patient values and preferences, DNR status, any advance health care directives, the presence or not of a power of attorney or guardian for health care decisions and financial matters, and the ability to communicate an informed choice (i.e., informed consent). In addition, it is important to:

- Determine the patient's and/or surrogate decision maker's current (and past) decision-making capacity as to healthcare, practical and financial matters.
- Acknowledge how patient culture, ethnicity, and religious/spiritual beliefs can impact values, preferences, and choice of desired treatments, *including no treatment.*
- Be aware that educational level and medical literacy can impact patient, caregiver, and family understanding and lead to misunderstanding.
- Obtain and review any advanced health care directives (e.g., "Living Will"), directive to physicians, power of attorney (whether durable or not), guardianship, and their limitations, if any.
- Remember such documents are often state-specific and may not be applicable to State law where the patient now resides.
- Inquire as to any previously written or orally expressed patient wishes.
- Remember the ethical principles of health care; *autonomy* (the right to patient self-determination); *beneficence* (the duty to do good); *nonmaleficence* (to avoid harm); *justice (to treat fairly, equally, and equitably)*; and *fidelity,* the duty of practitioners to be truthful, to support patient dignity, and to not abandon patients.

Symptom Assessment and Management

In persons with advanced illness, appropriate assessment is often challenging due to a patient's cognitive impairment, fatigue, and multimorbidities. Non-pain symptoms are prevalent, often greater than pain, even in persons diagnosed with cancer (see Table 2). For *any symptom* experienced by patients, a quasi-stepped approach can enable practitioners to intervene in a timely and effective manner.

First, recognize the presence of each symptom, then proceed to:

- Establish its intensity, temporal pattern, any exacerbating/relieving factors, location, and effect on function and cognition.
- Determine whether the symptom is acute, chronic, or intermittent.
- Identify any associated symptoms.
- Assess its impact on quality of life, ADLs, cognition, decisional capacity, sleep, mood, and dignity.
- Review previous and current treatment for the symptom.
- Perform an appropriate, timely, and *symptom-focused* physical exam.
- Ascertain, if possible, the likely pathophysiology underlying the symptom.
- Consider whether any medication could be causing or aggravating the symptom.
- Identify potentially reversible causes.
- If necessary, use the least invasive diagnostic testing, if any, to minimize patient pain, discomfort, or suffering.
- Given the above steps determine the most likely diagnosis, (if possible).

Table 2 Symptom assessment scales

Symptom	Assessment scales to consider
Anorexia	Functional Assessment Anorexia/Cachexia Therapy Scale
Anxiety	Hamilton Anxiety Rating Scale (HAM-A)
Cognition	Folstein MMSE, COGNISTAT, MOCA
Constipation	Modified Constipation Assessment Scale, Patient Assessment of Constipation Tool
Delirium	Confusion Assessment Method (CAM), Delirium Rating Scale
Depression	Beck Depression Inventory, Short Form Geriatric Depression Scale, Zung Depression Scale, Cornell Scale for Depression in Dementia, CES-D Boston Short Form
Dyspnea	Numerical Analog Scale (i.e., 0–10) Visual Analog Scale (VAS)
Fatigue	NAS, VAS, Fatigue Symptom Inventory
Nausea	VAS
Pain	Numerical Analog Scales (NAS), Visual Analog Scales (VAS), Verbal Descriptive Scale, Wong-Baker FACE Scale, FLACC Scale, Brief Pain Inventory (BPI), PAINAD
Spiritual pain	FICA Spiritual Assessment Tool, Herth Hope Index

RESOURCES: City of Hope Pain and Palliative Care Resource Center. http://www.cityofhope.org/prc. UNIPAC Series. American Academy of Hospice and Palliative Medicine. Fifth Edition. 2017

- Always evaluate for the presence of any psycho-emotional, spiritual, social, or practical factors that are contributing to the symptom.
- Initiate palliative **and** traditional treatment based upon the primary illness, phase of illness, prognosis, comorbidities, and patient/family preferences for care and care setting.
- Consider complementary and alternative therapies especially if requested by patients and families.

Any symptom can be complex and multifaceted, thus an *interdisciplinary* and *transdisciplinary* approach and treatment plan is more likely to be successful. Consider nonpharmacologic and practical interventions in an attempt to alleviate each symptom, i.e., change in body position, room temperature or ventilation, patient/ family, and staff education. Foremost consider timely pharmacologic treatment to palliate the distressful symptom. Finally, consider any medical and/or pharmacologic treatments directed at the *underlying cause of the symptom* (if known). The response to treatment and its outcomes, benefits, and burdens must be carefully balanced and the treatment adjusted accordingly, acknowledging that the *goals of care can change over time* as advanced care planning transitions to *terminal care planning*.

Keep in mind that interventions to relieve distressful symptoms can lead to unintended consequences (concept of *double effect*). For example, the use of opioids to treat pain can result in constipation and/or nausea, which in turn must be anticipated and addressed. Often, it is reasonable to continue the first-line treatment while initiating another treatment to alleviate the first is adverse effects. In the rare case of severe and intractable symptoms, including intolerable existential or psychological distress, the use of *palliative sedation* may be a consideration (NHPCO position statement 2010) [9], which states its use is "For the limited number of *imminently dying* patients who have pain and suffering that is **a)** unresponsive to other palliative interventions less suppressive of consciousness and **b)** intolerable to the patient………… palliative sedation is an important option to be considered by health care providers, patients and families."

At the practitioner and systems level, use of uni- or multidimensional tools may be helpful to assess a variety of symptoms (refer to Table 3) dependent upon ease of use and evidence-based palliative care. The Edmonton Symptom Assessment Survey (ESAS) is a scale that assesses for the presence and intensity of multiple symptoms and its score followed over time.

Several reviews have more thoroughly detailed the management of pain and other symptoms that occur in patients with advanced illness who reside in long-term care facilities [10, 11] and in general practice [12]. Other excellent resources include the "UNIPAC" Series, a publication of the American Academy of Hospice and Palliative Medicine, Fast Facts and Concepts (available at the Center to Advance Palliative Care website), the American Medical Directors Association Clinical Practice Guideline (CPG) on "Pain Management in the Long-Term Care Setting" and its respective CPG implementation manual, and the Palliative Care Formulary [13]. It should be noted that some medications are used "off-label" to palliate symptoms (i.e., not FDA-approved of the treatment of these symptoms), so practitioners should exercise due diligence and precaution when prescribing them.

Table 3 Major mechanisms of nausea/vomiting

Cause	Pharmacologic management
• Cortical:	
– tumor, increased intracranial pressure	Dexamethasone
– anxiety, situational stressors	Benzodiazepine
– pain response	Opioid, other pain medication/adjuvants
• Vestibular:	
	Meclizine
	Scopolamine
	Dimenhydrinate
• Chemoreceptor Trigger Zone:	
– medications	Decrease dose or discontinue, if possible
– metabolic (e.g., kidney/liver failure)	Haloperidol, olanzapine
– hyponatremia	Sodium chloride, demeclocycline
– hypercalcemia	Bisphosphonate, dexamethasone
• Gastrointestinal:	
– drug related	Stop drug, consider PPI
– tumor	Promethazine, metoclopramide, octreotide
– constipation	Bowel regimen
– cough-induced	Opioid, anticholinergic

Adapted from UNIPAC Four, 5th Edition, 2017, AAHPM

Anorexia/Cachexia

Anorexia is defined as a lack of appetite that may be associated with cachexia; the latter a catabolic state characterized by severe muscle loss with or without loss of adipose tissue. Either can occur during the late stages of advanced severe progressive illness.

Management Includes the Following:
- Assess for anorexigenic effects of medications such as chemotherapeutic drugs, antidepressants, NSAIDs, opioids.
- Evaluate whether either could be caused by or related to other symptoms such as nausea, constipation, or poorly controlled pain.
- Assess for any potentially reversible medical condition(s) such as a rectal fecal impaction, urinary retention, oral candidiasis, or other gastrointestinal causes such as GER, gastritis, or gastroparesis.
- Initiate practical interventions: small, frequent meals; administer medications separate from or with meals; encourage good oral care; try a variety of foods; improve the social and environmental aspects of eating.

Consider an Appetite Stimulant Such As:
- A corticosteroid: prednisone 5–20 mg/d; dexamethasone 4–8 mg/d.
- A progestin: megestrol, a maximum of 400–800 mg/d or less (trial 4–8 weeks).

- If anorexia is concomitant with depression, it may be reasonable to prescribe mirtazapine as an appetite stimulant (FDA off-label) and mood enhancer that may also improve sleep, recommended it be given at bedtime.

Note that the appetite stimulant effect of a corticosteroid often decreases after several weeks. Megestrol can cause lower limb edema and increase the risk of thrombophlebitis and thromboembolism. Consider oral nutritional supplements, though decreased appetite at meals may occur as a result of their use. If used, it is preferable to use nutritional supplements that are lactose free, especially in the elderly or African Americans who have a higher prevalence of lactose intolerance. There is insufficient evidence to recommend the use of cannabinoids (dronabinol), cyproheptadine, an androgenic steroid (oxandrolone), or thalidomide, though a therapeutic trial may be considered if refractory anorexia. A patient's advance directive for health care may either *request* or *preclude* artificially administered nutrition and hydration.

Dyspnea

Dyspnea is defined as discomfort in breathing that includes the sensation of breathlessness, shortness of breath, or an increased work of breathing. Often it is **not** associated with tachypnea or hypoxemia. Its assessment and management include the following:

- Rating of dyspnea is subjective and can be based on patient self-report and assessed on a numerical scale of 0–10.
- Initiate practical interventions such as the use of a fan to improve air circulation, ensure a comfortable ambient room temperature, eliminate respiratory irritants and strong odors such as perfumes, frequently reposition the person, encourage purse-lip breathing.
- Assess for potentially reversible causes, such as pneumonia, pleural effusion, pulmonary embolus, heart failure, anemia, bronchospasm.
- Recognize any associated symptoms such as cough, possible aspiration, excessive respiratory secretions, anxiety, social or financial concerns, and spiritual suffering.
- *First-line pharmacotherapy for palliation of dyspnea is an immediate-release opioid* administered every 3–4 h. For mild dyspnea and to minimize the risk of respiratory depression in an *opioid-naïve* patient, start with morphine sulfate 2.5–5 mg PO or the oral morphine equivalent (OME) of another opioid, (refer to OME interconversion Table 12 later in this chapter). Titrate the opioid dose upward 25–50% every 12–24 h to attain sufficient relief of dyspnea. Note that an *opioid-tolerant* patient is one who has been taking a consecutive oral daily MME (morphine milligram equivalent) of 60 mg or more for 7–10 days.
- For excessive oral or respiratory secretions consider hyoscyamine PO/SL; glycopyrrolate PO; atropine ophthalmic solution SL; scopolamine solution SL; or a

scopolamine patch every 3 days. To loosen thick respiratory secretions, consider guaifenesin.
- Optimize medical treatment of the primary respiratory or cardiac condition (i.e., COPD, heart failure).
- Consider prescribing a **low dose** benzodiazepine, preferably lorazepam given as either a tablet or sublingual concentrate for breakthrough or refractory dyspnea as anxiety can be a major contributing factor.
- Always gauge any medical treatment based upon its benefits versus burdens, phase of illness, prognosis, patient preferences, and advance health care directives.
- Remember that patients with dyspnea often do better with a *scheduled* dose of an opioid (and a benzodiazepine) rather than administered as needed (PRN) dosing. Opioids are effective in treating dyspnea in patients with COPD, though may be less effective relieving dyspnea in patients with cancer or heart failure. There is poor evidence as to the effectiveness of nebulized opioids, though it may warrant a therapeutic trial in refractory dyspnea. Though the use of oxygen may reverse hypoxemia, dyspnea may not improve. Be aware of the potential for oxygen therapy to cause hypercapnia and subsequent obtundation or respiratory arrest. When using an opioid for dyspnea it is prudent to aim for a respiratory rate between 14 and 20.
- Initiation or continuation of noninvasive ventilator (NIV) support as well as CPAP or BiPAP may be warranted under special patient circumstances in late stage COPD or ALS, though its associated physical discomfort and its hindrance to patients in communicating with family may preclude their use.

Not infrequently the family may request the use of oxygen for non-hypoxemic dyspnea. While there is no evidence to support this, at times it may alleviate either the discomfort of breathing that patients experience or the emotional distress that families may endure who observe breathlessness in their family member.

Nausea and Vomiting

The most rational approach to managing nausea and/or vomiting is to understand the four main pathophysiologic mechanisms and the neurotransmitters that mediate the emetic reflex in the brain (refer to Table 3). This will allow for a more effective choice of antiemetic drugs (i.e., antihistaminic, anticholinergic, antiserotonergic, antidopaminergic).

Management of Nausea/Vomiting Includes:
- Determine whether any medications are emetogenic such as chemotherapeutic agents, some antibiotics, bowel stimulants, opioids, NSAIDs.
- Identify potentially reversible causes such as GER, gastroparesis, constipation, rectal impaction, bowel obstruction, adynamic ileus, urinary retention, and UTI.
- Consider emotional and spiritual factors, including *anticipatory anxiety* that can occur prior to medical treatment.

- Initiate practical, nonpharmacologic interventions such as offering smaller, more frequent meals of blander food, relaxation techniques, appropriate body positioning when eating or while being fed, and attention both during and after PEG tube feeding.
- Prescribe pharmacologic treatment based on the major cause(s) of nausea/vomiting (refer to Table 3).

Combination pharmacotherapy (based on each medication's different antiemetic pharmacologic mechanism and neurotransmitter system) may be necessary especially when nausea/vomiting has multiple etiologies or is refractory. Note that dexamethasone, metoclopramide, and low dose antipsychotics also have central antiemetic effects. Be aware of the potential side effects of serotonin receptor antagonists such as ondansetron (headache, constipation, fatigue, xerostomia) and of anticholinergics and antihistamines (drowsiness, fatigue, confusion, dry mouth, constipation, urinary retention, blurred vision). Metoclopramide can cause extrapyramidal syndrome, dystonia, and tardive dyskinesia. Low dose haloperidol (0.5–2 mg) or olanzapine (2.5–7.5 mg) may be useful in alleviating nausea/vomiting.

Dronabinol can have an antiemetic effect though poor evidence of efficacy (start at 2.5 mg twice a day to a maximum of 20 mg/day). Though FDA approved for refractory chemo-related nausea/vomiting, practitioners may consider its off-label use yet must be prudent when prescribed in the elderly. High cost may preclude its use. Common adverse effects include somnolence, asthenia, paranoia, delirium, nausea, and vomiting. Opioid-induced nausea/vomiting may require either a dose reduction of the opioid or rotation to another opioid.

Constipation

Many patients who reside in a long-term care setting experience constipation, especially when terminally ill. Constipation can occur because of a combination of poor fluid intake, low dietary fiber, impaired mobility, as well as constipating drugs such as opioids, anticholinergics, iron, calcium preparations, and antihypertensive especially calcium channel blockers, diuretics and clonidine.

Management of Constipation Includes the Following:
- *Prevention* is paramount.
- Identify potentially reversible causes, including medication-induced and medical conditions such as a rectal fecal impaction; metabolic disturbances (hypercalcemia, hypothyroidism); GI causes (always consider if intestinal obstruction could be present); and neurologic causes (such as nerve root or spinal cord compression or, for example, visceral neuropathy that can occur in Parkinson's disease).
- Identify life-threatening causes such as malignant bowel obstruction or narcotic bowel syndrome.

Table 4 Stepwise regimen to prevent and treat constipation

"The Sixth Vital Sign"		
1. Begin with:	Senna with/without docusate	1–2 tabs/cap qd-bid
2. Titrate up to:	Senna	3–4 tabs bid
3. If needed *add*:	Sorbitol or lactulose or polyethylene glycol	30 cc qd-bid 17 g in 8 oz water qd-bid
4. Consider, *in addition*:	Glycerin rectal suppository with/without bisacodyl rectal suppository	scheduled qd -qod
5. If needed:	Mineral oil or soap suds enema	
6. If rectal impaction:	May need digital dis-impaction	

- Practical interventions include making toilets accessible, establishing a bowel routine, and encouraging increased fluid intake (if tolerated).
- Reduce the anticholinergic load of medications if possible.
- Establish an individualized bowel regimen according to each laxative's mechanism of action (refer to Table 4). Combination therapy is often required.
- Monitor for side effects of laxatives, which can include bloating, cramping, nausea/vomiting, and diarrhea.
- Bulk-forming laxatives are usually *not* recommended because they can exacerbate constipation in underhydrated and less mobile patients and often cause or worsen bloating, nausea, or vomiting.

Foremost remember to anticipate and prevent opioid-induced constipation, and second, *as the dose of the opioid is increased, so must the laxative regimen also be increased*. Stimulant laxatives such as senna are most effective for opioid-induced constipation. In severe constipation, consider oral lubiprostone or methylnaltrexone sc, though expensive.

Stool softeners are considered to have poor effectiveness but can be prescribed in some patients when initiating their bowel regimen, i.e., the "laxative ladder" (Table 4). Remember that some patients may also require a rectally administered lubricating agent (glycerin suppository) and/or stimulant (bisacodyl) to ensure defecation in addition to oral agents. Always consider the possible presence of a rectal fecal impaction. Note that a rectal fecal impaction can cause "paradoxical" diarrhea or urinary retention, either of which may not be evident on patient history, symptoms, or exam. This may require urinary bladder cauterization and manual dis-impaction, though PEG solution administered orally may be effective.

Delirium

Delirium is an acute confusional state that is characterized by a fluctuating course during the day/night, inattention, and disorganized thinking and speech. Delirium can be hyperactive, hypoactive, or mixed. A good caveat is to remember that any acute illness or any medication, regardless of when it was started, can precipitate delirium especially in those with advanced illness. Remember that even a gradual dose reduction or discontinuing an opioid, benzodiazepine, or alcohol can precipitate delirium.

Management of Delirium in Patients with Advanced, Serious Illness Includes the Following:

- Identify potential reversible causes, especially whether it may be medication-induced.
- Discontinue nonessential medications and reduce anticholinergic load.
- Initiate practical interventions: familiarize the patient to the environment, improve sleep and the sleep-wake cycle, reduce environmental stimuli, and optimize hearing and eyesight (i.e., hearing aids "in," eyeglasses "on"), and adequate hydration.
- Reduce immobility by removing/minimizing use of any physical restraints, including a Foley catheter, if possible.
- Determine whether pain could be contributing to the delirium, and if so, treat it appropriately.
- If delirium persists, consider as first-line medication therapy low-dose haloperidol (no more than 2–3 mg total/day), often in divided doses. Start low and go slow.
- Second-line medication may include a low-dose benzodiazepine, usually lorazepam 0.5–1 mg PO/SL every 6–8 h, more frequent if necessary; or valproic acid 125–250 mg every 6–8 to 12 h, the latter upon awaking in the morning and at bedtime, with a possible noontime or early afternoon dose.

Remember that even opioids and steroids can cause delirium. Also, haloperidol and lorazepam can cause paradoxical agitation or restlessness in which case their dose should be decreased (not increased!) or discontinued. It is not uncommon to use a combination of haloperidol and lorazepam to treat delirium. Be aware that **patients with dementia** are more sensitive to the adverse effects of antipsychotic medications that includes sedation and EPS, and that antipsychotics have a "black box" warning as they have been associated with an increased risk of sudden death and cerebrovascular events. Communication with the patient and their family about these risks and benefits must occur. Overall, judicious medication management as well as social, environmental, and practical interventions must all be implemented in an attempt to prevent and treat delirium. For further information, refer to the Chapter on "Dementia, Delirium, and Depression".

Fatigue/Weakness/Lack of Energy

These symptoms commonly occur in patients with advanced illness and will worsen during the last 6 months of life for patients whether on hospice or not. As discussed in previous sections, it is important to consider the adverse effects of medication as a contributing factor, to elucidate any associated clinical signs and symptoms, and to treat potentially reversible conditions. These symptoms often present with increasing daytime sleepiness/sleep with the patient eventually becoming bed ridden.

Fatigue can occur as a consequence of a patient's **primary** disease or secondary to other causes [5]. The pathophysiology of primary fatigue, though not well understood, may be a consequence of dysfunction of the reticular formation, the effects of proinflammatory cytokines, deregulation of the hypothalamic-pituitary-adrenal axis, and alteration of skeletal muscle metabolism. While **secondary** fatigue can be multifactorial and caused by anemia, infection/fever, dehydration/electrolyte imbalance, undiagnosed hypothyroidism or vitamin D and/or B12 deficiency, an untreated or unrecognized mood disorder/depression, poor sleep, inadequately treated chronic pain, side effects of medication including benzodiazepine and opioids, and unintended though anticipated adverse effects of disease-focused treatments such as chemotherapy and radiation. Whether primary or secondary fatigue, practitioners must balance each treatment/intervention's potential benefit versus risk burden.

Nonpharmacologic and Practical Considerations:
- Provide realistic prognostication and education to patient and family that these symptoms are in keeping with expected course in the advanced/terminal phase of his/her illness.
- Encourage the patient to better conserve energy by pacing activities and limiting social/family visits if contributing to their exhaustion, be it physical, emotional, and/or spiritual/religious.
- Consider psychosocial interventions or therapy.
- Encourage good sleep hygiene, nutrition, and pain control.
- Consider short-term physical therapy to improve safety of transfers and ambulation and to lessen fall risk.

Palliative Pharmacotherapy Considerations:
Once reversible etiologies of fatigue have been ruled out consider methylphenidate or modafinil, though the majority of trials have demonstrated little or no efficacy. However, under certain situations a trial may be reasonable, but with careful monitoring as to potential side effects.

- Methylphenidate: Start with low dose of 2.5 mg twice daily to be administered in the early and late morning; if tolerated, may increase to 5 mg twice daily, but not a higher dose (author's recommendation). Discontinue if no improvement in 1–2 weeks. Prudent use is advised in patients with heart disease or hypertension.
- Modafinil: Limited research: Expensive so unlikely to have costs covered by hospice.
- Corticosteroids: Consider prednisone 5–10 mg/day or dexamethasone 8–12 mg/day, the latter in divided doses. Beware that steroids can cause confusion and precipitate delirium, especially in the elderly and those with serious illness.
- Consider caffeinated beverages.

Depression/Anxiety

At end-of-life patients often suffer from anxiety and depression attributable to psychiatric, psychological, and spiritual or religious distress. These symptoms are thoroughly discussed in UNIPAC 2 published by the American Academy of Hospice and Palliative Medicine (AAHPM) [14]. While the use of anxiolytics and antidepressants is well known to practitioners this will not be discussed in this review. However, several factors can contribute to anxiety and depression. These include patient burden of non-pain and pain symptoms, loss of connectedness to family and community, loss of dignity, striving to find meaning (or not) to one's life, and leaving a legacy (or not), being forgiven (or not) by family and others. Palliative care must aim to balance a sense of hope *("hope for the best")* while helping the patient and family to transition through the last months, weeks, and days of life *("prepare for the worst").*

Practical Considerations:
- Provide empathic listening and supportive counseling to patient, family, and caregivers. It is the responsibility of all members of the interdisciplinary team to do so, including volunteers, practitioners, and at times the patient's community religious or spiritual leader.
- It is imperative to address the severity of depression and any suicidal ideation, as well as patient's access to means to commit suicide (or homicide) and to remove accessibility to these means. Psychiatric consultation, possibly inpatient evaluation, may be necessary.
- Encourage patient life review, the meaning of life and the search for meaning in dying.
- Facilitate social interaction and if tolerated, engage in recreational and distracting activities that provide individual patient meaning and satisfaction to every day.
- Consider holistic interventions such as guided imagery, aromatherapy, massage, sand therapy, and Dignity Therapy.
- Support family and caregivers in adopting positive coping skills.

For further information on the assessment and treatment of anxiety and depression in post-acute and long-term care, refer to the Chapter on "Dementia, Delirium, and Depression". It is important for practitioners to understand that depression can manifest differently in residents who face serious and life-limiting illness than residents who do not, so their assessment and treatment can differ for residents who have a greater life expectancy. For example, residents with a prognosis of less than 6 months to live may have a desire for hastened death due to overwhelming feelings of despair, hopelessness, and worthlessness and spiritual and existential distress. Though antidepressants such as an SSRI may be appropriate in residents with a longer life expectancy, psychostimulants may be preferred as first-line treatment for depression in patients with a prognosis of less than 6 months to live. Note that caution must be used to tapper the dose of most SSRI antidepressants (no need to taper fluoxetine due to its long half-life) when being discontinued in order to prevent a **discontinuation syndrome** (most likely to occur when discontinuing paroxetine due to its short half-life). The need to discontinue an SSRI is likely to occur when a resident is no longer able to swallow at end-of-life. As such the emergence of this syndrome should be anticipated. The discontinuation syndrome is characterized by signs and symptoms of headache, malaise, flu-like symptoms, agitation, restlessness, irritability, anxiety, and insomnia. An excellent palliative care resource on the assessment and treatment of depression and anxiety is UNIPAC 2 on Psychiatric, Psychological and Spiritual Care published by the American Academy of Hospice and Palliative Medicine (AAHPM) [14].

Pain Management

Effective pain management is essential to providing high quality palliative care in post-acute and LTC given the high prevalence of painful medical conditions in this patient population. The goals of pain control include:

- To relieve pain.
- To alleviate suffering.
- To prevent/minimize disability.
- To optimize function.
- To preserve decision-making capacity.

Practitioners need to assess every patient for the presence of pain and "total pain"; that is, the physical, psycho-emotional, social, and spiritual aspects of pain and how each can affect the other. Successful pain management entails proper evaluation and implementation of interventions that address each component of a patient's total pain. As with any distressful symptom, pain is more optimally managed if its cause and pathophysiologic mechanisms can be determined, together with an interdisciplinary approach and use of multiple treatment modalities, both nonpharmacologic and pharmacologic. The AMDA Clinical Practice Guideline on pain management [15] and its more recent pocket guide [16] and *Geriatrics at Your Fingertips* [17] published by the American Geriatrics Society are excellent resources that provide more in depth content than permits in this chapter. Also, the AGS guidelines on the pharmacologic management of persistent pain in older persons is a classic and noteworthy resource [18].

Key Components to the *Recognition and Assessment* of Pain Include the Following:
- If possible, **prevent** the occurrence of pain or a painful condition. For example, advanced osteoarthritis of one knee may result in contralateral hip pain: a total knee arthroplasty may prevent the latter happening. Another example is prophylactically prescribing an anti-inflammatory and analgesic in addition to an anti-viral in an attempt to prevent the occurrence of postherpetic neuralgia.

- **Anticipate** the occurrence of pain. For example, postsurgical incision pain; the pain associated with the occurrence of peripheral neuropathy in diabetics; or the onset of bone pain in cancer patients with known bone metastases.
- Identify the **presence** of pain or a painful condition. Remember to assess for nonverbal cues of pain such as guarding on movement or on transfers, rubbing and grimacing, and behaviors such as agitation, restlessness, withdrawn behavior, and sleeping poorly.
- Establish the pain's location, intensity, temporal pattern, any exacerbating and relieving factors and effect on (loss of) function and cognition. Consider using a pain assessment scale. Most can be converted to a scale of 1–10.
- Determine whether the pain is acute, chronic (duration of 1 month or more), new onset, intermittent, incidental (i.e., related to movement), breakthrough pain, and whether there are multiple causes and types of pain.
- Try to determine whether the pain is **nociceptive** (either somatic or visceral), **neuropathic,** or **inflammatory**, as suggested by the patient's description of the pain (see Table 5).
- Identify any associated signs and/or symptoms such as headache, dizziness, nausea/vomiting, constipation, decreased urination, a swollen joint, or painful extremity.
- Review any previous and current pharmacologic and nonpharmacologic treatments and their effectiveness, as well as any complementary and alternative medicine therapy.
- Assess **"total pain"** by elucidating any psycho-emotional, social, and spiritual dimensions to the physical pain, as well as the person's cultural beliefs as to the meaning of pain and his/her manner of expressing pain.
- Perform a **focused physical exam**, with particular attention to those body regions or organs systems that appear to be related to or contributing to the pain.
- Assess the need for diagnostic testing, if likely to be helpful in determining a diagnosis, always consider the pain or discomfort these tests may cause.
- Finally, determine the probable cause of the pain. Remember persons may have multiple and different types of pain. Always evaluate for potentially reversible causes of pain. For example, abdominal pain may be due to urinary retention, con-

Table 5 Classification of pain

Type of pain	Descriptors
Nociceptive	
• Somatic pain:	Sharp, tender
• Visceral pain:	Dull, cramping
• Bone pain:	Throbbing, aching
Neuropathic	Burning, tingling, stabbing shooting
Inflammatory	E.g., pleuritic, abdominal rebound, inflamed joints

Adapted from Von Roenn JH et al. Current Diagnosis and Treatment of Pain, Lange Series, McGraw Hill 2006

stipation, a rectal/fecal impaction, or caused by medication such as a bowel stimulant or bulk forming laxative. Prescribing an opioid analgesic in such a circumstance would be considered inappropriate and could result in harm to the patient.

- Remember that conditions such as bladder spasms, contractures, improper positioning, pressure ulcers, muscle strain, oral thrush, urinary retention, fecal impaction, or DVT can all cause pain.

Key Components to the *Treatment* of Pain Include the Following:

- Consider treatment options taking into account the patient's health status, prognosis, and known advance directives for health care. Conduct a thorough discussion to support informed choice (i.e., informed consent) by the patient and family or proxy decision maker.
- Establish an interdisciplinary treatment plan, part of which will be determined by the disciplines involved at the patient's care setting (i.e., nursing facility, SNF, residential/assisted living, home or hospital, and possibly hospice).
- Set goals for pain relief. For example, the desired or acceptable intensity of pain that can enable the achievement of positive functional outcomes in self-care, participation in desired personal and recreational activities, improved sleep, mood, and cognition. Also, it is important to assess whether a certain level of sedation would be acceptable to both patient and family in order to achieve effective pain control.

In up to 90% of persons with pain, practitioners can adequately control pain with orally administered medication guided by the World Health Organization (WHO) three-stepped analgesic ladder (see Table 6). The WHO recommends administering analgesic and co-analgesic (i.e., adjuvant) medication as follows:

- *By mouth:* Whenever possible, prescribe an oral analgesic. Avoid IM injections as they can be painful; subcutaneous injections are less painful and may not be practical in some care settings. Opioids in a concentrated liquid form can be administered sublingually or transbuccally.
- *Around-the-clock:* Prescribe scheduled dosing for continuous and persistent pain to minimize break through pain and choose an appropriate analgesic and dose for breakthrough pain.

Table 6 The WHO three-Step analgesic ladder

Step		3. Severe
	2. Moderate	Morphine
1. Mild	A/Codeine	Hydromorphone
ASA	A/Hydrocodone	Methadone
Acetaminophen	A/Oxycodone	Levorphanol
NSAIDs	A/Dihydrocodeine	Fentanyl
	Tramadol/apap	Oxycodone
±Adjuvants	±Adjuvants	±Adjuvants

Adapted from: Technical Report Series 804: Geneva WHO.1990

- *According to the ladder:* The initial choice of an analgesic and use of adjuvants is based on the severity of the pain. Using a numerical pain scale, 1 through 3 can be considered **mild** pain; 4 through 6 **moderate** pain; 7 through 9 **severe** pain, and 10 **excruciating pain**.
- *Adapted to the individual:* The choice of analgesic should be based upon the patient's condition, comorbidities (such as liver and kidney disease and coexistent dementia or delirium), drug safety and toxicity profile, ease of administration, and goals of both pain relief and the desired outcome in treating the pain.
- *With attention to detail:* ensure optimal dosing: Consider drug pharmacokinetics and pharmacodynamics, make appropriate dose adjustments in timely manner, and always monitor for potential benefit versus harm and adverse effects.

Optimal pain management also entails the choice of the most appropriate analgesic(s) based upon the patient's primary and comorbid diagnoses, the pathophysiologic mechanism underlying the type of pain (see Table 7), pain severity, diagnosis, the potential adverse effects of each medication and nonpharmacologic treatment, and the patient's individual characteristics that can alter a drug's metabolism, pharmacokinetics, and pharmacodynamics.

Caveats to Effective Pain Management Include:
- In most patients, prescribe at least one analgesic as scheduled, i.e., administered routinely, rather than just as needed (i.e., PRN).
- Choose an appropriate analgesic and dose for breakthrough pain.
- Remember that most types of pain respond, at least partially, to an opioid.
- The maximum recommended dose of acetaminophen is 3000–4000 mg/day, but 2000 mg/day may be prudent if either renal or hepatic insufficiency are present, and in older adults.
- Use caution when prescribing an opioid/acetaminophen combination drug as the ceiling dose of the acetaminophen may be reached before pain is adequately controlled by the opioid component.
- The maximum dose of tramadol is 300 mg/24 h; it may precipitate confusion, seizures, and serotonin syndrome. A lower daily dose should be prescribed in older adults.
- Conventional nonselective NSAIDs (e.g., ibuprofen, naproxen) should only be prescribed short term, that is days to no more than 3–4 weeks; precautions

Table 7 Select first and second line analgesics based on type of pain

Type of pain	Consider	
	First line	Second line
Nociceptive Pain:	WHO Step 1 or 2 drug	WHO Step 3 drug
Neuropathic Pain:	TCAs, anticonvulsants	WHO Step 2 or 3 drug
Bone Pain:	NSAIDs, corticosteroids	WHO Step 2 or 3 drug
Intracranial Pain:	Corticosteroids	WHO Step 2 or 3 drug
Visceral Pain:	Anticholinergic, opioid	Steroids, opioids

Source: UNIPAC Three. AAHPM 2017

include risk for gastrointestinal bleeding, renal impairment, platelet dysfunction, edema, increased blood pressure, and worsened heart failure.

- Long-term use of a NSAID would be appropriate when prescribed for bone pain due to cancer metastases, but may need to be discontinued during the last days of life when pills can no longer be swallowed.
- Selective COX-2 inhibitors (e.g., celecoxib) still have a significant risk of a GI bleed and renal insufficiency.
- Consider holding or discontinuing ASA chemoprophylaxis when administering a conventional or COX-2 NSAID.
- Consider prescribing a proton pump inhibitor or H-2 blocker in patients to lower the risk for a GI bleed when prescribing a NSAID.
- Never prescribe a NSAID when a patient is taking warfarin as the risk for a GI bleed is high.
- Consider a topical analgesic such as capsaicin cream, diclofenac gel, or a lidocaine patch for persons with one or two localized areas of musculoskeletal, arthritic, or neuropathic pain.
- Remember the use of the lidocaine patch is *non*continuous, to be applied for only 12 h during a 24-h period, while off the remaining 12 h, and applying no more than three patches at one time.
- Avoid use of meperidine because of its potential to cause undesirable CNS side effects such as confusion and seizures due to the accumulation of its toxic metabolite normeperidine.
- Opioid with partial agonists activity such as butorphanol, pentazocine, buprenorphine and nalbuphine are not recommended because of their analgesic ceiling effects and ability to counteract the analgesic effect of **pure agonist** opioids, which can then precipitate an opioid-withdrawal pain crisis.

Opioid Analgesics

Opioids are both appropriate and effective for the treatment of moderate to severe acute or chronic pain not relieved by other analgesics or modalities. Judicious prescribing can provide effective pain relief in patients in post-acute and LTC, with a low risk of psychologic dependency or addiction. Scheduled low doses of opioids can be very effective in the treatment of chronic pain associated with various chronic musculoskeletal conditions that often afflict the elderly. Note that physical dependency, characterized by withdrawal symptoms, can occur when regularly scheduled opioids are abruptly discontinued. The gradual dose reduction of the opioid can prevent this when being discontinued.

General Guidelines to the Use of Opioids Include:
- *For acute pain:* Start by prescribing an immediate-release (IR) opioid (see Table 8 for suggested equianalgesia **starting doses**).
- *For chronic pain:* Consider starting a low dose of a *sustained-released* opioid (LA/ER), with a sufficient dose and dosing interval of an *immediate release* of

Table 8 Suggested equianalgesic starting doses for selected oral opioids

Frail or elderly opioid-naïve patients	
The practitioner may choose from the following suggested starting doses:	
Morphine 2 mg PO or SL	0.1 cc morphine 20 mg/cc (Roxanol®)
Oxycodone liquid 2 mg PO or SL	0.1 cc oxycodone 20 mg/cc (Oxyfast®)
Oxycodone 2.5 mg	• ½ tablet 5 mg oxycodone • ½ tablet oxycodone 5 mg/acetaminophen 325 mg (Percocet ®)
Hydromorphone 0.5 mg PO	0.5 cc hydromorphone 1 mg/cc (Dilaudid®)
Hydrocodone 2.5 mg PO	½ tablet hydrocodone 5 mg/acetaminophen 500 mg (Vicodin®)
Adult Opioid-Naive Patients	
The practitioner may choose from the following suggested starting doses:	
Morphine 5 mg PO or SL	0.25 cc morphine 20 mg/cc (Roxanol®)
Oxycodone liquid 5 mg PO or SL	0.25 cc oxycodone 20 mg/cc (Oxyfast®)
Oxycodone 5 mg	• 5 mg oxycodone • 1 tablet oxycodone 5 mg/acetaminophen 325 mg (Percocet®)
Hydromorphone 1 mg	½ of 2 mg tablet PO (Dilaudid®) 1 cc of hydromorphone 1 mg/cc SL
Hydrocodone 5 mg	1 tablet (Vicodin®) 5/500

Source: Permission granted by The Society for Post-Acute and Long-Term Care Medicine. Palliative Care in the Long-Term Care Setting (LTC Physician Information Tool Kit Series). Columbia, MD: 2012

the same opioid for breakthrough pain. *OR* start with an IR opioid and when adequate analgesic is obtained, convert to an equianalgesic dose of same opioid in its sustained-release formulation.

- Remember that the total dose of a mixed opioid (i.e., an opioid with acetaminophen) is limited by its 24-h accumulative dose of acetaminophen.
- Once the total daily dose of an immediate release opioid has been able to adequately control the patient's pain, consider converting it to an equivalent dose of a sustained-release opioid (see Table 9 on the different formulations of sustained-release opioids).
- Note that the duration of analgesia for all immediate-release morphine preparations is 3–4 h whether administered PO, SL, SC, or IV, while the onset of action and its peak analgesic effect do vary (see Table 10).
- The suggested opioid dose for breakthrough pain is 10–15% of the total daily opioid dose usually given every 3–4 h, though for a severe pain crisis it can be administered as often as every 1–2 h *if* needed.
- The total daily dose of an opioid can usually be safely uptitrated by 25–50% for mild to moderate pain and 50–100% for moderate to severe pain in an **opioid tolerant** patient
- When starting a patient on an opioid, *ALWAYS start the patient on a bowel regimen to prevent constipation.* A stimulant and/or osmotic agent are preferable.
- The use of an *adjuvant* analgesic may allow use of a lower dose of an opioid and accordingly lessen the likelihood of opioid adverse effects.

Table 9 Available formulations of sustained-release oral opioids

Morphine sulfate ER (MS Contin®)[a]	q 8h–12h	15,30,60,100,200 mg ER
Morphine sulfate ER (Kadian®)[a,b]	q 12h–24h	10,20,30,50,60,80,100,200 ER
Morphine sulfate ER (Avinza®)[a,b]		Discontinued in USA
Oxycodone ER (Oxycontin®)[a]	q 8h–12h	10,15,20,30,40,60,80 ER
Oxymorphone (Opana ER®)[a]		Discontinued in USA

[a]Formulation must not be crushed
[b]Capsules can be opened and contents administered in pudding or applesauce or per PEG

Table 10 Pharmacodynamics of immediate release morphine

Administered	Peak analgesic effect	Duration of analgesia
Oral/sublingual	45–60 min	3–4 h
Subcutaneous	15–30 min	3–4 h
Intravenous	5–15 min	3–4 h

Table 11 Common and less common side effects of opioids

Common	Less common
Constipation (almost always)	Hypotension
Somnolescence	Diaphoresis
Nausea/vomiting	Urinary retention
Dizziness	Confusion, delirium
Sweating	Bradycardia
Dry mouth	Seizures
Asthenia	Respiratory depression, apnea
Dysesthesias	Paralytic ileus
Pruritus	Paresthesia, hyperesthesia
	Shock, cardiac arrest

In contrast to *non*opioids and NSAIDs, opioids commonly used for the treatment of pain have no analgesic ceiling. However, adverse drug effects may limit further dose increases (see Table 11) or require "rotating" to another opioid, especially if adequate pain relief is not being achieved (see below).

Use of meperidine should be avoided because of its high potential to cause CNS toxicity. Codeine is too constipating in relation to the dose required for an adequate analgesic effect. It is NOT recommended to use three or more different opioids because of the potential for adverse drug– drug or opioid–receptor interactions (either unknown or unrecognized by practitioners). Different opioids interact to different degrees at the mu, delta, and kappa opioid receptors. For a patient on a transdermal fentanyl patch, an immediate release opioid such as morphine or oxycodone will need to be prescribed for breakthrough pain. Transmucosal oral fentanyl (i.e., Actiq®) is only indicated for severe breakthrough **cancer pain** and its use should be *avoided* in the post-acute and LTC setting.

Table 12 Oral Morphine
Milligram Equivalents (MME)

	Oral	Parenteral
Morphine	30	10 (1/3 oral dose)
Oxycodone	20–30	N/A
Oxymorphone	10	1 (1/10 oral dose)
Hydromorphone	7.5	1.5 (1/5 oral dose)
Meperidine	300	100 (1/3 oral dose)
Hydrocodone	30	N/A
Codeine	200	100 (1/2 oral dose)

(25 microgram fentanyl patch = 50 mg oral morphine/24 h, ×3 days); N/A = not available as a parenteral formulation)
Source: Adapted from Principles of Analgesic Use. 7th edition. 2016. American Pain Society

When changing from one opioid to another, whether because of inadequate pain relief or unmanageable adverse effects of the opioid, use *oral morphine milligram equivalents (MME)* as a common denominator for opioid dose conversion in order to avoid either under-dosing or over-dosing and to maintain effective pain relief (see Table 12 on oral morphine milligram equivalents). In order to adjust for incomplete cross-tolerance, the relative conversion of the total daily dose of the new opioid should be decreased by 25–50%. When converting from one opioid to another it is prudent to do so over 2 or 3 days, with down titration of the opioid being discontinued coupled with the uptitration of the newly prescribed opioid, especially if the patient is on a high dose of an opioid. This can avoid a withdrawal pain crisis.

Caution is warranted when prescribing opioids in an *opioid-naïve* patient where the dictum, "start low and go slow" is advisable. A suggested starting dose of oral morphine is 2–5 mg every 3–4 h or the equianalgesic dose of another opioid. The use of a fentanyl patch when initiating opioid treatment in the frail elderly **opioid-naïve patient** is *not* advised as the lower strength patches of 12 mcg/h and 25 mcg/h provide an oral morphine milligram equivalent approximate dose of 25 mg and 50 mg, respectively, *every 24 h*. Such doses will cause excess fatigue, sedation, loss of appetite, and increase fall risk. Though expensive, the fentanyl patch has an ease of use and can provide excellent analgesia in some patients, but is likely ineffective in thin patients and those who weigh less than 105 lbs due to an inadequate subcutaneous fat depot necessary for fentanyl absorption through the skin for eventual release into the blood. A patient is considered to be **opioid-tolerant** when having taken 60 MME daily for 7–10 consecutive days.

Morphine, oxycodone, and hydromorphone should be used cautiously in patients with moderate to severe renal failure (GFR 30–50 mL/min or less) because of the risk of neurotoxic metabolite accumulation. Methadone and fentanyl are safe to use for patients with advanced renal failure or on dialysis, though neither is dialyzable. Non-opioid medications safe to use for patients with renal failure include acetaminophen and tramadol with the maximal daily dose of tramadol reduced to no more than 50–100 mg twice a day.

Morphine and codeine doses may need to be reduced in patients with liver disease, especially those with cirrhosis. Fentanyl may be optimal to use in such patients, unless there is inadequate subcutaneous tissue to enable its absorption.

Methadone is gaining popularity in the treatment of chronic musculoskeletal pain as well as for the treatment of cancer pain and neuropathic pain. Other indications for its use include refractory pain, intolerance to other opioids, or clinician concern about patient diversion of opioids. Methadone has several mechanisms of action, is extensively metabolized in the liver and is minimally renally excreted, and has a cost advantage of being cheap. However, its prolonged and variable metabolism (half-life may vary from 45–180 h) is such that its steady state plasma concentration may not be reached until 10 days. It has complex drug–drug interactions and has been associated with prolongation of the QT interval and an increasingly higher cause of opioid related deaths. Thus, methadone should only be used by (or in consultation with) a physician who is experienced with its use. When treating frail elders, starting at a low dose of methadone between 2.5 mg and 5 mg, two or three times a day would be prudent. *Methadone should never be used for the treatment of acute or breakthrough pain,* as the risk of respiratory depression is high. For more complete information on methadone use in long-term care, refer to Appendix 4 of the AMDA Clinical Practice Guideline on Pain Management in the Long-Term Care Setting [15]. For guidelines on the use of patient controlled analgesia (PCA), refer to References [19] (UNIPAC Three) and [20].

Eligibility Guidelines for Hospice

Practitioners in post-acute and LTC should consider, offer, and facilitate resident access to hospice care as residents transition into the terminal phase of advanced illness when residents would be eligible for the Medicare Hospice Benefit (MHB). Hospice is an underutilized benefit with many patients being referred too late in their illness to be able to fully benefit from its services. The National Hospice and Palliative Care Origination (NHPCO) reports that the proportion of hospice stays of 7 days or less to be 35% of hospice admissions, while long stays greater than 180 days account for 10% of admissions. The Office of the Inspector General (OIG) periodically audits hospice agencies that have a high number of long stay patients as to their eligibility to have remained on hospice or not.

Practitioner knowledge of the *general eligibility guidelines* and *disease-specific guidelines* (see Table 13) for hospice can help prognosticate whether a resident with advanced illness may have a prognosis less than 6 months to live if the resident's condition would likely follow its natural progression ending in death. Such a determination can provide the opportunity to open a frank discussion with the resident and family on advance care planning in order to decide upon a more palliative approach to care whether or not the resident and family opt for life-sustaining treatment or not.

Table 13 Disease-specific eligibility guidelines for hospice

Cancer
Widespread metastatic disease
Palliative Performance Scale (PPS) ≤70%
No longer seeking curative care
Dementia (e.g., Alzheimer's disease)
Inability to ambulate due to dementia (FAST 7c)
No consistent meaningful speech
Life-threatening infections, multiple stage 3 or 4 skin ulcers
Inability to maintain sufficient fluid and calorie intake
Heart disease
Poor response or intolerant to optimal medical treatment
NYHA Class IV CHF
EF ≤20% (helpful, not required)
Unexplained or cardiac-related syncope
HIV/AIDS
CD 4 count <25
Persistent viral loads >100,000/mL
Major Aids-defining refractory infections or other medical conditions
Significant functional decline in ADLs
Neurologic diseases
(PD, ALS, MS, MD, Myasthenia gravis)
Rapid disease progression and critical nutritional state
Life-threatening infections in preceding 12 months
Stage 3, 4 decubitus ulcers
Critically impaired breathing capacity, declines ventilator
Pulmonary disease
Disabling dyspnea at rest or with minimal exertion
Increasing visits to ER, hospitalizations
Hypoxemia on room air (<88%); hypercapnia of $_pCO_2$ >50 mmHg
FEV 1 <30% (helpful, not required)
Renal failure
Not seeking dialysis, not a candidate.(or refusing further dialysis)
Calculated creatinine clearance <10 (<15 for diabetics)
Creatinine >8 (>6 for diabetics)
Stroke
Coma (acute phase)
Dysphagia with insufficient intake of fluids and calories
Post stroke dementia (See Dementia criteria)
Liver disease
INR >1.5 not on Warfarin
Serum albumin <2.5 gm/dL

(continued)

Table 13 (continued)

Refractory ascites
Previous spontaneous bacterial peritonitis
Hepatorenal syndrome
Recurrent variceal bleeding

Adapted from: National Hospice and Palliative Care Organization

General indicators (i.e., general eligibility guidelines for hospice) that a chronic illness *may* have progressed to its *terminal phase* include the following:

- Frequent transfers to the ER.
- More frequent hospitalizations.
- Significant weight loss (5% in 1 month; 10% in the past 6 months).
- Multiple stage 3–4 decubitus ulcers/injuries.
- Serum albumin less than 2.5 g/dL.
- Recurrent life-threatening infections such as pneumonia, pyelonephritis, or sepsis.
- Resident has a progressively declining functional status as determined by either a Karnofsky Performance Scale (KPS) score of <70% or an increasing dependency in 2 or more of 6 Basic Activities of Daily Living or Tasks of Daily Living. The Palliative Performance Scale (PPS) is similar to the KPS and takes into account ambulation, physical activity, ability for self-care, oral intake of food and fluids, and level of consciousness.
- Use of these scales can help practitioners better prognosticate how far advanced is a resident's illness.
- The *F*unctional *A*ssessment *S*taging (FAST) is a scale (scored 1–7) used to determine the severity of loss of function in dementia, 1 being no functional difficulty and 7 presence of significate loss of ability to speak, ambulate, smile, and hold their head up independently.
- The KPS, PPS, and FAST [21] scales are readily available from any hospice.

When the *guidelines* for *disease-specific eligibility* for hospice are not fully met, the presence and severity of comorbid medical conditions and/or psychosocial factors may support eligibility. For example, advanced COPD or dementia may further support eligibility for hospice in a resident with late-stage heart failure. Finally, there is excellent predictive value in the "surprise question": "Would you be surprised if a certain patient died in the next 12 months?"; if so, then it would be appropriate to consider hospice care. Note that the diagnoses of failure to thrive, generalized debility, and nonspecific terminal illness are no longer accepted as a terminal condition under the MHB.

Certification for hospice requires that two physicians, usually the hospice medical director and the attending or referring physician, sign a statement certifying that the patient's medical prognosis supports a life expectancy of 6 months or less if the individual's illness follows its natural and expected progression. Once on hospice, a patient must be *recertified* for each benefit period. Recertification requires a narrative statement by the hospice medical director as to continued eligibility. With the

MHB, the first two hospice certification periods are each 90 days and all subsequent periods are 60 days with no limit as to the number of 60 day periods. However, continued eligibility for hospice requires that the eligibility parameters present on admission to hospice continue to be met *and* that physical, functional, and/or nutritional *decline continues* to support that life expectancy is 6 months or less if the individual's illness follows its natural course. Note that every 60-day recertification period after 6 months now requires a *face-to-face* visit by the hospice medical director or a nurse practitioner contracted by the hospice, to determine and verify continued eligibility for hospice. Every patient on hospice has the right to *revoke* their hospice benefit at any time in order to seek life-sustaining or curative treatment. In such circumstances, if the treatments are of no further benefit, these patients can be readmitted to hospice if the hospice eligibility guidelines are still met.

Billing by practitioners for services rendered to patients on hospice can be confusing and dependent upon the Local Medicare Intermediary (now called Medicare Administrative Contractors). It is recommended that practitioners clarify hospice billing practices with their Medicare Administrative Contractor (MAC) or the hospice.

End of Life Care

As patients with advanced serious and life-limiting illness enter the last months and weeks of life, practitioners need to recognize this terminal phase and to inform patients and family accordingly. If not already done, goals of care need to be reviewed and modified through advanced care planning to determine whether the patient and family want to continue to pursue life-prolonging treatments or are amenable to hospice care, *with palliative care integrated into either choice.* Care must be taken to establish clear and medically appropriate goal-concordant care that ensures a shared understanding between practitioners, patients, and family [22]. Irrespective of where a patient resides, interdisciplinary management is essential to maintaining hope, dignity, and the best possible quality of life until the patient dies. Eventually however, continuing life-sustaining treatments (such as IV fluids, PEG tube feeding, blood transfusions, antibiotics, pacemakers, ICDs, and hemodialysis) during the last weeks and days of life can become overly burdensome, and cause more harm, pain, and suffering than benefit to both the patient *and* the family. As such, consideration will need to be given as to discontinuing such treatments.

The physiologic changes of dying, although complex, can be effectively managed if practitioners and the interdisciplinary team understand the etiologies and underlying pathophysiology of each distressful symptom and use appropriate non-pharmacologic and pharmacologic interventions. Given each patient's terminal illness and comorbidities, palliative drugs, equipment, and supplies should be available in *anticipation of the emergence of distressful symptoms* that are likely to occur at the end of life.

As death approaches, patients and families should be advised that fatigue and weakness will increase while the desire for food and fluid intake is reduced due to the loss of both appetite and thirst. Reduced cardiac output and intravascular volume depletion result in tachycardia, hypotension, peripheral cooling, cyanosis, and mottling. Urine output will diminish with eventual anuria. Neurologic dysfunction will occur, leading to a decreased level of consciousness and eventual coma. Note that 10% of dying patients may experience an agitated delirium during the last days of life. When this occurs satisfactory symptom management can be very challenging.

Practical interventions to maintain patient comfort include periodic repositioning; decreasing food and fluid intake to prevent choking or aspiration; maintaining a moist oral mucosa; and providing moisture and lubricating agents to the conjunctiva and lips. Family members should be encouraged to participate in this care as it can often provide them with a sense of fulfillment in having helped to comfort their loved one at end of life.

Nonessential drugs (e.g., aspirin, multivitamins, calcium supplements, lipid-lowering agents) should be discontinued. Practitioners should also consider the benefits and risks of continuing drugs such as antidepressants, antihypertensives, warfarin, antiarrhythmics and thyroid replacement. Other drugs, such as diuretics, ACE inhibitors, and hypoglycemic agents (even insulin) may require a dosage reduction or even discontinuation. Be aware that reduced hepatic function and renal perfusion can precipitate an *opioid-induced terminal delirium*. If this occurs, consider (1) reducing the opioid dosage while ensuring that pain is still adequately controlled and (2) prescribing a low dose antipsychotic and gradually uptitrating until an effective outcome is achieved.

During the last few days of life, medication reconciliation is essential to avoid polypharmacy and its potential sequelae, especially as "comfort medications" are administered to manage pain and distressful symptoms and suffering. Polypharmacy can become a major issue that must be addressed.

Remember that a peaceful death is just as important to the *family* as to the patient, perhaps even more so. Practitioners should be wary for the potential for surveyor citation under F-Tag 757 that each resident's drug regimen be free from unnecessary drugs. For example, the prescription of either an opioid or an antipsychotic for anxiety could be construed as unnecessary.

General guidelines on the use of comfort-directed pharmacologic treatment during the last days of life include:

- **For tachypnea or breathlessness:** Use low doses of an immediate release opioid with or without a benzodiazepine, each administered sublingually or transbuccally.
- **For excessive respiratory or oral secretions:** Consider an anticholinergic agent administered sublingually (e.g., hyoscyamine or an ophthalmic solution of atropine) or topically (e.g., transdermal scopolamine patch). It is beneficial to educate the family and staff to minimize use of suction as it can paradoxically stimulate the production of even more secretions.
- **For pain:** Use a concentrated oral formulation of either morphine (e.g., Roxanol® 20 mg/cc) or oxycodone (Oxyfast® 20 mg/cc). Either can be administered sublin-

gually or transbuccally. Avoid IM or SC injections if possible as these can be painful.

- **For anxiety or agitation:** Use a benzodiazepine or an opioid, possibly an antipsychotic. Remember any of these can cause paradoxical agitation.
- **For restlessness or delirium:** Perform a careful medication review and rule out a rectal fecal impaction or urinary bladder retention. The former will require disimpaction while the latter, placement of a Foley catheter. Ensure adequate pain control. If needed, consider treatment with an antipsychotic, with or without a benzodiazepine. Remember that either can cause paradoxical agitation.
- **For fever:** If distressing to the patient, schedule doses of acetaminophen administered orally, per rectum or per PEG (if present).
- **If excessive sweating:** Review medications, consider cooling the room, use a fan, and consider an opioid dose reduction (as opioids can cause sweating) and even cause a fentanyl patch to no longer adhere to skin.

Compounded formulations applied topically on the skin may be effective for restlessness, though evidence is lacking. For example, compounded ABH gel contains *A*tivan/lorazepam, *B*enadryl/diphenhydramine, and *H*aloperidol. Review of compounded topicals is beyond the scope of this chapter so practitioners are encouraged to contact a local compounding pharmacy or hospice agency.

Pearls for the Practitioner
- Integrate palliative care into the traditional care provided to patients throughout the post-acute and long-term care continuum irrespective of whether they choose to continue disease-directed or curative therapies.
- Support informed patient and family decision making through advance care planning consistent with patient values and preferences for care.
- Determine, if possible, the pathophysiologic and clinical factors underlying each pain and non-pain symptom in order to choose the most appropriate nonpharmacologic and pharmacologic treatment.
- Treat pain with the use of multiple modalities, both nonpharmacologic and pharmacologic as well as complementary and alternative therapies (the latter if requested by patient/family).
- Choose the most appropriate analgesic based on the type of pain, pain severity, potential adverse effects, and the patient's individual characteristics.
- Always initiate a bowel regimen to prevent constipation when prescribing an opioid and remember to intensify the bowel regimen as the dose of the opioid is increased.
- Consider education on Risk Evaluation and Mitigation Strategy (REMS) on the use of opioid analgesics.
- Anticipate which symptoms are most likely to occur during the patient's illness trajectory in addition to identifying, assessing, treating, and monitoring for distressful symptoms, and if possible, preventing their emergence.
- Consider both the general and disease-specific guidelines as a prognostic tool when evaluating patients for hospice.

- Consider palliative sedation to alleviate intractable and intolerable pain or suffering that persists despite aggressive palliative care.
- Use resources in your community offered by health care professionals who have an expertise in palliative care and hospice, including the PA and LTC facility medical director!

Suggestions for Further Reading
- AMDA White Paper on Palliative Care and Hospice in Long Term Care. (last accessed online August 4, 2021)
- Essential Practices in Hospice and Palliative Medicine. Fifth Edition. 2017. AAHPM. Chicago, IL

    – UNIPAC 1: Medical Care of People with Serious Illness
    – UNIPAC 2: Psychiatric, Psychological and Spiritual Care
    – UNIPAC 3: Pain Assessment and Management
    – UNIPAC 4: Nonpain Symptoms Management
    – UNIPAC 5: Communication and Teamwork
    – UNIPAC 6: Ethical and Legal Practice
    – UNIPAC 7: Pediatric Palliative Care and Practice
    – UNIPAC 8: COPD, Heart failure, and Renal Disease
    – UNIPAC 9: HIV, Dementia, and Neurological Conditions

- Equianalgesic Guide for Adults and Children. Revised 2019. AAHPM. (a four-paged fold out)
- Pain Management in the Post-Acute and Long-Term Care Setting: Clinical Practice Guideline. 2021. The Society for Post-Acute and Long-Term Care Medicine. Columbia, MD
- Pain Management in the Post-Acute and Long-Term Care Setting. Pocket Guide. 2018. The Society for Post-Acute and Long-Term Care Medicine. Columbia, MD (A spiral bound concise 27-page pocket size guide printed in thin cardboard)
- Primer of Palliative Care. 7th edition. 2019.
- Periyakoil VS, Denney-Koelsch EM, White P, Zhukovsky DS, Quill TE. Chicago, IL.
- Emanual LL and Librach SW. (Editors). Palliative Care: Core Skills and Clinical Competencies. 2nd edition. Elsevier Saunders. 2011.
- McPherson ML. Demystifying Opioid Conversion Calculations: A Guide for Effective Dosing. American Society of Health-System Pharmacists. 2nd ed. 2018.
- Chochinov HM. Dignity Therapy: Final Words for Final Days. Oxford University Press Inc. 2012.
- Matzo M. and Sherman D. (Editors). Palliative Care Nursing Education: Quality Care to the End of Life, Fourth Edition. Springer Publishing Company, New York. 2015.
- Winn P. Essentials of Hospice: What Every Practitioner Needs to Know but Are Afraid to Ask. Internal Medicine Review, Vol 5, Issue 1. 2019

- Nonopioid Drugs for Pain. The Medical Letter on Drugs and Therapeutics. Volume 64. Issue No. 1645.2022
- Sheikh F, Brandt N, Vinh D, Elon R. Management of Chronic Pain in Nursing Homes: Navigating Challenges to Improve Person-Centered Care. J Am Med Dir Assoc 2021; 119–1205.

References

1. Currow DC, Wheeler JL, Glare PA, et al. A framework for generalizeability in palliative care. J Pain Symptom Manage. 2009;37(3):373–86.
2. Kristler CE, Sloane PD, Zimmerman S. New findings on palliative care issues near the end-of-life. J Am Med Dir Assoc. 2021;22(2):265–7.
3. Aronow WS. Clinical causes of death in 2372 older persons in a nursing home during 15-year follow-up. J Am Med Dir Assoc. 2000;1:95–6.
4. Goldberg TH, Botero QA. Causes of death in elderly nursing home residents. J Am Med Dir Assoc. 2008;9:565–7.
5. Periyakoil VS, Denney-Koelsch EM, White P, Zhukovsky DS, Quill TE. Primer of palliative care. 7th ed. Chicago, IL: American Academy of Hospice and Palliative Medicine; 2019.
6. Flacker JM, Kiely DK. Mortality-related factors and 1-year survival in nursing home residents. J Am Geriatr Soc. 2003;51:213–21. eprognosis.ucsf.edu/flackernew@php. Accessed 18 July 2021.
7. Wilner LS, Arnold R. The palliative projnostic score. Fast fact #124. Palliative Care Network of Wisconsin. https://www.mypcnow.org/fast-fact/the-palliative-prognostic-score/. Accessed 18 July 2021.
8. Anderson F, Downing GM, Hill J, et al. Palliative Performance Scale (PPS): a new tool. J Palliative Care. 1996;12(1):5–11.
9. Kirk TW, Mahon MM. National Hospice and Palliative Care Organization (NHPCO). Position statement and commentary of the use of palliative sedation in imminently dying terminally ill patients. J Pain Symptom Manage. 2010;39(5):914–23.
10. Winn PA, Dentino AN. Quality palliative care in the long-term care setting. J Am Med Dir Assoc. 2005;6:589–98.
11. Winn PA, Dention NA. Effective pain management in the long-term care setting. J Am Med Dir Assoc. 2004;5:342–52.
12. Rodgers PE, Ross JS, Tatum PE, Vandekieft GK. End-of-life care. FP Essentials, vol. 498. Leawood, KS: AAFP Home Study, American Academy of Family Physicians; 2020. p. 1–48.
13. Wilcock A, Howard P, Charlesworth S. Palliative Care Formulary PCF7. London, UK: Pharmaceutical Press; 2020.
14. Irwin SA, Fairman N, Hirst J, et al. Essential practices in hospice and palliative medicine, UNIPAC 2. Psychiatric, Psychological and Spiritual Care. 5th ed. Chicago, IL: AAHPM; 2017.
15. Pain management in the long-term care setting. Clinical practice guideline. American Medical Directors Association; 2012.
16. Pain Management in the post-acute and long-term care setting. Pocket guide. The Society for Post-Acute and Long-Term Care Medicine; 2018.
17. Dr R, Herr KA, Pacola JT, et al. Geriatrics at your fingertips. 23rd ed. New York: The American Geriatrics Society; 2021.
18. American Geriatrics Panel on the Pharmacologic Management of Persistent Pain in Older Adults. Pharmacologic Management of Persistent Pain in Older Adults. J Am Geriatr Soc. 2009;57(8):1331–46.

19. Essential Practices in Hospice and Palliative Medicine. UNIPAC 3. Pain Assessment and Management. American Academy of Hospice and Palliative Medicine. Chicago, IL; 2017.
20. Principles of analgesic use. 7th ed. American Pain Society, Chicago, IL; 2016.
21. Reisberg B. Functional Assessment Staging (FAST). Psychopharmacol Bull. 1988;24:653–9.
22. Klement A, Marks S. The pitfalls of utilizing "goals of care" as a clinical buzz phrase: a case study and proposed solution. Palliat Medicare Reports. 2020;1(1):216–20.

Weight and Nutrition in Post-Acute and Long-Term Care

Todd H. Goldberg and Joel A. Levien

Introduction

The nutritional needs of older adults are influenced by many factors. Changes associated with normal aging, individual behavior, as well as drugs and progressive disease all increase nutritional risk. As with persons of all ages, maintaining proper nutrition and a healthy weight are important for persons who reside in the community, assisted living facilities, and nursing homes. Ideally, optimal nutrition can improve health, function, quality of life, and reduce the risk of morbidity, mortality, and conditions such as osteoporosis, weakness, pressure sores, frailty, sarcopenia, and lack of resistance to infection. Weight loss is both a facility quality measure and a risk factor for poor outcomes, while survival can improve with better nutrition. Maintaining appropriate nutrition, hydration, oral intake, and weight can pose a challenge especially for those who have dementia, depression, and gastrointestinal, neurological, musculoskeletal, or psychiatric disorders. Also, drugs can affect appetite, chewing, swallowing, digestion, and bowel function that can predispose to weight loss.

Older adults who require long-term care often reside in residential care (personal care/assisted living) or nursing home care facilities for a variety of reasons: ranging from *temporary disability* such as due to a hip fracture, to *chronic disability* from COPD, CHF, or dementia. As such persons with chronic illness and disability

T. H. Goldberg (✉)
Department of Internal Medicine/Geriatrics, Jefferson Abington Hospital, Abington, PA, USA

J. A. Levien
Gastroenterology, Jackson, TN, USA

Table 1 Recommended intakes for key nutrients in older adults

Nutrient	Typical recommended intake/DRI[a]	Comments for geriatrics/LTC
Calories/energy	1800+ calories	Varies by body size and activity level and desired weight loss or gain
Protein	46 g/day Females >18 (0.36–0.66 g/kg/day) 56 g/day Males >18 10–35% of calories	Increased protein to 1–1.2 g/kg/day suggested for geriatric LTC patients
Fat	20–35% of calories	
Carbohydrate	130 g/day, 45–65% of calories	
Water	2.7–3.7 L/day	Includes total water, all beverages, in average temperate climate
Vitamin A	700–900 mcg/day	Higher doses associated with increased toxicity and mortality.
Vitamin B_{12}	2.4 mcg/day. Typical oral supplement dose 100–1000 mcg.	Common deficiency in elderly; measure levels. Often malabsorbed requiring supplements
Vitamin C Zinc	75–90 mg 11 mg	Larger doses often recommended for pressure sores but not evidence-based
Vitamin D	800 IU (20 mcg) for adults over 70 (2011 IOM Update ref. [3]).	Older adults often deficient. Consider measuring 25-OH vitamin D levels and adding supplements if deficient
Vitamin E	15 mg (22.5 IU)	Supplementation >200 IU no longer recommended due to meta-analysis showing increased mortality [4]
Calcium	1200 mg/day	Calcium + vitamin D supplements should be considered for all older adults at risk for osteoporosis
Iron	8 mg/day	Doses >325 mg/day ineffective and cause increased constipation

[a]Adapted from various sources, chiefly "Dietary Reference Intakes" from the Institute of Medicine, and US Department of Agriculture, Food and Nutrition Information Center (Ref. [2]). What were formerly called Recommended Daily Allowances (RDA's) are now called Dietary Reference Intakes (DRI's). Not all vitamins and minerals are included; for more complete lists see the full sources cited

require diligent nutritional assessment. There is a strong correlation between low body mass index (BMI), low serum albumin, and increased mortality for months even years after discharge from the hospital. When nutritional deficiencies are recognized, interventions are often suboptimal, leading to poor outcomes and possible ethical and legal issues [1].

Detailed dietary guidelines and Dietary Reference Intakes are beyond the scope of this review, but are widely available at many websites including that of the US Dept. of Agriculture Food and Nutrition Information Center https://www.nal.usda.gov/legacy/fnic/dietary-reference-intakes [2]. Table 1 summarizes the recommendations for key nutrients.

Risk Factors

Normal aging generally is accompanied by modest changes in appetite, metabolism, intestinal function, and absorption of nutrients. Older patients may experience less hunger than younger patients after a period of underfeeding. Various physiological functions that assure appropriate nutrition; ingestion, digestion, assimilation, and absorption of nutrients will be affected by the patient's medical, psychosocial, and functional status. A good bowel regimen and adequate fluid intake are important (see AMDA's Dehydration/Fluid Maintenance Guideline) [5]. Inadequate intake of food and fluids can increase the risk of dehydration, constipation, slow gastric emptying, regurgitation, cognitive impairment, aspiration, infection, decubiti, and sepsis.

Most if not all patients admitted to a post-acute/long-term care (PALTC) facility will have some *nutritional risk factors* such as:

- A history of weight loss or loss of appetite
- Oral/dental problems (edentulousness)
- Reduced mobility and functional disability
- Skin breakdown or pressure injury
- Disease: depression, dementia, and chronic or terminal illness
- Symptoms: fluid retention/edema, nausea, vomiting, or a change in bowel habits
- Multiple medications

Medication

Numerous drugs can cause GI disturbances, anorexia, and weight loss. These include: NSAID's, opioids, anticholinergics (which reduce salivary and gastric secretions, and GI motility); diabetic drugs such as metformin, digoxin, and dementia drugs such as cholinesterase inhibitors. Psychotropics, particularly TCAs, can cause worsened cognition, poor oral intake, and constipation. ACE inhibitors and antibiotics may distort normal smell and taste. Antiacid drugs, especially proton pump inhibitors, may reduce absorption of nutrients such as calcium and vitamin B_{12}. Many drugs cause constipation, including analgesics and antihypertensives (especially calcium channel blockers). Opioids and antidiarrheals such as loperamide may decrease peristalsis and potentially result in toxic megacolon. Some drugs cause weight gain, such as the antidiabetic agents and antipsychotics. Polypharmacy can compromise appetite, weight, and nutrition. Recent surgery or trauma may result in immobility, ileus, and constipation. One of the most critical tasks of the admitting practitioner is to review and verify the list of medications patients are taking, to discontinue unnecessary medications, while ensuring a safe transition between health care settings (see AMDA's Transitions of Care Guideline) [6].

Disease

Numerous disease-related factors can cause changes in weight, appetite, swallowing, and gastrointestinal function, such as: hyperthyroidism or hypothyroidism; diabetes; neurologic and psychiatric disorders such as Parkinson's, dementia, and depression; alcohol and other substance abuse; oral/dental problems; numerous GI disorders such as achalasia, malabsorption, peptic ulcers, and irritable or inflammatory bowel disease; and systemic conditions such as scleroderma, CHF, AIDS, cancer, and infection. Physiologic stress due to acute or chronic illness can increase protein and energy requirements and result in weight loss.

In community dwelling elderly, the ability to obtain, prepare, and eat food may be impeded by psychosocial and functional problems, sensory deficits, limited mobility, or inadequate income. Paradoxically being admitted to a LTC facility where three good meals a day are provided may actually improve nutrition and reverse weight loss.

Assessment of Nutritional Status

Evaluation of nutritional status and weight loss/gain entails a good medical history, physical examination, with a nutritional and laboratory assessment. Facility staff often observe problems with eating or note weight loss. Body weight and BMI is a basic screen of nutritional status. Thus, serial weights are a simple means for recognizing a change in nutritional well-being. Obtaining accurate weights may be challenging, especially with bedridden or immobilized patients. A calibrated bed or chair scale can be used for these patients.

Monitoring for *significant weight loss* is required for all LTC patients and is part of the MDS (Minimum Data Set), and the facility's CMS Quality Measures. According to federal nursing home Federal regulations ("OBRA," Omnibus Budget Reconciliation Act of 1987), staff must recognize and address *significant weight loss*. This is *defined as 5% weight loss over the past 30 days, or >10% weight loss over the past 6 months* [1].

General medical history questions should be asked of the patient or caregiver such as "Is there any difficulty with eating, chewing, swallowing, elimination, or maintaining weight?" No single test exists that identifies all patients at risk [7]. Brief tools for nutritional assessment include the Subjective Global Assessment [8], the Mini Nutritional Assessment (MNA) [9], and the abbreviated MNA-SF (Short Form) [10]. Weight loss alone is one of the best indicators of nutritional compromise and a proven risk factor for increased morbidity and mortality [11]. Another test to assess nutritional status is the Instant Nutritional Assessment (INA) (Table 2) [12]. The INA consists of measuring the serum albumin and total lymphocyte count, which help to identify a patients at nutritional risk.

Table 2 Instant nutritional assessment

Laboratory result	Abnormal
Serum albumin	Less than 3.5 mg/dL
Total lymphocyte count	Less than 1500/mm^3

Several other laboratory parameters can be monitored in patients who present with weight loss, fatigue, or signs and symptoms of undernutrition or inadequate hydration. These include a CBC, comprehensive metabolic panel, lipids, and a TSH. Obtaining blood levels of vitamin B_{12} and 25-Hydroxy-vitamin D should also be considered. Low serum albumin is the most commonly used indicator of protein malnutrition and is correlated with increased mortality in older persons [13]. These labs should be ordered not only when nutritional concerns arise but also periodically in those at risk for poor nutrition.

Screening for dementia and depression is an important component in the management of malnutrition in LTC [14]. Depression and dementia can impact food intake and weight, and may be the most common cause of weight loss. Medications prescribed for these conditions (antidepressants and cholinesterase inhibitors) may further decrease appetite and cause GI upset and decrease food intake. Mirtazapine and nortryptyline can be of therapeutic benefit as they tend to increase appetite and cause weight gain more than other antidepressants [14]. In one study of older adults depression was one of the most common causes of weight loss (30%) followed by cancer [15]. However, use of antidepressants solely for appetite/weight gain in the absence of depression is not validated.

Weight Management

Achieving an ideal healthy weight in LTC patients is controversial. Patients should be counseled and provided nutritious and well-balanced meals and activities in order to maintain a reasonably healthy weight. Obese patients should be put on a healthy diet with perhaps mild caloric restriction, but dramatic weight loss would not be expected in older persons who cannot participate in vigorous exercise. A too restrictive diet may decrease the patient's quality of life and lead to nutritional deficiencies [16, 17]. The optimal weight range for assisted living and nursing home patients has not been clearly defined but is presumably the same as the general population. It has been reported that overall mortality rates were lowest with a "normal" BMI in the range of 22.5–25 kg/m^2 [18]. A longitudinal study of Canadian obese adults indicated that mortality was lowest in *moderately overweight individuals (BMI 25–30)* [19], indicating that older adults may benefit from extra body weight and protein stores when illness occurs; *while those underweight (BMI <20)* had an increased risk of illness and mortality. Therefore, an optimal weight range for older adults, including LTC residents, appears to be a BMI of 25 ± 5 (i.e., 20–30).

A more common and concerning problem in the nursing home is *underweight*. Underweight residents commonly have anorexia, leading to excessive weight loss, malnutrition, frailty, depression, low energy and activity, and poor skin integrity. Those who lose at least 5% of their body weight have been reported to be 5–10 times more likely to die [20]. Even those who regain weight still have increased mortality. A workup for potentially reversible causes of weight loss should consider GI and other diseases, medication side effects, and depression. If no specific cause is found, one might then diagnose anorexia of aging, terminal stage of dementia or *failure to thrive*, and the weight loss subsequently determine as being *unavoidable*. It is difficult to determine how aggressive to be with nutritional interventions in those patients with a limited prognosis and poor quality of life. The facility staff and family should provide residents with ample enjoyable food that includes a liberalized diet and appropriate supplements. Be aware that some calorie dense supplements may actually suppress appetite at meals and lead either to failure to gain weight or further weight loss.

AMDA's Clinical Practice Guideline (CPG) on Altered Nutritional Status recommends a process of over 20 steps to evaluate and treat nutritional issues in long-term care, beginning with a baseline evaluation of the patient's nutritional status, weight, height and BMI, and dietary preferences [1]. Risk factors for poor nutritional status include a history of recent weight or appetite change and impaired functional status, as well as any related medical complications such as pressure injuries should all be documented. The presence of terminal illness, depression, or medications affecting taste or appetite should be noted. The CPG states that treatment should address the underlying issues that have been identified, tailor meals/food to individual preferences and function, limit unnecessary dietary restrictions, and add supplements when necessary. Appetite stimulants should be considered as a last resort and on an individual basis. Tube feedings should only be used in appropriate patients (see "Indications and Usage of Feeding tubes" later in this chapter as well as the chapter on "Ethical and Legal Issues" for further discussion). The AMDA CPG recommends that practitioners and facilities continually monitor nutritional status. The "feed.ME" (Medical Education) Global Study Group has published a Nutritional Care Pathway suggesting hospitals and LTC facilities "screen, intervene, and supervene" for the nutritional care of all patients in health care facilities [21].

Nutritional Interventions

Fluids

Recommended fluid intake for the average adult is approximately 3.7 L/day for males and 2.7 L/day for females [2]. This assumes a temperate climate and includes total daily consumption of water, all beverages, and the water content derived from foods. Those with illness, fever, or experiencing a humid/high ambient temperature may require additional fluids. Oral intake is preferred; IV therapy may be available in SNF's but often not available in other LTC settings. An alternative means of hydration is *hypodermoclysis* (subcutaneous infusion of isotonic fluids) as a short-term option [22]. Note that lab abnormalities of electrolytes or renal function do not necessarily indicate true "dehydration" [23]. A diagnosis of dehydration may be judged as an indicator of inadequate care and is considered a *sentinel event* by regulatory agencies, so it should not be diagnosed with caution.

Supplements

"Food first"—nutritious food is always preferable to any artificial formula or supplement. In addition to offering and providing sufficient fruits, vegetables, starches, healthy fats, dairy products, and fluids, recent position papers have suggested that increased protein intake is generally beneficial in order to maximize muscle and bone health and to minimize the development of sarcopenia and osteoporosis [24, 25]. Increasing the daily intake of protein to 1–1.2 g/kg/day has been recommended. Some studies have reported that a higher protein diet was beneficial in adults over 65 in terms of lower cancer incidence, improved function, and decreased total mortality [26–28].

Nutritional supplements such as Ensure[R] (Abbott Laboratories) are tasty, safe, and beneficial for those who can eat and drink but cannot consume sufficient quantities of calories and nutrients via "normal" meals. One can of Ensure[R] Plus contains 350 calories, nutrition equal to about half of an average modest meal. Various brands of supplements exist with different ingredients/properties, e.g., low glucose, added fiber, or higher fat for pulmonary patients. For details on ingredients and which products are available in your local facility, consult the facility dietary services supervisor or dietician. In order to minimize appetite suppression supplements they should be given between meals [1]. An additional option is to provide a *nutritional supplement drink* rather than water when administering medication, e.g., MedPass 2.0[R] (Hormel Health Labs).

Vitamin and mineral supplements are generally reserved for those who have specific nutritional deficiencies or medical conditions. However it may be reasonable to provide a "senior" multivitamin to all LTC patients. Most women and many men should be encouraged to consume foods rich in calcium and/or receive a calcium supplement to obtain a total daily intake of 1200–1500 mg. Due to hypochlorhydria commonly occurring in the elderly, calcium *citrate* is preferred due to its better absorption than calcium carbonate.

Studies have shown that even those taking a multivitamin and a calcium/vitamin D supplement may still be vitamin D deficient [29]. Vitamin D deficiency has been associated with numerous health concerns besides osteopenia and osteoporosis [30]. The Institute of Medicine has updated the Dietary Reference Intakes for vitamin D (to 800 IU daily) for adults over 70 [3]. Three meta-analyses have shown a benefit of vitamin D supplementation of at least 800 IU/day on falls [31], fractures

[32], and total mortality [33]. Consideration should be given to supplementing all elderly LTC patients with vitamin D, or at least measuring 25-OH-vitamin D levels and supplementing those who do not have sufficient levels (defined as ≥ 30 ng/mL) [34]. The latest studies in 2022, however, have questioned the value of vitamin D measurement and supplementation (https://www.nytimes.com/2022/07/27/health/vitamin-d-bone-fractures.html).

Avoiding excessive/unnecessary medication has always been a principle of good medical and long-term care. This issue became particularly important during the Covid-19 pandemic, when staff were overwhelmed and needed to lessen in-person staff time during med passes. In a recent (08/22) commentary in AMDA's "Caring for the Ages" newsletter, nutritional supplements have been highlighted as a good example of potentially unnecessary pills, since recent evidence has failed to support the value of many supplements in patients without a clear deficiency [35].

Appetite Stimulants

All patients with difficulty eating should be evaluated by a dietitian and a language speech therapist to evaluate for the presence of a swallowing problem and to provide recommendations on diet and consistency [36]. Those with oral/dental or swallowing problems may require special textures such as mechanical soft, pureed, or thickened liquids. However, such diets may not be palatable and appealing to patients and can result in loss of appetite and decreased food intake. Feeding assistance should be provided when needed, and an appealing "mealtime social ambience" can be of benefit [37].

If patients are still unable to ingest adequate nutrition, cautious use of an "appetite stimulant" or orexigenic medication may be considered, such as megestrol acetate, but it is expensive (up to $500 a month) and of questionable efficacy, and has safety concerns (e.g., fluid retention, edema, and an increased risk of DVT in up to 32%) [38]. Orexigenic drugs are FDA approved only for AIDS and cancer, and their use off-label in patients with dementia, failure to thrive, and endstage disease. Despite lack of evidence-based support for use in the elderly, they are often tried. Both megestrol and cyproheptadine (another medication used off-label to stimulate appetite) are included in the AGS Beers list of potentially inappropriate medication use in older adults [39].

Other drugs sometimes used to stimulate appetite include mirtazapine (Remeron[R]), as it has been noted to cause weight gain (1–6 lbs) in depressed patients. There is little or no evidence that mirtazapine is effective for weight gain in the absence of depression. Dronabinol (Marinol[R]) is a cannabinoid derivative also FDA approved for anorexia and nausea in cancer and AIDS patients. It has been tried in the elderly, with little evidence of efficacy. However it can cause somnolence and seizures and precipitate delirium [40].

The American Geriatrics Society, in its "Choosing Wisely" campaign, stated the following: "Avoid using prescription appetite stimulants or high-calorie supplements for treatment of anorexia or cachexia in older adults; instead, optimize social supports provide feeding assistance, and clarify patient goals and expectations" [41].

Indications and Use (or Not) of Feeding Tubes

Artificial nutrition with a feeding tube may be needed if a patient presents with esophageal obstruction; postoperative head and neck cancer or GI surgery; severe protein/calorie deprivation/depletion; moderate to severe weight loss, hyper-metabolic or hyper-catabolic state; choking or otherwise unable to swallow safely, which result in the inability to maintain sufficient oral intake [1]. Nasoenteric or oroenteric tubes are a short-term and temporary means of accessing the GI tract. A more permanent access with a gastrostomy or jejunostomy tube may be needed if enteral support is required for more than a few weeks. A patient's advance directive or stated wishes may preclude artificial feeding.

Evidence-based literature suggests that the use of feeding tubes is ethically debatable and not proven effective in preventing complications such as aspiration, pressure sores, and death in elderly demented patients [42, 43]. A recent article reported that while about 5% of demented nursing home residents had a feeding tube inserted over a 1-year period, the median survival was only 56 days with a 1 year post-insertion mortality of 64%, with many patients requiring multiple hospitalizations for complications related to tube placement and replacement [44]. Thus, insertion of a feeding tube should only be considered when there is reasonable expectation or hope of recovery from a temporary condition such as an acute stroke.

Not eating can be a natural and inevitable sign of impending death. When considering the need for a feeding tube this recognition should trigger a discussion with the health care proxy that the patient is at high risk to die within the next few months, and that palliative care or hospice care could best serve the patient. Both AMDA [45] and the American Geriatrics Society [46] as part of the ABIM Foundation's *"Choosing Wisely"* initiative, have stated, *"Don't insert percutaneous feeding tubes in individuals with advanced dementia. Instead, offer oral assisted feedings."* AGS has also published a position paper recommending against insertion of feeding tubes in patients with advanced dementia [47].

If a feeding tube is decided upon, many different formulas are available. Standard formulas have low residue, supply 1 kcal/mL, with 13–17% of calories as protein (*Ensure HN* and *Osmolite HN* are examples). A high fiber formula, such as *Jevity*, contains 10–14 g of fiber per liter, 1 Kcal/mL and about 14–18% Kcal as protein. High protein formulas, such as *Replete* or *Promote* contain 20–25% of calories as protein. Some products have added fiber, vitamins, and minerals. When patients have a problem with an increased gastric residual, they may require a lower volume (i.e., more concentrated) formula such as *Two-Cal HN* or *Magnacal*. Lower volume formulas have up to 2 kcal/ml of which 14–17% is protein and 68–78% water.

Vivonex Plus and *Vital HN* are *hydrolyzed formulas* that are available for postpyloric or jejunal feeding. Some hydrolyzed formulas have added glutamine and arginine, which are important for bowel integrity. Medium chain triglycerides (MCT) are used to replace long chain triglycerides in these postpyloric formulas. *Renal* and *hepatic formulas* are necessary in the presence of renal and hepatic impairment. *Suplena* and *Nepro* are examples of renal formulas that are restricted in water, sodium, potassium, magnesium, and vitamin A. Hepatic formulas have limited aromatic amino acids and methionine, and are higher in branched chain amino acids. Immune formulas such as *Immune-Aid* are recommended in patients who suffer severe physiologic stress, such as those who are on ventilators. They contain increased amounts of omega-3 and decreased omega-6 fatty acids as well as enriched with arginine and glutamine. A number of other additives are also available including glucose polymers, protein powder, and vegetable oil or medium chain triglycerides.

Ethical and Legal Issues Related to Feeding

The consensus in the medical and ethical literature is that withholding or withdrawing *natural feedings* (when unsuccessful, futile, or inappropriate), is no different than not initiating tube feeding or other medical treatments based on the patient's clinical condition and patient wishes. Again, *not eating* is an expected and natural part of advanced dementia and the dying process. Tube feedings unfortunately do **not** reduce the risk of aspiration, pneumonia, pressure sores, or infections, and *decrease rather than increase quality of life* due to tube-related complications, mobility restrictions, and discomfort. The provision of food and fluids is considered basic caring and should never be withheld (unless overt aspiration or discomfort is evident). Remember that artificial tube feeding is a medical intervention that has both risks and benefits and may be refused, not begun, or withdrawn when deemed inappropriate. Under either scenario, patients and families should provide informed consent. When patients can no longer eat or swallow safely or sufficiently, careful hand feeding should be offered as tolerated. Palliative care and hospice may be most appropriate for patients nearing the end of life due to advanced illness (see Chapter "Integrating Palliative Care into Practice").

Updated Regulations Related to Nutrition and Tube Feeding

Federal regulations for nursing homes originated from the Omnibus Budget Reconciliation Act of 1987, commonly known as "OBRA." The CMS regulations were recently updated in 2016, and published in the Federal Register and in the CMS State Operations Manual Guidance to Surveyors. The regulations contain many provisions relating to nutritional status, including several newly renumbered "F-Tags."

- **F692** (Nutrition/Hydration Status)
- **F693** (Tube Feeding Management) relating to nutrition and hydration status
- **F694** (Parenteral/IV Fluids)
- **F800-814** relates to food and nutrition services.
- **FTag 692** (CFR 483.25g) specifically mandates that the facility, based on a resident's comprehensive assessment, must ensure that each resident ... :

> ... *maintains acceptable parameters of nutritional status, such as usual body weight or desirable body weight range and electrolyte balance, **unless the resident's clinical condition demonstrates that this is not possible or resident preferences indicate otherwise;***
> ... *is offered sufficient fluid intake to maintain proper hydration and health; and*
> ... *is offered a therapeutic diet when there is a nutritional problem and the health care provider orders a therapeutic diet."*
> ***F-Tag 693*** *further provides that in reference to enteral nutrition (tube feedings):*
> *A resident who has been able to eat enough alone or with assistance is not fed by enteral methods unless the resident's clinical condition demonstrates that enteral feeding was clinically indicated and consented to by the resident; and*
> *A resident who is fed by enteral means receives the appropriate treatment and services to restore, if possible, oral eating skills and to prevent complications of enteral feeding including but not limited to aspiration pneumonia, diarrhea, vomiting, dehydration, metabolic abnormalities, and nasal-pharyngeal ulcers.*

Summary

It should be understood that malnutrition and weight loss, though sometimes judged as signs of poor care or neglect, are in many instances actually a natural and inevitable process despite the best efforts of clinicians, and attributable to the patient's advanced age, loss of functioning, and underlying medical multimorbidities. To avoid claims of negligence or liability, a thorough evaluation should be performed and interventions fully documented that are consistent with the patient's condition and wishes. The patient, family, or proxy decision maker should be duly informed. If weight loss or other nutritional conditions continue to worsen and prove to be *unavoidable*, then this and its discernable causes and consequences should be clearly documented in the medical record.

Pearls for the Practitioner
- All adults in LTC require careful attention to nutrition and hydration as both are a clinical, quality of life, and legal-ethical issue.
- Frequent causes of weight loss in elderly patients include dementia and other neurologic disorders (e.g., Parkinson's), depression; drug effects/side effects, malignancies, and GI problems such as swallowing disorders and malabsorption syndromes.
- Optimal health and longevity in the elderly are achieved with a BMI of 25 ± 5.

- Innumerable drugs and diseases affect nutritional status.
- Weight and labs should be monitored periodically in all patients.
- Some patients will benefit from vitamin supplements (such as multivitamins and/ or calcium/vitamin D and/or vitamin B12), especially if blood levels indicate deficiency, but also consider *deprescribing* these and supplements that may not be necessary.
- Nutritional drinks such as Ensure can supplement inadequate calorie and protein intake.
- Hypodermoclysis may be used short term to supplement oral fluid intake and avoid dehydration.
- Restricted diets are generally not advisable or tolerated in patients and should be avoided when not absolutely necessary.
- Tube feedings are ineffective in reducing morbidity and mortality in demented patients and should be limited to carefully selected patients who need short-term nutritional support during a potentially reversible illness such as stroke.
- Federal "OBRA" regulations require nursing home facilities to ensure that each resident maintains acceptable parameters of nutritional status. AMDA's *Synopsis of Federal Regulations* [48] provides a concise tabulation of all medically related federal regulations for long-term care facilities. Note that the F-Tag numbers were updated in 2016.
- Incorporate patient preferences regarding nutrition and hydration when discussing advance directives and advance care planning.

References

1. American Medical Directors Association (AMDA). Altered nutritional status in the long-term care setting. Columbia, MD: American Medical Directors Association (AMDA); 2010, Rev. Available for purhase from AMDA at https://paltc.org/?q=product-store/altered-nutritional-status-cpg. Available online at https://fliphtml5.com/zlds/aalp. Accessed 17 July 2022.
2. Dietary Reference Intakes (DRI). https://ods.od.nih.gov/HealthInformation/Dietary_Reference_Intakes.aspx. Accessed 17 July 2022.
3. Ross AC, Manson JE, Abrams SA, Aloia JF, et al. The 2011 report on dietary reference intakes for calcium and vitamin D from the Institute of Medicine: what clinicians need to know. J Clin Endocrinol Metab. 2011;96(1):53–8. https://pubmed.ncbi.nlm.nih.gov/21118827/. Accessed 17 July 2022.
4. Miller ER, Pastor-Barriuso R, Dalal D, et al. Meta-analysis: high dosage vitamin E supplementation may increase all cause mortality. Ann Intern Med. 2005;142(1):37–46.
5. American Medical Directors Association (AMDA). Dehydration and fluid maintenance in the long-term care setting. Columbia, MD: American Medical Directors Association (AMDA); 2009, Rev. Available for purchase at https://paltc.org/product-store/dehydration-and-fluid-maintenance-cpg. Accessed 17 July 2022.
6. American Medical Directors Association (AMDA). Transitions of care in the long-term care continuum. Columbia, MD: American Medical Directors Association (AMDA); 2010. Available online at https://paltc.org/?q=product-store/transitions-care-cpg. Accessed 17 July 2022.

7. Van Bokhorst MAE, Guaitoli PR, Jansma EP, De Vet HCW. A systematic review of malnutrition screening tools for the nursing home. J Am Med Dir Assoc. 2014;15:171–84.

8. Detsky AS, McLaughlin JR, Baker JP, et al. What is subjective global assessment of nutritional status? JPEN J Parenter Enteral Nutr. 1987;11:8–13. https://pubmed.ncbi.nlm.nih.gov/3820522/. Tools available free at https://nutritioncareincanada.ca/resources-and-tools/hospital-care-inpac/assessment-sga. Accessed 17 July 2022.

9. Guigoz Y. The mini-nutritional assessment (MNA). J Nutr Health Aging. 2006;10:466–87. Tools available online at https://www.mna-elderly.com/sites/default/files/2021-10/mna-mini-english.pdf. Accessed 17 July 2022.

10. Messinger-Rapport BJ, Gammack JK, Little MO, Morley JE. Clinical update on nursing home medicine, 2014. J Am Med Dir Assoc. 2014;15:786–801.

11. Morley JE, Thomas DR, Kamel H. Nutritional deficiencies in long-term care. Ann Long Term Care. 1998;6(5):183–91.

12. Seltzer MH, Bastidas A, Cooper DM, et al. Instant nutritional assessment. JPEN J Parenter Enteral Nutr. 1979;3:157–9.

13. Corti MC, Guralnik JM, Salive ME, Sorkin JD. Serum albumin level and physical disability as predictors of mortality in older patients. J Am Med Dir Assoc. 1994;272:1036–42.

14. American Psychiatric Association practice guideline for the treatment of patients with major depressive disorder, 3rd ed. 2010. https://psychiatryonline.org/pb/assets/raw/sitewide/practice_guidelines/guidelines/mdd.pdf. Accessed 17 July 2022.

15. Wilson MM, Vaswani S, Liu D, et al. Prevalence and causes of undernutrition in medical outpatients. Am J Med. 1998;104:56.

16. Thomas DR, Ashmen W, Morley JE, et al. Nutritional management in long-term care: development of a clinical guideline. J Gerontol A Biol Sci Med Sci. 2000;55A:M725–34.

17. Bucker DA, Kelber ST, Goodwin JS. The use of dietary restrictions in malnourished nursing home patients. J Am Geriatr Soc. 1994;42:1100–2.

18. Prospective studies collaboration. Body mass index and cause specific mortality in 900000 adults: collaborative analysis of 57 prospective studies. Lancet. 2009;373:1083–96.

19. Orpana HM, Berthelot JM, Kaplan MS, Feeny DH, et al. BMI and mortality: results from a national longitudinal study of Canadian adults. Obesity. 2010;18(1):214–8.

20. Thomas DR. But is it malnutrition? J Am Med Dir Assoc. 2009;10(5):295–7.

21. Correia MI, Hegazi RA, Higashiguchi T, Michel JP, et al. Evidence-based recommendations for addressing malnutrition in health care: an updated strategy from the feed. ME Global Study Group. J Am Med Dir Assoc. 2014;15:544–50.

22. Mei A, Auerhahn C. Hypodermoclysis: maintaining hydration in the frail older adult. Ann Long Term Care. 2009;17(5):28–30.

23. Thomas DR, Tariq SH, et al. Physician misdiagnosis of dehydration in older adults. J Am Med Dir Assoc. 2003;4:251–4.

24. Bauer J, Biolo G, Cederholm T, Cesari M, et al. Evidence-based recommendations for optimal dietary protein intake in older people: a position paper from the PROT-AGE Study Group. J Am Med Dir Assoc. 2013;14(8):542–59.

25. Gaffney-Stomberg E, Insogna KL, Rodriguez NR, Kerstetter JE. Increasing dietary protein requirements for elderly people for optimal muscle and bone health. J Am Geriatr Soc. 2009;57:1073–9.

26. Levine ME, Suarez JA, Brandhorst S, Priya B, et al. Low protein intake is associated with a major reduction in IGF-1, cancer, and overall mortality in the 65 and younger but not older population. Cell Metab. 2014;19(3):407–17.

27. Imai E, Tsubota-Utsugi M, Kikuya M, Satoh M, et al. Animal protein intake is associated with higher-level functional capacity in elderly adults: the Ohasama study. J Am Geriatr Soc. 2014;62(3):426–34.

28. Morley JE, Thomas DR. Cachexia: new advances in the management of wasting diseases. J Am Med Dir Assoc. 2008;9(4):205–10.

29. Goldberg TH, Hassan T, Grant R. High prevalence of Vitamin D deficiency in elderly nursing home patients despite vitamin supplements (abstract). J Am Med Dir Assoc. 2008;9(3):B15.
30. Holick MF. High prevalence of Vitamin D inadequacy and implications for health. Mayo Clin Proc. 2006;81(3):353–73.
31. Bischoff-Ferrari HA, Dawson-Hughes B, Willett WC, et al. Effect of Vitamin D on falls: a meta-analysis. JAMA. 2004;291(16):1999–2006.
32. Bischoff-Ferrari HA, Willett WC, Wong JB, et al. Fracture prevention with Vitamin D supplementation: a meta-analysis of randomized controlled trials. J Am Med Dir Assoc. 2005;293(18):2257–64.
33. Autier P, Gandini S. Vitamin D supplementation and total mortality: a meta-analysis of randomized controlled trials. Arch Intern Med. 2007;167(16):1730–7.
34. Morley JE. Should all long-term care residents receive Vitamin D? J Am Med Dir Assoc. 2007;8:69–70.
35. Famularo P. Deprescribing: what about vitamins, minerals, and other nutritional supplements? Caring for the Ages. 2022;23(6):10–20. https://www.caringfortheages.com/article/S1526-4114(22)00273-6/fulltext. Accessed 9 April 2023.
36. Vitale CA, Monteleoni C, et al. Strategies for improving care for patients with advanced dementia and eating problems: optimizing care through physician and speech pathologist collaboration. Ann Long Term Care. 2009;17(5):32–9.
37. Nijs K, Graaf C, Staveren W, et al. Malnutrition and mealtime ambience in nursing homes. J Am Med Dir Assoc. 2009;10:226–9.
38. Yeh S, Lovitt S, Schuster MW. Pharmacological treatment of geriatric cachexia: evidence and safety in perspective. J Am Med Dir Assoc. 2007;8(6):363–77.
39. 2019 AGS Beers Criteria Update Expert Panel. American Geriatrics Society 2019 Updated AGS Beers Criteria for potentially inappropriate medication use in older adults. J Am Geriatr Soc. 2019;67(4):674–94. https://pubmed.ncbi.nlm.nih.gov/30693946 or https://agsjournals.onlinelibrary.wiley.com/doi/10.1111/jgs.15767. Accessed 17 July 2022.
40. Miller LJ, et al. Pharmacological treatment of undernutrition in the geriatric patient. Consult Pharm. 2002;17:739–47.
41. AGS Choosing Wisely Workgroup. American geriatrics society identifies another five things that healthcare providers and patient should question. J Am Geriatr Soc. 2014;62(5):950–60. https://pubmed.ncbi.nlm.nih.gov/24575770/. Accessed 9 April 2023.
42. Finucane TE, Christmas C, Travis K. Tube feeding in patients with advanced dementia: a review of the evidence. J Am Med Dir Assoc. 1999;282:1365–70.
43. Gillick M. Rethinking the role of tube feeding in patients with advanced dementia. N Engl J Med. 2000;342:206–10.
44. Kuo S, Rhodes R, Mitchell SL, et al. Natural history of feeding tube use in nursing home residents with advanced dementia. J Am Med Dir Assoc. 2009;10:264–70.
45. AMDA—The Society for Post-Acute and Long-Term Care Medicine. Fifteen things physicians and patients should question in post-acute and long-term care. https://paltc.org/choosing-wisely. Accessed 9 April 2023.
46. AGS Choosing Wisely Workgroup. American Geriatrics Society identifies five things that healthcare providers and patient should question. J Am Geriatr Soc. 2013;61:622–31. https://pubmed.ncbi.nlm.nih.gov/23469880/. Accessed 17 July 2022.
47. AGS Ethics Committee and Clinical Practice and Models of Care Committee. American Geriatrics Society feeding tubes in advanced dementia position statement. J Am Geriatr Soc. 2014;62(8):1590–3. https://pubmed.ncbi.nlm.nih.gov/25039796/. Accessed 17 July 2022.
48. American Medical Directors Association. Synopsis of Federal Regulations in the nursing facility: implications for attending physicians and medical directors. Available for purchase online from AMDA at https://paltc.org/?q=synopsis-federal-regulations. Accessed 9 April 2023.

Wound Assessment and Management

Richard G. Stefanacci

Introduction

The medical and psychosocial complexities of wound care highlight the challenges that face practitioners in long-term care (LTC). Understanding wound formation and healing is critical to the prevention and treatment of wounds. Treatment plans must not only address the wound itself but also comorbidities and medications that may hinder healing or predispose patients to acquiring wounds. The psychosocial and ethical principles of caring for patients who are no longer able to participate in their own care subsume a critical role in treatment success or failure. Though wounds may have more than one etiology, the four most common types of wounds will be reviewed: pressure, diabetic, ischemic or arterial, and venous. Pressure injuries are emphasized due to their implications on quality of care in the LTC environment. The occurrence and poor management of wounds is a major area of liability for facilities and practitioners.

Upon admission to a nursing facility 17–35% of patients have pressure injuries while the prevalence of pressure injuries ranges from 7% to 23% among nursing home residents. Among high-risk patients, (bedridden or nonambulatory) the incidence of pressure injuries is estimated to be 14/1000 patient-days [1]. The most recent data on the prevalence of pressure wounds reported by the CDC and extracted from the National Nursing Home Survey, reported that 159,000 current nursing home residents (11%) had pressure injuries. Stage 2 pressure injuries were the most common [2]. Note that the terminology for a pressure ulcer has changed to that of *pressure injury* by the National Pressure Ulcer Advisory Panel (NPUAP).

R. G. Stefanacci (✉)
Thomas Jefferson University, Jefferson College of Population Health, Philadelphia, PA, USA

© The Author(s), under exclusive license to Springer Nature
Switzerland AG 2023
P. Winn et al. (eds.), *Post-Acute and Long-Term Care Medicine*, Current Clinical
Practice, https://doi.org/10.1007/978-3-031-28628-5_13

Morbidity associated with pressure injuries is significant with residents experiencing a 6-month mortality rate as high as 77.3% [3]. And 55.7% residents who die with a pressure injury do so within 6 weeks of the onset of the pressure injury [4].

The Centers for Medicare and Medicaid Services (CMS) has established a payment system, which ceases paying hospitals for "preventable complications," or "never events" that occur during a hospitalization. This includes Stage III and IV pressure injuries [5]. The term "Never Event" was first introduced in 2001 by Ken Kizer, MD, former CEO of the National Quality Forum (NQF), in reference to avoidable and severe medical errors. Hospitals typically care for patients for very short lengths of stay, the average length of stay being 4–5 days, Thus the occurrence of a pressure wound is considered to be unlikely and should "never" occur. SNFs like hospitals have a responsibility to prevent pressure injuries. This includes assessing patient risk to acquire a pressure injury from which the resident care plan can be developed and implemented with ongoing monitoring and adjustments to the treatment plan.

The basic premise in prevention is *pressure off-loading*. In addition, the degree of pressure and its duration are major attributing factors. Due to longer stays of residents in nursing facilities, facilities must focus on the prevention of these wounds. Prevention of a pressure injury is critical as once it has occurred these wounds become more difficult to heal [6]. Complications include increased mortality and morbidity such as cellulitis, osteomyelitis, and sepsis, even limb amputation. Accordingly, skilled nursing facilities' staff must carefully exam all admitted patients to identify *wounds present on admission* (POA) *having started during the preceding hospital admission.*

In the "Guidance to Surveyors for Long Term Care Facilities," CMS acknowledges that some pressure injuries are "unavoidable" [7]. If a pressure injury develops despite the facility's best efforts to prevent it, the pressure injury is determined to be unavoidable. Evidence from the literature suggests that many of the known risk factors to the development and failure of wounds to heal are unmodifiable so *management of modifiable factors is essential*. CMS surveyor guidelines F686 on skin integrity *recognize that pressure injuries as "unavoidable" when appropriate assessment and interventions were implemented and treatment documented*. To be considered unavoidable the nursing home staff must demonstrate that the pressure wound developed in the presence of the standard of care in risk assessment, prevention, and the treatment provided (in the context of resident needs and goals of care and life).

The most recent guidelines from the National Pressure Ulcer Advisory Panel (NPUAP) multidisciplinary conference on wound management were updated in 2019 [8]. AMDA has also updated the Pressure Ulcers and Other Wounds Clinical Practice Guideline to now include information regarding arterial and venous ulcers [9].

Wound care should be guided and focused on the following domains: Management, Prevention, Treatment and Care.

1. Management

    (a) Pressure wound risk assessment
    (b) Care plan development and implementation
    (c) Monitoring and adjustment of the care plan

2. Prevention

   (a) Pressure off-loading
   (b) Skin protection
   (c) Nutrition and overall health maintain (smoking cessation, diabetes, hypertension, COPD)

3. Treatment and Basic Care

   (a) When wet make dry, when dry make wet
   (b) Treat infections
   (c) Remove dead tissue

Risk Assessment

Wounds develop when causative factors increase a patient's susceptibility to developing a wound, or persist when factors impair the healing of an existing wound [10]. These risk factors are listed in Table 1. Relieving pressure on the wound area is a cornerstone to wound prevention and treatment. Because pressure is a primary causal factor, a plan for patient repositioning needs to be implemented and tailored to the needs of each patient. Wounded skin has only about 80% of the tensile

Table 1 Risk factors

Risk factor	Examples	Notes
Comorbid conditions	Diabetes, end-stage renal disease, thyroid disease	Conditions that increase risk of wounds by affecting patient's immune response, skin integrity, or environment risks
Drugs	Steroids, antimetabolites	Drugs that hinder proliferation of fibroblasts and collagen synthesis
History of healed ulcer History of Stage III or IV ulcer		Patient may still have risk factors that predispose to these ulcers
Impaired blood flow	Atherosclerosis, lower extremity arterial insufficiency	Decrease blood flow for wounds to heal
Impaired or decreased mobility and functional ability	Bed bound, decreased lower extremity use, altered mental status (e.g., dementia)	Environmental risk of developing wounds due to increased pressure on skin, friction, or shear during transfer or repositioning
Malnutrition and hydration deficit		Protein–calorie malnutrition and deficiencies of vitamins A, C, and zinc impair normal wound-healing mechanisms

Adapted from AMDA Pressure Ulcers in the Long-Term Care Setting. Clinical Practice Guideline 2008 (last updated 2012)

properties of intact skin and thus is at an increased risk of breakdown. Patients with a history of pressure injuries are five times more likely to develop another pressure injury [11]. Dermatologic conditions and limb contractures also increase the occurrence of wounds.

Peripheral arterial disease hinders wound healing by depriving the injured area of oxygen and nutrients. Diabetics are at additional risk of foot wounds due to the triad of peripheral neuropathy, microvascular disease, and suboptimal glycemic control. It is estimated that among patients with diabetes, 15% will develop a foot wound, and 12–24% of those will eventually require amputation. Even with successful wound healing, the recurrence rate of a diabetic foot wound is 66% [12].

End-stage renal disease and thyroid disease are also risk factors for skin injury. Steroids and anti-metabolites hinder proliferation of fibroblasts and collagen synthesis that are integral to wound healing.

Cognitive impairment, seen in 45–67% of assisted living residents and 69% of nursing facility residents, increases the risk for skin breakdown [13]. Risks include functional disability, poor nutritional status, and a higher incidence of skin exposure to pressure, friction, and shear. Moisture-related skin breakdown is often associated with excess perspiration, heavy wound exudates, and urine and/or fecal incontinence. Diarrhea is caustic and urine contains urea and ammonia, both of which damage normal skin. With prolonged exposure, these fluids soften the outer protective layer of skin and result in skin breakdown [14]. Data also suggest an association between fecal incontinence and skin injury likely related to skin exposure to bile acid and gastrointestinal enzymes [15].

Poor nutritional status frequently seen in patients with advanced dementia is another risk factor for wound development. Dehydration, deficiencies of arginine, vitamins A, C, and zinc, as well as protein–calorie malnutrition have all been implicated in wound development and impaired wound healing [16]. With dehydration, skin integrity and wound healing are impaired due to decreased tissue perfusion. Severe protein–calorie malnutrition hinders tissue regeneration, the inflammatory reaction, and immune function. Albumin and prealbumin levels are indicators of protein–calorie nutritional status (see Chapter "Weight and Nutrition in Post-Acute and Long-Term Care" for further discussion). Obesity places patients at risk for skin breakdown under the pannus or in skin folds [16]. The warm and moist environment in skin folds promote the growth of yeast and bacteria that further increase the risk for wounds to occur.

An initial skin assessment should be performed immediately upon admission of a resident to the LTC facility to note any and all skin issues described as Present on Admission (POA). An ulcer can develop after only a few hours of pressure. Discovered wounds should prompt thorough patient assessment and a treatment plan that includes a timeline for wound reassessment. This assessment involves a complete medical evaluation of the patient including careful attention to conditions that may predispose to wound development and delay healing. A comprehensive wound history should be obtained, if possible.

Wound Assessment

Assessment of the patient's living and personal environment is also important. Frequency of repositioning, surfaces, turning schedules, transferring techniques, and durable medical equipment (such as assistive devices, trapeze, bed rails, and padding) can all impact wound development and healing. *Use of risk assessment scales* may increase awareness, but have limited predictability and effectiveness in pressure injury prevention [17]. A meta-analysis of 33 studies demonstrated a lack of evidence for risk assessment scales in decreasing pressure injury incidence, *but the scales did increase preventive interventions* [18]. The two most commonly used tools are the Braden and Norton scales. No conclusive evidence demonstrates that one is superior to the other.

- **The Braden scale** evaluates six categories: sensory perception, moisture, activity, mobility, nutrition, friction, and shear for predicting pressure injury development. Research has shown that patients with scores of 18 or less are at risk for the development of pressure sores [19].
- **The Norton Score** is another commonly used tool for assessing pressure injury risk that evaluates five categories: physical condition, mental condition, activity, mobility, and incontinence.

Most nursing facilities use a pressure injury report to document identified wounds: location, stage, measurement, and description. Pressure injury reports fulfill standardized documentation as mandated by both state and federal (F686) regulations. Practitioners should document the number, location, and size (length, width, and depth **in centimeters**) of wounds and assess for the presence of an exudate, odor, sinus tracts, necrosis or eschar formation, tunneling/undermining, infection, healing signs (granulation and epithelialization), and wound margins. **For a pressure injury**, determine the stage of the ulcer according to the National Pressure Injury Advisory Panel (NPIAP) Staging System (Table 2).

Risk of developing a pressure injury is significantly high within the first 4 weeks after admission to a long-term care facility [20]. After the initial assessment, a weekly reassessment should occur during the first 4 weeks, followed by at least a quarterly assessment and when there is a change in patient status [21]. The patient's overall clinical condition should be reassessed whenever a pressure injury fails to show evidence of healing within 2–4 weeks of any intervention. Every nursing facility is required to develop and implement its own comprehensive wound care plan in accordance with CMS regulations.

Some patients develop a pressure injury 2–3 days before death. These are referred to as **Kennedy terminal ulcers** and are markers of imminent death. The Kennedy ulcer develops suddenly over the sacrum as a blister or Stage 2 and rapidly progress to Stage 3 or 4. These ulcers can be pear-, horseshoe-, or butterfly-shaped with irregular borders. Kennedy terminal ulcers are initially

Table 2 National Pressure Injury Advisory Panel Staging System

Stage	Definition	Comment
Suspected deep tissue injury (SDTI)	Pressure-related necrosis of soft tissue with intact overlying skin	Discoloration (crimson→purple), changes in temperature, texture, tenderness. May progress rapidly
Stage I	Localized nonblanchable erythema. Skin intact. Compressed between bony prominence and external surface	Clinically similar to SDTI. May be difficult to detect with deepened skin pigmentation
Stage II	Exposed dermis characterized as either a shallow ulcer with a crimson wound bed (without slough or bruising) or as an intact or ruptured fluid-filled blister	Do not use to describe skin tears, tape burns, dermatitis, maceration, or excoriation
Stage III	Full thickness skin loss. Adipose tissue may be visible, but bone, tendon, or muscle not exposed	Tunneling or undermining may occur. Depth may vary by location
Stage IV	Full thickness skin and tissue loss characterized by exposed bone, tendon, or muscle. Rolled edges, undermining and/or tunneling often occur	Slough or eschar if present may obscure the extent of tissue loss
Unstageable	Full thickness skin and tissue loss which cannot be staged until slough or eschar is removed from the ulcer bed	Do not remove eschar present on heels

Adapted from Edsberg, L. E. et al J Wound Ostomy Continence Nurse 2016:43(6):585–597

red/purple, then turn to yellow, and finally turn black. The etiology is unclear, but is thought to be part of multiorgan failure. Treatment is the same as that for pressure injuries.

Types of Wounds

There are four main categories of wounds (pressure injury, diabetic, arterial, and venous), and those of mixed etiology. The type of wound can usually be determined by its location, inspection of the wound, and the patient's clinical history. If the wound type remains uncertain, laboratory and/or radiographic studies may help. For example, with a lower extremity wound, an ankle-brachial index or a Doppler arterial study can help determine whether the ulcer is caused by vascular insufficiency, pressure or both.

Pressure Injury

- 95% of wounds develop on the lower body, 65% over the sacrum and pelvic area, and 30% in the lower extremities. Other common pressure sites include the coccyx, heels, ischium, iliac crest, lateral foot, lateral malleolus, and greater trochanter.
- There are three mechanical factors that can produce tissue damage: pressure, friction, and shear. Shearing occurs between shifting of tissue plains beneath the

skin. A friction (or rubbing) injury is superficial and easily discernible (e.g., as may occur with a Parkinson tremor). Shear and friction usually occur together to cause skin injuries.

- A pressure injury is a localized area of damaged or necrotic tissue that develops when soft tissue is compressed between a bony prominence and an external surface for a prolonged period of time.
- In 2009, NPUAP-EPUAP *redefined* a pressure "ulcer" as "*a compressive tissue injury*" that is caused by pressure alone *or* by pressure combined with shearing. Friction alone is not a direct cause of a pressure injury, but it does contribute shear strain in tissue.
- Pressure injuries can range from *nonblanchable erythema* of intact skin (Stage 1) (or in dark-skinned persons, the skin may have a deep blue or purple hue), to deep ulcers extending down to the bone (Stage IV).
- The skin failure at the end of life is not considered to be a pressure injury. Skin tears, abrasions, or lacerations are not pressure injuries.

Diabetic Wounds

- Commonly occur over the metatarsal heads.
- Due to vascular compromise of the lower extremities coupled with a decreased potential for healing and peripheral neuropathy.
- Typically painless, thus the wound is often not noticed until symptoms of infection occur (malodor, fever or chills).
- When examining the wound it should be probed with a sterile implement to assess its depth and to determine whether undermining or osteomyelitis could be present [22].

Ischemic Wounds

- Typically occur in the lower extremities, but can also occur in the upper extremities.
- Diabetes mellitus and smoking have been implicated as contributing factors due to their decreasing arterial blood flow causing peripheral vascular disease.
- Clinical signs of arterial insufficiency often precede development of an ischemic wound. These include a cold, pale or cyanotic foot, absence of digital and lower extremity hair, and thin atrophic skin of the legs.
- Present either as a painful wound with discrete borders (a "punched out" appearance), or "wet" or "dry" gangrene.
- The base of the ulcer may be covered with a dry black or brown eschar, or appear pale pink and fibrous.

Venous Wounds

- Commonly seen in the lower extremities.
- Caused by peripheral edema due to venous insufficiency/stasis, and may be associated with organ dysfunction (i.e., heart, liver, and kidney) [23].
- Less painful than ischemic wounds.
- Have irregular borders and often seen with hyperpigmented changes of the surrounding skin.

Prevention of Wounds

Paramount to wound care management is prevention. In 2014 the Agency for Health Care Policy and Research (AHCP) had developed guidelines and recommendations on the prediction, prevention and early treatment of pressure injuries in adults [24], that are still widely utilized today as they remain applicable in many health care settings. *The first step* recommended for the prevention of pressure injuries by the Institute for Healthcare Improvement (IHI) is to *identify patients at risk,* and then implement prevention strategies in these patients [25]. The *"six essential elements of pressure injury prevention"* include:

- "Conduct" a *pressure injury assessment* on *admission* for all patients.
- *"Reassess risk"* for all patients daily
- *"Inspect"* skin *daily*
- "Manage" *moisture*
- "Optimize" *nutrition and hydration*
- "Minimize" *pressure*

The IHI recommends that prevention measures include a comprehensive treatment plan with risk factor reduction, multidisciplinary interventions, functional adaptation, environmental modifications, and a psychosocial evaluation. Evaluating and optimizing residents' *predisposing conditions* and *comorbidities* can help prevent the development of wounds. Inspecting the skin daily during bathing or personal care, as well as scheduled turning and positioning of patients, has been shown to help prevent wounds. Provide *support surfaces* with special mattresses and overlays to help eliminate friction, shear, and moisture. *Minimize pressure over bony prominences. Seats* should be padded with air, foam, or gel cushioning and avoid use of donut-shaped devices. Residents at highest risk (those who completely compress a static surface, or have pressure injuries that fail to heal), should be placed on *a dynamic surface.* A patient should never be directly positioned on the greater trochanter for more than momentary positioning. *Use padding* (i.e., heel or "bunny" boots, egg crates, heel lifts, suspension devices, etc.) for *off-loading of heels and elbows.* Patients should have a static support surface such as a *foam overlay or gel mattress placed on their standard mattress.* A supine patient should be maintained at the *lowest head elevation below 30° as tolerated*; head elevation ≥30° provides as much pressure as being in a seated position. *Repositioning* every 4 h has been shown to be as effective as 2-h intervals in wound healing, but this *repositioning or partial turning does not always remove pressure from the sacrum or heels.* Care should be taken to *minimize shearing or friction during repositioning.* If necessary, *lift devices* should be used to prevent soft tissue injury. *Slow gradual turns should be used in patients with hemodynamic instability.*

The 2-h turning schedule was established through research done in 1946 on spinal cord injury patients [26]. However, the actual *interval for optimal turning* in prevention has *not been established.* This interval can be shortened or lengthened by a host of intrinsic and extrinsic factors. For example, in a study using healthy volunteers, intervals of 1–1.5 h rather than the traditional 2-h schedule were required to prevent skin erythema on a standard mattress [27].

Nutritional and hydration status are intrinsic factors that affect pressure wound development and healing. Hospitalized patients who are undernourished are twice as likely to develop pressure injuries as compared to non-undernourished patients [28]. Inadequate hydration and nutrition predispose to pressure injury development [16]. The daily caloric intake of 30–35 kcal/kg and *daily protein intake* of 1.2–1.5 g/kg of body weight is recommended for nutritionally compromised patients who either have or are at risk of pressure injuries. *Adequate fluid hydration* is provided by 30–35 mL of fluid per kg body weight per day, or 1 mL of fluid per calorie for persons receiving enteral tube feeding. *Enteral nutritional support* can significantly reduce the risk of developing pressure injuries in selected patients by up to 25% in some studies. The benefit of nutritional support in promoting wound healing is still debated [29]. Use of vitamin C supplementation in wound healing is disputed. Two well-designed randomized controlled trials compared high dose vitamin C with either low dose vitamin C or placebo and had contradictory results [30]. (For a more in-depth discussion on nutrition refer to the Chapter on "Weight and Nutrition in Post-Acute and Long-Term Care.")

Under clinical circumstances such as metastatic cancer, multiple organ failure, cachexia, severe vascular compromise, and terminal illness, **unavoidable wounds** may develop [31]. The clinician should judiciously document the reasons why preventive interventions were not appropriate, untreatable, or unsuccessful, such as frequent repositioning causing discomfort or severe pain.

Unavoidable Pressure Ulcers/Injuries

Pressure ulcers/injuries are considered to be a quality measure of care in LTC. There are many factors that are responsible for "unavoidable" pressure injuries. According to the National Pressure Ulcer Advisory Panel (NPUAP) a pressure injury is considered to be unavoidable if it developed despite the following interventions.

1. The patient's clinical condition and risk for pressure injuries were evaluated.
2. Interventions were consistent with the patient's needs and goals, as well as recognized standards of practice that were assessed and implemented.
3. The impact of the interventions was monitored, evaluated, and revised as necessary.

A pressure injury is considered to be avoidable if the facility failed to implement these interventions. Many LTC residents are either bed or chair-bound, which significantly limits pressure off-loading and places them at risk for pressure injury. Residents with hemodynamic instability can make turning or repositioning at risk to develop bradycardia, hypotension, or hypoxemia. In addition, some patients are comfortable in a particular body position and may move themselves back into the previous position after being turned. Vasoconstrictive medication to counter low blood pressure can predispose to skin ischemia. An advanced directive for health care that defers artificial nutrition and hydration can put the patient at risk for malnutrition and skin ulcer development. Refusal of basic personal care is a common issue, especially in residents who are confused and cognitively impaired. This can frustrate staff who are attempting to offload tissue pressure.

Staging of Pressure Ulcers/Injuries

AMDA—The Society for Post-Acute and Long-Term Care Medicine follows the guidelines set forth by the National Pressure Ulcer Advisory Panel (NPUAP) that define, classify, and stage pressure injuries as summarized in Table 2. Staging is based on the extent of observable tissue damage [32]. The latest version of these guidelines describe Stages I–IV along with two adjunctive terms, "suspected deep tissue injury and "unstageable," utilized to more accurately classify these wounds (see website http://www.npuap.org). *Reverse staging should not be used.* For example, a lesion may be referred to as a, "healing stage IV" but it cannot be described as progressing from a Stage IV to a Stage III. If a healed Stage IV pressure injury reopens at the same anatomical site, it is always considered as Stage IV. A wound covered by eschar should be categorized as a Stage IV until the eschar has been debrided or self-debrides. *Do **not** debride wounds over the heal as this can expose the calcaneum and result in osteomyelitis.*

Serialized staging of wounds can help monitor wound progression and healing. The *Pressure Ulcer Scale for Healing (PUSH)* tool was developed by the NPUAP to help monitor pressure wound healing over time. It evaluates wound surface area, exudate, and the type of tissue seen in the wound bed. This scale has been adopted by many institutions [33]. Despite the theoretical simplicity of the PUSH tool, confusion regarding its use and interpretation still exists leading to inter-practitioner variability in staging ulcers [34]. The NPUAP guidelines have been used (at times inappropriately) as "quality of care" indicators or to identify suboptimal wound management.

Management of Wounds

The *burden of wound care* treatment should be weighed against its *intended benefit*. Communication with the patient and family/caregivers is important and concerns should be clarified and discussed. However, it is imperative to establish realistic expectations for wound healing. As with any medical treatment, if a patient with decision-making capacity declines or does not adhere to the recommended plan of treatment, the practitioners should offer alternatives and document them in the medical record. A palliative approach should always be considered when wound healing is unlikely. With good care many Stage 1 or 2 wounds can heal in persons on hospice.

Treatment of Wounds

Numerous factors impede healing. An interdisciplinary team approach is essential. Table 3 provides commonly encountered challenges to optimal wound care.

Principles of Treatment for Wound Care in Long-Term Care [35].

1. Assess risk factors, preexisting wounds, pain, and quality of life.
2. Consider an analgesic medication prior to and after wound care/dressing changes and, if needed, prescribe scheduled pain medicine for chronic wound pain.
3. Clean the wound surface with an isotonic solution (normal saline) to remove debris and to decrease bacterial load.
4. Debride necrotic tissue—sharp, autolytic, mechanical, biologic, and enzymatic debridement.

Table 3 Wound care challenges

Wound type	Challenge to wound care	Standard approach	Treatment
Pressure	Excess pressure and shear/friction forces	Pressure relief	Topical: packing with hydrogel or saline. Devices: Pressure reduction mattresses, padding overlying bony prominences
Ischemic	Inadequate blood flow	Revascularization or surgical removal/correction	Topical: dry or antimicrobial
Venous	Venous insufficiency causing edema	Correct incompetent valves, reduce edema	Topical: moist environment
Diabetic	Peripheral neuropathy causing pressure points on feet	Offload pressure, careful routine evaluation of feet	Topical: pack with antimicrobial solution or hydrogel

5. Fill dead space (undermining, tunnels) with loose absorbent wound packing.
6. Decrease bacterial load/infection.
7. Keep the wound moist to promote granulation with appropriate dressings—films, foams, alginates, hydroactives, hydrogels, and hydrocolloids.
8. Support the wound healing process with adjunctive treatments—vacuum-assisted closure, electric stimulation, skin grafts, and growth factor treatment.
9. Prevent further injury by relieving pressure and providing proper surface support to protect the surrounding skin.
10. Improve the patient's overall condition with proper nutrition and hydration.
11. Manage risk factors and comorbidities—diabetes, ESRD, anemia, PVD, malnutrition.
12. Address complications—psychosocial issues, malodor, exudates.
13. Accurately track wound-healing progress using tools—PUSH, Sussman Assessment Tool.

Causal factors should continue to be identified and addressed, including systemic factors and comorbidities. Optimize nutritional status. Address psychosocial issues. Manage pain and infection; both are crucial for effective wound care. If necrotic tissue exists, it should be debrided in order to allow viable granulation and wound healing to occur. Wounds should be cleansed and irrigated to remove necrotic debris at each dressing change. Necrotic tissue impedes the healing process and may represent a nidus for infection. Saline should be chosen for wound irrigation rather than cytotoxic antiseptic agents such as Dakin's solution, iodine, and acid- and alcohol-based solutions that can retard healing.

There are five methods of debridement—sharp or surgical, autolytic, mechanical, biologic, and enzymatic debridement. Any *dry black eschar on the heels* should **not** be debrided **unless** it is tender, fluctuant, erythematous, or suppurative. Wounds with no surrounding local infection can have an occlusive hydrocolloid dressing placed over them, allowing the eschar to autodigest itself via autolytic debridement. Hydrocolloids and hydrogels are used as autolytic debridement and help to maintain moisture in the dressing. Enzymatic debridement involves applying a topical debriding agent such as collagenase or papain-urea to devitalized tissue. This may cause some degree of pain but is more tolerable than surgical debridement. Biological debridement uses live, disinfected larvae, or maggots. Mechanical debridement uses dressings that are allowed to dry and then removed, peeling off nonviable adherent tissue. This mode of debridement has fallen into disfavor as it also removes new healing tissue!

When a wound is exceptionally large, malodorous, or has a large amount of necrotic tissue, more aggressive measures may be required. If all other methods of debridement have failed and/or timing is critical because of worsening infection and imminent sepsis, surgical debridement may be necessary. Obviously, the risks of an invasive procedure with sharp debridement, albeit relatively low, must be weighed against the intended benefits.

Major categories of dressings that cover wounds include films, foams, alginates, hydroactives, hydrogels, and hydrocolloids. Many products exist in combinations. A chosen dressing must be able to maintain a moist wound bed, keep surrounding skin dry, and limit contamination of the wound. The ideal wound bed is not too moist or dry. The wound characteristics as well as the wound coverings' cost, ease of use, and made of action should be considered when choosing a product. Wound care also includes the use of transparent, impermeable films on wounds that could be contaminated by urinary or fecal incontinence. These dressings need to be attached with waterproof tape to intact skin. Deep wounds and wounds with tunneling or undermining should be lightly packed with moist gauze or other filler. Packing should be changed regularly to avoid contamination with bacteria. Hydrogels are useful for deep wounds with little exudate whereas alginates help absorb tissue fluid and significant exudate. Overly dry intact skin should be protected with moisturizers. Silver impregnated dressings provide broad-spectrum antimicrobial coverage in lesions that are colonized or particularly susceptible to becoming infected based on location, mechanism, or clinical context. Collagen dressings promote the development of new granulation tissue.

Several novel modalities have recently been developed with mixed. These include growth factors (fibroblast growth factor, platelet-derived growth factor, and nerve growth factor); electrotherapy; and negative pressure wound therapy. One type of negative pressure therapy is vacuum-assisted closure (VAC). A wound VAC is a closed system that uses negative pressure to drain wound fluid and approximate wound edges, thereby promoting wound healing. Although this therapy may improve healing, it has not been shown to be cost effective [36]. Hyperbaric oxygen therapy increases oxygen tension at the wound site and has demonstrated improved healing rates in selected patients. Its use has been limited by high cost and lack of availability. Other novel therapies that have proven successful are noncontact normothermic wound therapy, ultrasound/ultrasonic misting, as well as infrared and ultraviolet light therapy.

Complications of Wounds

Pressure injuries are associated with a multitude of short- and long-term medical and psychosocial complications [37]. These may have a significant and damaging impact on a person's sense of well-being by worsening quality of life with isolation, increased dependence, pain, and disfigurement [38]. Odor, drainage, and pain from the wound are common. Infection is a major complication that spans the spectrum from clinically insignificant bacterial colonization to cellulitis, deep tissue infection, osteomyelitis, and sepsis. Treating infected wounds can be difficult because they may be chronically contaminated and/or colonized and topical antibiotic agents are often caustic to cells and growth factors required for healing. Osteomyelitis is more common in this population as pressure sores frequently occur over bony prominences [39].

Wound odor and heavy exudates can distress patients and result in significant feelings of embarrassment and/or depression. This can then lead to decreased social interaction and poor quality of life. Adequate wound cleaning, debridement, and proper disposal of used dressings can significantly control odor. Topical metronidazole can help control odor by eradicating anaerobic bacteria. Other products to decrease bacterial count and odor include cadexomer iodine, Dakin solution, medical-grade honey, and silver dressings. Excessive wound exudates can lead to maceration, breakdown, and itching. Foams and alginate dressings are good choices to reduce these exudates. However, excessive dryness in a wound causes delayed wound healing by inhibiting epithelialization. An absorptive dressing should not excessively dry the wound.

Pressure injuries in long-term care residents have been shown to increase morbidity and mortality especially from sepsis. Osteomyelitis is associated with high levels of morbidity related to the need for several weeks of IV antibiotics, extra radiographic imaging, and surgical debridement. These occurrences contribute to side effects, discomfort, and immobility. Because skin breakdown can be a portal for bacteremia, nursing facility residents have been shown to have a high risk of sepsis with mortality rates as high as 50% [40]. In one study, nursing facility residents with pressure injuries were shown to be two to three times more likely to die (as compared to their cohort who have no pressure injuries) with a 1-year mortality rate of 50%. The length of hospitalization for nursing facility residents with pressure injuries is two to three times greater than those without [41]. Anyone with a large wound or large amount of drainage should be monitored for dehydration and metabolic derangements. Any nonhealing wound should be evaluated for fistula formation, heterotopic calcification, and squamous cell carcinoma.

Wound prevention and management have financial implications. Estimates have shown that the cost of care triples for a nursing home resident with a pressure injury. The Centers for Medicare and Medicaid Services (CMS) periodically revises the Interpretive guidance and investigative protocol for Surveyors for use in assessing wound care in nursing facilities. As of 2014 the CMS guidelines under Federal Tag F686 state that a nursing facility may be cited if they fail to prevent new pressure injury development; fail to promote healing of previously identified injury; fail to prevent ulcer progression; fail to treat an infectious complication of a pressure injury; or there is development of a Stage 4 ulcer, unless the wound is deemed unavoidable [42].

Accurate and complete documentation of wound care is vital. Wound parameter and description are reviewed in Table 4. For optimal wound care, AMDA The Society for PA and LTC Medicine recommends standardized timelines for assessment, descriptions, care plans, and treatments of wounds. A timeline should include reevaluations based on the severity of the wound. As previously discussed, a thorough skin examination should occur on admission to LTC that identifies and documents any existing wounds. Scheduled 2–3 week reevaluations should be performed by trained staff members that know how to follow a consistent approach to wound care and its documentation. In community-based home care or in assisted living wound care can be improved when the physician and facility engage the services of a home health care agency.

Table 4 Components for documentation of wounds

Parameter	Description
Type	Pathology or disease etiology Duration of wound If applicable, what setting it occurred
Size	Measurement in centimeters: length, width, depth
Color	Define in percentage, with red indicating amount of granulation tissue, yellow indicating amount of slough present, and black indicating necrotic tissue or eschar
Exudates	Describe absence or presence of exudates If exudates present, describe if serous, serosanguinous, sanguineous, or purulent
Odor	Determine after wound is cleaned, if odor is present or absent
Peri-wound tissue	Describe if viable, macerated, inflamed, or hyperkeratotic
Undermining	Describe absence or presence of tunneling or sinus tracts

Adapted from American Medical Directors Association Pressure Ulcers in the Long-Term Care Setting Clinical Practice Guideline

IDT Member Roles/Responsibilities for Wound Management

In post-acute and long-term care, skin care involves many disciplines. Each discipline has a key role to ensuring effective wound care.

Certified Nurses Aid (CNA)—identification of skin issues as observed while providing routine bathing and toileting with notification of any and all concerns to the nursing staff for assessment.

- Nurse—Identification of skin concerns, bringing these to the attention of the attending PCP, as well as following skin orders and care plan.
- PCP—Working with SNF staff to identify skin issues, assist in development of the care plan, write appropriate orders, and consider referral to the wound care team and/or specialist.
- Consultant Pharmacist—During monthly drug regimen review assure appropriate use of wound treatments especially antibiotics to prevent inappropriate antibiotic use.
- Dietitian—Assess and assure essential nutritional support to assure appropriate skin care.
- Medical Director—Develop, implement, and track the progress of a comprehensive skin care program. This can be part of a Quality Assurance and Performance Improvement Program (QAPI).
- Administrative—Assure availability of needed staff, specialist, and supplies including specialty beds.
- Admission Coordinator—Assess incoming residents to assure that their wound care needs can be met by the SNF.
- Wound Care Team—Provide comprehensive skin care management including assessment and prevention of patients at high risk for skin breakdown.

- Transitionist/Discharge—In transitioning patients from a subacute stay to the community assure continuation of care plan through patient adherence, caregiver support, and use of home care services including durable medical equipment services.
- Homecare Services—To continue the skin care plan for patients returning home following a subacute stay.
- Hospice—That the required written agreement that each hospice agency must have with each nursing facility includes the separation of role and responsibilities between the hospice organization and the nursing facility as to whether the facility or the hospice is to provide wound care.

CMS Wound Management Guidance (F686)

The Centers for Medicare and Medicaid Services (CMS) has an F-tag focused on Wound Management. F686 Treatment/Services to Prevent/Heal Pressure Ulcers.

This regulation states that based on the comprehensive assessment of a patient, the facility must ensure that:

(i) A patient receives care, consistent with professional standards of practice, to prevent pressure injuries and does not develop pressure injuries unless the individual's clinical condition demonstrates that they were unavoidable
(ii) A patient with pressure injuries receives necessary treatment and services, consistent with professional standards of practice, to promote healing, prevent infection, and prevent new ulcers from developing.

The intent of this requirement is that the patient does not develop pressure ulcers/injuries (PU/PIs) unless clinically unavoidable and that the facility provides care and services consistent with professional standards of practice to:

- Promote the prevention of pressure ulcer/injury development.
- Promote the healing of existing pressure ulcers/injuries (including prevention of infection to the extent possible).
- Prevent development of additional pressure ulcer/injury.

Factors that CMS considers as part of wound management that are extracted from the Minimum Data Set (MDS), include the following:

- Turning and repositioning the patient every 2 h
- Assisting with toileting and/or providing incontinence care every 2 h and as needed
- Using a pressure relieving mattress to decrease pressure on bony prominences
- Application of heel protectors
- Promoting adequate nutritional intake
- Providing nutritional supplements as ordered
- Ensuring adequate hydration

– Using proper lifting and transfer techniques to avoid trauma due to shearing or friction

These regulations and guidance are important for nursing facilities and practitioners to appreciate and establish as a foundation for wound care management.

Summary

The need for assessment and management of wounds in LTC residents has increased along with the increasing geriatric demographic of advanced age and morbidity. Wounds represent a geriatric syndrome with significant medical, psychosocial, and economic implications. Given the increase in morbidity, mortality, and costs related to wounds, they have become a top priority in LTC regulation at the national and state levels. LTC residents are more susceptible to developing pressure injuries due to impaired mobility and compromised nutrition status, as well as multi-morbidities including diabetes, cardiovascular disease, and dementia. If prevention through risk factor modification has failed or a resident is found to have a wound present on admission (POA), the admission assessment should include a thorough and timely evaluation of the resident and their environment and the need to document wound characteristics and proper staging. Wound management requires an interdisciplinary and multidisciplinary approach based on frequent assessment and use of wound-specific treatment modalities. The functional status of the resident, goals of care, and risk-benefit ratio of any treatment should all factor into the treatment plan. Pain should always be assessed and treated. Care should be taken to reduce pressure, friction, shearing forces, moisture, exposure to bacteria, and pain. Preventing and treating wounds can reduce medical and psychosocial complications, decrease morbidity and mortality, and improve the quality of life of LTC residents.

Pearls for the Practitioner
- As the complexity of residents in long-term care has increased, the prevalence of wounds has also increased.
- An interdisciplinary and multidisciplinary team in conjunction with the patient and family should develop a holistic wound care treatment plan that considers resident factors into the goals of care, as well as appropriate wound-specific care and adequate pain control.
- All wounds are not pressure injuries. Thus, the NPUAP guidelines cannot be applied to traumatic, ischemic, venous, or diabetic wounds.
- As pressure injuries heal, reverse staging is **not** used.
- All wounds covered by eschar should be categorized as a suspected deep tissue injury (SDTI).
- Any dry, black eschar on the heel should not be debrided if it is nontender, nonfluctuant, nonerythematous, and nonsuppurative.

- Not all ulcers are avoidable. Some pressure injuries are unavoidable due to the overwhelming burden of risk factors, multiple diseases, and advanced life-limiting illness.

Websites
- Home of the Braden Scale—http://www.bradenscale.com
- National Pressure Ulcer Advisory Panel—http://www.npuap.org/
- American Medical Directors Association (AMDA)—www.amda.com/http://www.amda.com/tools/library/ref-pressureulcers.cfm
- Institute for Healthcare Improvement—http://www.ihi.org/IHI/Programs/Campaign/PressureUlcers.htm
- Centers for Medicare & Medicaid Services. "Guidance to Surveyors for Long Term Care Facilities"—http://www.cms.hhs.gov/transmittals/Downloads/R4SOM.pdf
- Wound, Ostomy and Continence Nurses Society—http://www.wocn.org/index.php
- Wound Research—http://www.woundsresearch.com
- "Push tool"—http://www.npuap.org/resources/educational-and-clinical--resources/push-tool

Acknowledgment This chapter was updated and revised from Ganesh Merugu MD & Andrew Rosenzweig MD, CMD, FACP published in the second edition. Assistance in the formatting of this chapter was provided by Drs. Nader Tavakoli and Amrit Parhar and editing assistance by Peter Winn MD, CMD.

References

1. https://pubmed.ncbi.nlm.nih.gov/7639444/
2. https://www.cdc.gov/nchs/products/databriefs/db14.htm
3. Michocki R, Lamy P. The problem of pressure sores in a nursing home population: statistical data. J Am Geriatr Soc. 1976;24(7):323–8.
4. Kennedy K. The prevalence of pressure ulcers in an intermediate care facility. Decubitus. 1989;2(2):44–5.
5. Centers for Medicare & Medicaid Services (CMS), HHS. Medicare program: changes to the hospital inpatient prospective payment systems and fiscal year 2008 rates. Fed Regist. 2007(72):47379.
6. Thomas DR. Prevention and treatment of pressure ulcers. JAMDA. 2005;10:46–59.
7. Centers for Medicare and Medicaid Services. Guidance to surveyors for long term care facilities. CMS manual. Washington, DC: CMS; 2004.
8. https://npiap.com/page/2019Guideline
9. https://paltc.org/topic/pressure-ulcers
10. Moore ZEH, Patton D. Risk assessment tools for the prevention of pressure ulcers. Cochrane Database Syst Rev. 2019;1
11. Horn SD, Bender SA, Ferguson ML, et al. The national pressure ulcer long-term care study: pressure ulcer development in long-term care residents. J Am Geriatr Soc. 2004;52(3):359–67.
12. Singh N, Armstrong DG, Lipsky BA. Preventing foot ulcers in patients with diabetes. JAMA. 2005;293(2):217–28.

13. American Health Care Association. Medical condition-mental status CMS OSCAR data current surveys; 2009.
14. Diane KL, Joyce B. Pressure ulcers in individuals receiving palliative care: a National Pressure Ulcer Advisory Panel White Paper. Adv Skin Wound Care. 2010;23(2):59–72.
15. Wishin J, Gallagher TJ, McCann E. Emerging options for the management of fecal incontinence in hospitalized patients. J Wound Ostomy Continence Nurs. 2008;35(1):104–10.
16. Saghaleini SH, Dehghan K, Shadvar K, Sanaie S, Mahmoodpoor A, Ostadi Z. Pressure ulcer and nutrition. Indian J Crit Care Med. 2018;22(4):283–9. https://doi.org/10.4103/ijccm. IJCCM_277_17.
17. Schoonhoven L, Haalboom JR, Bousema MT, et al. Prospective cohort study of routine use of risk assessment scales for prediction of pressure ulcers. BMJ. 2002;325(7368):797.
18. Pancorbo-Hidalgo PL, Garcia-Fernandez FP, Lopez-Medina IM, Alvarez-Nieto C. Risk assessment scales for pressure ulcer prevention: a systematic review. J Adv Nurs. 2006;54(1):94–110.
19. Ayello E, Lyder C. A new era of pressure ulcer accountability in acute care. Adv Skin Wound Care. 2008;21(3):134.
20. Lyder CH, Ayello EA. Pressure ulcers: a patient safety issue. In: Hughes RG, editor. Patient safety and quality: an evidence-based handbook for nurses. Rockville, MD: Agency for Healthcare Research and Quality (US); 2008, Chapter 12.
21. Ratliff CR. WOCN. WOCN's evidence-based pressure ulcer guideline. Adv Skin Wound Care. 2005;18(4):204–8.
22. Morales Lozano R, González Fernández ML, Martinez Hernández D, Beneit Montesinos JV, Guisado Jiménez S, Gonzalez Jurado MA. Validating the probe-to-bone test and other tests for diagnosing chronic osteomyelitis in the diabetic foot. Diabetes Care. 2010;33(10):2140–5. https://doi.org/10.2337/dc09-2309.
23. Takahashi P. Chronic ischemic, venous, and neuropathic ulcers in long-term care. Ann Long Term Care. 2006;14(7):26–31.
24. https://www.ahrq.gov/patient-safety/settings/hospital/resource/pressureulcer/tool/index.html
25. http://www.ihi.org/resources/Pages/Tools/HowtoGuidePreventPressureUlcers.aspx
26. Kenedi RM, Cowden JM, Scales JT. Bedsore Biomechanics. Baltimore: University Park Press; 1976.
27. Know DM, Anderson TM, Anderson PS. Effects of different turn intervals on skin of healthy older adults. Adv Wound Care. 1994;7:48–56.
28. Dr T, Goode PS, Tarquine PH, Allman R. Hospital acquired pressure ulcers and risk of death. JAGS. 1996;44:1435–40.
29. Heyman H, Van De Looverbosch DE, Meijer EP, Schols JM. Benefits of an oral nutritional supplement on pressure ulcer healing in long-term care residents. J Wound Care. 2008;17(11):476–8.
30. Galley H. Vitamin C and pressure sores. J Dermatol Treatment. 1995;6(3):195–8.
31. Witkowshi A, Parish L. The decubitus ulcer: skin failure and destructive behavior. Int J Dermatol. 2000;39:894.
32. Black JM, National Pressure Ulcer Advisory P. Moving toward consensus on deep tissue injury and pressure ulcer staging. Adv Skin Wound Care. 2005;18(8):415–6.
33. Duncan SM. Preventing & managing pressure sores. http://www.amda.com/publications/caring/march2003/policies.cfm#refs
34. Defloor T, Schoonhoven L. Inter-rater reliability of the EPUAP pressure ulcer classification system using photographs. J Clin Nurs. 2004;13(8):952–9.
35. Takahashi P, Chandra A, Kiemele L, Targonski P. Wound care technologies: emerging evidence for appropriate use in long-term care. Ann Long Term Care. 2008;16(12). http://www.annalsoflongtermcare.com/content/wound-care-technologies-emerging-evidence-appropriate-use-long-term-care
36. Hopkins A, Dealey C, Bale S, Defloor T, Worboys F. Patient stories of living with a pressure ulcer. J Adv Nurs. 2006;56(4):345–53.

37. Bates-Jensen BM, Guihan M, Garber SL, Chin AS, Burns SP. Characteristics of recurrent pressure ulcers in veterans with spinal cord injury. J Spinal Cord Med. 2009;32(1):34–42.
38. Smith DM. Pressure ulcers in the nursing home. Ann Intern Med. 1995;123(6):433–42.
39. Bryan CS, Dew CE, Reynolds KL. Bacteremia associated with decubitus ulcers. Arch Intern Med. 1983;143(11):2093–5.
40. Allman RM, Goode PS, Burst N, Bartolucci AA, Thomas DR. Pressure ulcers, hospital complications, and disease severity: impact on hospital costs and length of stay. Adv Wound Care. 1999;12(1):22–30.
41. Lyder CH. Implications of pressure ulcers and its relation to federal tag 314. Ann Long Term Care. 2006;14(4):19–24.
42. Ayello EA, Braden B. How and why to do pressure ulcer risk assessment. Adv Skin Wound Care. 2002;15(3):125–31.
43. Bergstrom N, Braden B. A prospective study of pressure sore risk among institutionalized elderly. J Am Geriatr Soc. 1992;40(8):747–58.
44. US Department of Health and Human Services, Centers for Medicare and Medicaid Services. Nursing home data compendium; 2008.

Dementia, Delirium, and Depression

Pamela A. Fenstemacher, Brandon Cantazaro, Daniela Hernandez, Andres Suarez, Krishna Suri, and Andrew Dentino

Introduction

Dementia, delirium, and depression will affect many residents at some point during their stay in a post-acute or long-term care (PA/LTC) facility. Cognitive disorders can either be chronic as in dementia, acute as in seen in delirium, or subacute as in depression [1]. Understanding the similarities and differences between the clinical features of dementia, delirium, and depression is paramount to evaluating the resident with a change in mentation. Assessment by the clinician is challenging when determining which of these frequently seen conditions is present as residents may be suffering with one or more of them at the same time. Careful observation by staff and providers can help the interdisciplinary team to recognize and assess any mental status changes and to initiate appropriate interventions in a timely manner. Clinical aspects of these three conditions are summarized in Table 1, while Table 2 details the clinical evaluation of depression, delirium, and dementia.

P. A. Fenstemacher
The University of Pennsylvania, Jenkintown, PA, USA

B. Cantazaro · D. Hernandez · A. Suarez
University of Texas Rio Grande Valley School of Medicine, Edinburg, TX, USA

K. Suri
University Hospitals, Cleveland, OH, USA

A. Dentino (✉)
Rio Grande Valley Graduate Medical Education Consortium, Edinburg, TX, USA

© The Author(s), under exclusive license to Springer Nature Switzerland AG 2023
P. Winn et al. (eds.), *Post-Acute and Long-Term Care Medicine*, Current Clinical Practice, https://doi.org/10.1007/978-3-031-28628-5_14

Table 1 Comparison of the clinical features of depression, delirium, and dementia

Clinical feature	Depression	Delirium	Dementia
Onset	Gradual, may be recurrent	Sudden	Gradual, progressive
Course	Chronic	Acute	Chronic
Mood	Low	Variable	Variable
Apathy	Present	May be present or absent	May be present or absent
Attention	Intact or impaired	Impaired	Intact early; impaired later
Memory	Intact or impaired	Usually impaired	Impaired
Hallucinations or delusions	Absent[a]	Present	Variable
ADLs[b]	Intact or impaired	Intact or impaired	Intact early; impaired later
IADLs[c]	Intact or impaired	Intact or impaired	Intact early; impaired before ADLs
Signs of other illness	Present	Present	Usually absent

[a]Except in depression with psychotic features
[b]Activities of daily living
[c]Instrumental activities of daily living

Table 2 Clinical evaluation of depression, delirium, and dementia[a]

Evaluation	Depression	Delirium	Dementia
History or interval history and physical examination	x	x	x
Screening tool	GDS, SIGECAPS Cornell Scale for Depression in Dementia	CAM	Folstein MMSE, SLUMS
CBC with differential	x	x	x
Complete metabolic panel	x	x	x
Vitamin B_{12} level	x		x
Medication review and medication level	x	x	x
Thyroid-stimulating hormone	x	x	x
RPR			x
Lyme titer			x
Urinalysis with culture		x	x
Chest X-ray		x	
Arterial blood gas		x	
Electrocardiogram		x	
Brain imaging		x	x
Lumbar puncture		x	x
Electroencephalogram		x	

[a]The clinical evaluation of dementia, delirium, and depression should **always** be guided by presentation and goals of care

Dementia

Dementia is a syndrome of chronic, irreversible, progressive global decline in cognition with associated loss of memory. It is one of the most common impairments in older adults in PA/LTC and while it occurs with a clear sensorium, in its early stages it frequently complicates the evaluation of a resident with an acute change in mental status [2–4]. Dementia occurs when an abnormality in the structure and function of the brain disrupts cognition. Symptoms of dementia may be noted by the clinician, observed by the staff, or reported by the patient and/or family. Although dementia is often associated with a disrupted sleep–wake cycle, disturbances in language, recall, and memory may be the most evident findings [5]. Other psychiatric disorders and medical conditions that cause cognitive dysfunction may accompany dementia making it more challenging to diagnose and treat. The ongoing COVID-19 pandemic was shown to have a profound impact on people with dementia, causing an increase in morbidity and mortality. Ongoing studies are currently underway to evaluate the effect of the causative agent, SARS-CoV-2, on the central nervous system, and its risk of causing cognitive decline.

Differential Diagnosis

Alzheimer's Disease (Dementia of Alzheimer's Type or DAT), vascular dementia (multi-infarct dementia or MID), Dementia with Lewy Bodies (LBD), frontotemporal dementia (FTD), and dementia due to HIV/AIDS are the most commonly seen types of dementia. Dementia can be categorized as cortical or subcortical, with DAT being a classic example of a cortical dementia. *Cortical dementias* are typically characterized by amnesia, disorientation, and relatively preserved personality. Whereas *subcortical dementias* show relatively preserved memory with difficulties in executive function, attention, and concentration. Dementia associated with Parkinson's disease is an example of subcortical dementia. It is important to remember that with increasing age persons more frequently suffer from more than one type of dementia, and this is referred to as *mixed dementia* [6].

DAT is the most common cause of dementia and is estimated to account for 55–75% of all cases [1, 3, 7] and classified as a neurocognitive disorder (NCD) due to Alzheimer's Disease in *DSM-5* [8]. In DAT, personality and attention are preserved in the early stages of disease as opposed to other types of dementia where a more rapid deterioration of personality may occur. Executive functioning declines progressively over time in DAT, but progression of behavioral symptoms is the most common reason for admission to a memory care unit or nursing facility.

The second most common etiology for dementia is vascular disease (Vascular NCD in *DSM-5*) and accounts for 13–16% of affected individuals [1, 3, 7]. Vascular or multi-infarct dementia (MID) is characterized by early onset of decreased attention accompanied by blunting of affect and memory disturbances. Patients usually have known risk factors for vascular disease (e.g., hypertension, diabetes mellitus, hyperlipidemia) and behavioral risk factors (e.g., smoking, obesity, sedentary lifestyle). Vascular dementia frequently progresses in a stepwise fashion as opposed to the gradual progression seen in DAT. Microcirculatory deficits accumulate over time as a result of the vasculopathic nature of the underlying disease process. On physical exam evidence of arterial vascular compromise is commonly seen as well as focal neurologic abnormalities.

Lewy Body Disease (LBD) is the third most common dementia seen and accounts for 20–25% of all dementia, LBD NCD in *DSM-5*. LBD usually occurs at an earlier age and has a faster progression than DAT. LBD is also associated with psychiatric symptoms, fluctuations in level of alertness, and an increased sensitivity to antipsychotic medications [9]. Unfortunately, psychiatric symptoms are very common and include anxiety, depression, and perceptual disturbances. Perceptual disturbances are characterized by hallucinations that are usually visual and delusions or fixed false beliefs that are frequently paranoid. LBD is closely associated with Parkinson's disease and is characterized by many of the features of the Parkinson's disease. These features include a *motor syndrome* (bradykinesia, rigidity, tremors, and gait difficulties leading to falls) and *autonomic dysfunction* (constipation and orthostatic hypotension leading to syncope). Loss of smell and sleep disturbances are frequently seen as well. Sleep disturbances include excessive daytime drowsiness and nighttime difficulty not only staying asleep but also REM sleep behavior disorder (RBD). RBD manifests as the patient acting out his or her dreams, a symptom often first recognized by a caregiver. Persons diagnosed with Lewy body dementia are also sensitive to antiparkinsonian drugs that can increase confusion and problematic behaviors. Therefore, when prescribing these medications, it is important to weigh the risk of worsening cognition versus the potential benefit of improving function.

Some dementias are rapidly progressive such as *Creutzfeldt–Jakob disease* (Prion disease NCD), which is caused by a prion or infectious protein. Symptoms of this dementia develop quickly often accompanied by myoclonic jerks and eventually seizures [10]. The progression of symptoms is less obvious in frontotemporal lobe dementias (FTDs), classified as frontotemporal lobar degeneration NCD in *DSM-5*. FTD manifests as mood swings and impulsivity, with personality coarsening as well as a concomitant deterioration in functional status. Affected individuals also demonstrate inattention and affective flattening. A more unusual cause of dementia is Huntington's disease, which is inherited and begins at a very young age (e.g., 35–45). Huntington's disease causes subtle mood changes and cognitive problems that progress fairly rapidly to dementia with behavioral disturbances, which are accompanied by a lack of coordination and chorea (i.e., involuntary writhing movements).

Other etiologies of dementia to consider in the differential diagnosis include HIV disease, Parkinson's disease (where the Parkinson's motor symptoms will *precede* cognitive decline by several years), Wilson's disease, traumatic brain injury (i.e., from falling in older adults), or other neurological conditions (e.g., ALS, multiple sclerosis, Korsakoff's syndrome/alcoholic encephalopathy). Medical conditions that can cause cognitive dysfunction include obstructive sleep apnea, metastatic disease, neurosyphilis, and substance abuse. The possibility of substance abuse or prescription medications influencing cognition should always be considered in anyone presenting with memory complaints, even if the medication had been taken for many years [8]. *Remember to look for the more common potentially reversible causes of dementia*: B_{12} deficiency, thyroid disease, subdural hematoma, normal pressure hydrocephalus, and primary tumors of the brain.

One important etiology of the developing and worsening of dementia that has gained our attention recently is infection. One episode of any kind of infection in the elderly population, for example, pneumonia or urinary tract infection, can accelerate cognitive decline, especially if the individual is predisposed to cognitive problems. Respiratory viruses also seem to have a detrimental effect on the central nervous system (CNS). During the influenza pandemic in 1918 an increase in cognitive decline, psychosis, Parkinson disease, and encephalitis lethargica was seen. Influenza is now suspected to be the underlying cause of encephalitis lethargica. Outbreaks like the SARS (severe acute respiratory distress syndrome) outbreak in 2002 and the MERS (Middle East Respiratory Syndrome) outbreak in 2012 showed that one in five recovered patients reported memory impairment. Coronaviruses are known to invade the CNS and cause symptoms like headache, hypogeusia, and anosmia that precede the onset of respiratory symptoms. People with coronaviruses have also presented with ataxia and altered mental status. SARS-CoV2 RNA has been found in the CSF of patients with encephalopathy and meningoencephalitis. Cerebrovascular accidents are also commonly seen within 2 weeks of the onset of symptoms of COVID-19. Immune response to the virus is thought to accelerate the progression of brain inflammatory neurodegeneration and hence worsen dementia and cause severe outcomes after COVID-19 infection. Ongoing research on the current COVID-19 pandemic is focusing on understanding the long-term impact of COVID-19 on the CNS, and how it may impair cognition and functioning. Research is also seeking to understand the underlying biology of COVID-19 and how it contributes to the different kinds of dementias.

Diagnosing Dementia

When the staff in the PA/LTC facility is trained and experienced in caring for persons with dementia, those residents who develop early symptoms of dementia are more readily recognized. In nursing facilities (NFs) MDS evaluations can be compared to determine changes in resident cognition, memory, and other manifestations such as:

- Inability to perform activities or tasks of daily living
- Changes in hygiene
- Altered interactions with staff and other residents

The diagnosis of dementia starts with a patient history, often obtained from a family member and/or staff in PA/LTC. It is important to determine if the onset of the condition was insidious and difficult to pinpoint in time or if the progression was gradual or stepwise (i.e., DAT vs. MID). Any specific neurologic and psychiatric symptoms that have occurred also need to be considered [3]. The diagnosis can then be refined on the basis of the neurologic signs and symptoms, mental status, physical examination and the results of neuropsychologic testing (though often not needed), brain imaging, and laboratory studies.

According to the DSM-5 the criteria to diagnose dementia (major neurocognitive disorder) include:

- Evidence from the history and clinical assessment that indicate significant cognitive impairment in at least one of the following:
  - Learning and memory
  - Language
  - Executive function
  - Complex attention
  - Perceptual-motor function
  - Social Cognition

- The impairment must be acquired and represent a significant decline from a previous level of functioning
- The cognitive deficits must interfere with independence in everyday activities
- The disturbances are not occurring exclusively during the course of delirium and are not accounted by another mental disorder

Screening for Dementia

Research on the routine screening of asymptomatic adults has not shown enough evidence for or against routinely screening for dementia. Currently we do not perform routine screening for cognitive impairment in asymptomatic patients. When a family member, patient, or staff member notices any cognitive changes, then a thorough evaluation is recommended. It is important to completely evaluate a resident with suspected dementia, as many medical conditions can cause or worsen dementia, some of which can be reversed (See Table 3). In particular, a patient presenting with new symptoms of memory or cognitive impairment should be evaluated for depression as well. Depression can cause a form of cognitive impairment referred to as *pseudodementia* (for further discussion see section on depression).

Table 3 Medical conditions that can cause or worsen dementia	Delirium
	Developmental disability
	HIV/AIDs
	Hyperglycemia or Hypoglycemia
	Mental Retardation (i.e., neuropsychological impairment)
	Normal Pressure Hydrocephalus
	Sequelae of traumatic brain injury
	Subdural Hematoma
	Tertiary Syphilis
	Vasculitides
	Vitamin B12 deficiency

Evaluation of the Resident with Cognitive Impairment

The *"gold standard" for the diagnosis of dementia is **clinical***, based upon the patient history and physical assessment, with ancillary information such as formal neuropsychologic testing [11] and brain imaging performed as needed. A basic evaluation of the resident with new cognitive impairment includes a medication history, laboratory tests such as a complete blood count with differential, comprehensive metabolic panel, vitamin B_{12} level, thyroid function panel including a TSH, and possibly blood levels of medication such as digoxin, lithium, theophylline, anticonvulsants (e.g., phenytoin, valproic acid), and tricyclic antidepressants (e.g., amitriptyline). It is imperative to do complete medication use history including nonprescription drugs. Everyday drugs used by the elderly population including analgesics, anticholinergics, psychotropic and sedative-hypnotics have been shown to impair cognition. Reducing polypharmacy is a crucial step when evaluating dementia. Other tests to consider when evaluating dementia are HIV, RPR, or perhaps a test for Lyme disease (depending on local prevalence and other risk factors) as possible causes for a change in cognition [3, 4].

It is also necessary to evaluate underlying medical conditions and to optimize their management. Medical conditions commonly implicated in cognitive dysfunction include: recent coronary artery bypass grafting, hypertension, nutritional deficiencies including B vitamins, diabetes mellitus, stroke, Parkinson's disease, and diseases that cause hypoxia such as COPD and obstructive sleep apnea [4].

Quantifiable scales that may be used as benchmarks for diagnosing and monitoring dementia progression include the Montreal Cognitive Assessment (MOCA), the Folstein Mini Mental Status Exam (MMSE), the St. Louis University Mental Status Exam (SLUMS), or other commercially available instruments [11, 12]. The MMSE is a simple 30-point screening tool frequently used to evaluate for cognitive impairment. Recently, the official form has been copyrighted and must be purchased (www.minimental.com.). Because of this expense, some practitioners have chosen instead to use the SLUMS (https://www.slu.edu/medicine/internal-medicine/geriatric-medicine/aging-successfully/assessment-tools/mental-status-exam.php) or the MOCA assessment tool (https://www.mocatest.org). More tools can be found in "Other Resources" at the end of this chapter. Keep in mind that the MDS in skilled nursing facilities will also provide an evaluation of the resident's cognitive status (Brief Interview for Mental Status or BIMS) and functional status.

Finally, neuroimaging of the brain may be performed to rule out structural lesions such as a neoplasm or other potentially reversible conditions such as normal pressure hydrocephalus or a subdural hematoma. A neuroimaging study should be considered especially when the onset of the dementia has occurred within the past 6–12 months, is rapidly progressive, or is following an unpredictable course.

If there is a question of diagnosis, or if the resident or their family has difficulty accepting the diagnosis of dementia, neuropsychologic testing may be done to more definitively diagnose the resident's cognitive status. Not only may neuropsychologic testing help determine the type of dementia, but it can also help to delineate the patient's strengths and weaknesses; to identify particular areas of cognitive dysfunction in order to suggest compensation strategies, and to aid in behavioral management [5]. The diagnosis of dementia can aid in the care of the resident. Its diagnosis will provide a framework for prognostication and will aid in health care decision-making by both resident and family. Although dementia is a chronic, progressive, and ultimately terminal illness, it is often unrecognized in its early stages. The goals of care in the management of dementia are to provide a safe environment, educate caregivers and family, and provide emotional support for the healthcare team, patient, and family.

Prognosis

Different types of dementia have varied manifestations at onset, with the common pathway being one of progressive loss of ability to perform daily tasks of living (i.e., ADLs and IADLs). Residents eventually develop advanced dementia and become unable to care for themselves, incontinent of bowel and bladder, and unable to safely swallow and to maintain sufficient nutrition to sustain life. Observational studies do not show any benefit of tube feeding in these patients. Even when carefully hand fed, the resident with end stage dementia will eventually develop progressive weight loss and be at high risk for developing pressure ulcers. The demented resident may also develop urinary retention, constipation, and repeated urinary or respiratory infections (the latter due to aspiration of food and secretions) [5]. Patients also develop profound memory deficits and sometimes are unable to recognize their family members. It is imperative that the family be educated on the disease process of dementia and its course. This may be difficult for families to accept, as many do not understand that dementia is a terminal illness. Given how hard it is to predict life expectancy in patients with advanced dementia there should be access to palliative care, which should be focused on comfort care that is based on prognostic estimates. (See Chapters "Integrating Palliative Care into Long Term Care" and "Weight and Nutrition in Post-Acute and Long-Term Care" for further reading).

Pharmacologic Treatment

Pharmacologic treatment of dementia should focus on the underlying medical and psychological condition(s) affecting the individual, with the goal being maximization of his or her functional well-being. For example, in those with coexistent depression, the use of antidepressants with serotoninergic activity may improve both depressive symptoms and cognition [3].

Alzheimer's Disease (DAT)

In Alzheimer's disease, the mainstay of treatment is neurotransmitter modulation to lessen the symptoms of the disease. Although it is an area being avidly researched, no medication has yet been found that slows the progression of DAT.

Specific treatment for DAT includes the use of two major classes of medications, *cholinesterase inhibitors* and the *NMDA receptor antagonists* [13, 14]. The most widely used cholinesterase inhibitor is donepezil (Aricept) but other medications include rivastigmine (Exelon) and galantamine (Razadyne). Cholinesterase inhibitors are currently indicated for mild (MMSE >19), moderate (MMSE 19–10), or severe (MMSE <10) DAT. The only currently available NMDA receptor antagonist is memantine (Namenda). Memantine is currently indicated for moderate to severe AD either in conjunction with a cholinesterase inhibitor or as monotherapy [3, 4]. Monitoring for and management of potential common side effects of these two classes of medications should be as much a part of patient care as their prescribing. Because *these medications are not curative but palliative* decisions about whether to continue them must be individualized as the benefits and risks are weighed on an ongoing basis.

Other medications and treatments have not been shown effective in treating or preventing AD. These include anti-inflammatory medications such as NSAIDs, hormone replacement therapy such as estrogen, and ginkgo biloba. Research in this area continues predominantly investigating the prevention of CNS inflammation and the formation of beta-amyloid plaques, both hallmarks of DAT [3].

Non-DAT Dementias

The mainstay of treatment for non-DAT dementias is preventing progression of the underlying disease process (as in the case of vascular dementia) and treating the symptoms that arise in the course of the disease (as in the case of hallucinations in LBD.) Donepezil has been tested (off label) in other cognitive disorders, including LBD and MID, but it is not currently FDA approved for these diagnoses.

Challenging Behaviors in Dementia

Pacing, wandering, hoarding, agitation, insomnia, aggression, hypersexuality, perseveration, hallucinations, paranoia, and emotional lability are challenging behaviors seen in dementia [4, 15]. Agitation frequently is seen with "sundowning," which is a syndrome of disorientation, confusion, and agitation that often starts in the middle to late afternoon and progressively worsens through the evening into the night. An environment and medical evaluation often give insight into ways in which these behaviors can be mitigated or prevented. Frequently, these behaviors are a natural manifestation of the dementing process, but they may be exacerbated by stimuli in the environment or a medical illness. On one hand, commonly seen environmental causes of disruptive behavior include a new caregiver, an absent family member, or another disruptive resident. On the other hand, commonly seen medical causes of disruptive or changed behaviors include pain, constipation, urinary retention, drug effect(s), dehydration, or infection. It is important to first evaluate any reversible environmental and/or physical stimuli that may be implicated in precipitating the behavior before initiating any treatment interventions for the behavior [4]. Communication becomes increasingly difficult for patients as their dementia progresses. Often what may be deemed as "agitation" or other abnormal behavior might be reformulated to questions of, "What is this behavior attempting to communicate?" "What are their unmet needs, if any?" "What is this behavior attempting to convey?" Whether it is pain or discomfort due to constipation or inability to urinate, boredom or hunger, attempting to identify and address the ante- cedents to these underlying behaviors should be a first-line intervention rather than prescribing a pharmacologic agent for "agitation."

Psychosocial interventions constitute a mainstay for the creation and promotion of a sense of well-being for those with progressive dementia. Learning about and acknowledging individual resident preferences and personhood, as well as providing care with dignity can help establish a fulfilling and meaningful activity program. Physical activity, even if limited to the upper extremity for wheelchair-bound residents, may be a welcomed and enjoyable part of the day. Social activities such as listening to reading, singing, or reminiscing and reality orientating may bring solace and peace to patients, families, and staff. Respect for privacy, sleep, and meal preferences, and effective verbal, visual, and tactile cueing may further benefit the resident with dementia and others at the end of life [16].

Treatment of Behaviors in Dementia

Behaviors in dementia may be addressed using non-pharmacologic and/or pharmacologic treatment.

Non-Pharmacologic Treatment

An adjustment of environmental factors (both physical and human) may lesson or resolve distressing behaviors. For example, although providing areas in the facility with more home-like furnishings and wall decorations did not reduce wandering and pacing, residents were kept safe and were easier to monitor because they preferred to remain in the home-like areas [15].

Suggested Interventions Include:
- Establish a daily routine for personal care and meals while maintaining some flexibility to accommodate the resident's needs and preferences. If the resident is resistant, re-approach the resident a short time later and they may then be more willing to allow care or eat.
- Reduce isolation; segregate noisier or disruptive residents from quieter ones.
- Maintain adequate and appropriate lighting at all times.
- Provide pleasant experiences, such as ethnic foods and other culturally oriented activities, pet therapy, or stuffed animals [4].

Interventions for Disruptive or Challenging Behavior:
- For inappropriate sexual behavior use clothing that reduces access to genitalia, provide care from same-sex caregivers, seat away from residents of the opposite sex [15].
- Redirect with individual and group activities.
- Know the resident's social history and preferences, which will often give insight into behaviors and preferred activities. For example, the resident who continuously moves tables and chairs in the dining room may be repeating his former motor activity of returning grocery carts from the parking lot to the supermarket. When staff observed him moving furniture safely, he was allowed to continue this activity with supervision and his agitation was reduced.

The ongoing COVID-19 pandemic restricted the possibility of tackling the behavioral changes in dementia because environmental factors and family interactions needed to be adjusted. These restrictions also caused changes in routines and isolation of in-patients with a positive test for COVID-19, which were shown to worsen patients' severity of dementia as well as their morbidity and mortality. Because of these restrictions, there has been an overall worsening of cognitive symptoms in nursing facility patients with dementia, particularly their memory, orientation, and behavior. This experience has showed us that non-pharmacological measures have a major impact on the treatment of patients with dementia.

Pharmacologic Treatment

If modifying the environment cannot alleviate distressing behaviors, medication management may need to be considered. As with other changes to a resident's plan of care, the risks and benefits of any medical treatment need to be carefully considered. The staff and family should be advised of the issues and interventions that have been tried before instituting medical therapy. There has not been a great deal of consensus on which medications to treat challenging behaviors in dementia, or research to prove efficacy [15]. *One must also take into consideration State regulations and facility policies regarding medications that are considered chemical restraints.* The following may be considered:

- Residents who exhibit agitation with psychotic features such as hallucinations, delusions, or preservative behaviors such as pacing or hoarding may respond to treatment with antipsychotic medication.
- Residents with sundowning or insomnia may improve with a medication that promotes sleep (trazodone) or reduces confusion (antipsychotic).
- Residents who exhibit behaviors with an anxiety component may benefit from a serotonergic reuptake inhibitor or trazodone.
- Residents with hypersexual behaviors may respond to antipsychotic medication or to antiandrogenic hormone therapy such as estrogen (in male residents).
- Residents with anger or aggression may respond to the use of serotonergic agents, mood stabilizing agents such as divalproex, carbamazepine, gabapentin, or antipsychotic medication such as risperidone and olanzapine [15].

Medication regimens must be reviewed on a regular basis to evaluate their effectiveness. This includes periodic attempts to reduce dosing or discontinue medications. For example, 3–6 months after admission to a facility, it is not uncommon that a resident is able to have medications that were necessary at the time of admission be reduced or even discontinued. *Beware that antipsychotics and benzodiazepines can cause paradoxical agitation and/or worsen confusion.*

Medication Management in Cognitive Impairment

The average nursing facility resident takes seven medications, and nearly a third of residents take nine or more medications [16]. Therefore, when evaluating cognitive impairment, it is crucial to consider medications and medication interactions that can alter cognitive function. Medications that are commonly implicated include antiarrhythmics, hypnotics, psychotropics, sedatives, analgesics, and medications with significant anticholinergic properties such as those used for urinary urge incontinence. Toxicity from certain medications such as digoxin can also cause changes in cognition. In 1991, Dr. Mark Beers created a list of *potentially inappropriate* medications used in the geriatric population. The Beers list continues to be updated and is used for guidance by practitioners in PA/LTC and by state surveyors (See Chapter "Medication Management in Long-term Care" for further discussion) [13].

Delirium

Delirium is a medical emergency. Its differential is vast, and maintaining patient safety is paramount. Because undiagnosed or untreated delirium can increase morbidity and mortality, a timely and prudent workup is essential. In contrast to dementia and depression, delirium is a medical condition that can be either acute or subacute, with its onset frequently unrecognized. It is caused by an imbalance in brain acetylcholine that occurs either because of changes in the body's homeostatic internal environment (e.g., fever) or changes in the metabolic milieu (e.g., ischemia, hypoxia), which then disrupt standard neuronal circuitry [17, 18]. *It is so common that it should be anticipated* whenever an older adult undergoes surgery, is hospitalized, or suffers an acute medical illness. Long term, delirium is associated with cognitive and functional decline and represents a financial burden to society [19].

Nevertheless, regardless of its pathophysiology, the behavioral manifestations of delirium include symptoms of abnormal attention, arousal, and awareness [20]. Most striking is the patient's inability to maintain attention for all but extremely short periods of time, frequently changing topics mid-sentence. The patient will also experience a change in cognition, including perceptual impairments such as illusions, delusions, or hallucinations [21]. Delirium can be described according to the level of psychomotor activity manifested by the patient, either *hyperactive* or *hypoactive* or *mixed*. A patient with *hyperactive delirium* experiences increased psychomotor activity and may appear anxious or agitated. In contrast, *hypoactive delirium* causes reduced psychomotor activity. It is often under-recognized due to the "absence of a complaint" or the attribution of the apathy to another illness such as depression. The staff will describe patients with hypoactive delirium as "quiet and requiring little or no attention." This may lead to delirium being overlooked and therefore untreated. The third type of delirium is a *mixed delirium*, and the resident exhibits fluctuating levels of psychomotor activity ranging from immobility to extreme agitation [4, 22].

Any resident who has an acute change in sensorium or behavior (i.e., suspected delirium) warrants an immediate review of the antecedents and consequences of the behavior with consideration as to its possible etiology. Delirium is likely to occur in a vulnerable resident who develops an acute illness, affecting at least one-third of hospitalized elders [23]. It may last for weeks to months and has been associated with poor health outcomes, including increased in-hospital mortality, a longer length of stay, functional decline, and risk of institutionalization. When associated with dementia, the odds of walking dependence, institutionalization, and 1-year-mortality are also increased [24]. As pressure increases to discharge individuals sooner from acute inpatient facilities, many of these acutely confused elderly transitions from hospital to a post-acute facility, where they remain delirious and can experience potentially life-threatening complications [22, 25]. Many of the residents in PA/LTC facilities are at risk of developing delirium due to multiple risk factors (see Table 4). Delirium occurs more frequently in women in LTC settings and was found in 18% of patients with an acute illness [24]. In PA/LTC, the identification, assessment, and management of delirium are urgent as delirium may signify an underlying medical emergency. Delirium is frequently the presenting

Table 4 Delirium risk factors

Dementia
Older age
Functional impairment
Multiple comorbidities
Dehydration
Malnutrition
Sensory impairment
History of depression
History of substance abuse
Frailty
Polypharmacy
Restrain Use

symptom of a resident's change in condition. If hospital admission or readmission is going to be prevented, quickly addressing any acute change in mental status is essential (see Chapter "Preventing Hospital Admissions and Readmissions" for further discussion). Consider how frequently delirium occurs when a NF resident develops an infection or dehydration with underlying dementia, multi-morbidities, and a complicated medication regimen. Patients admitted to PA facilities had worsened outcomes with a 6-month mortality rate of 25.0%, as compared to a mortality of 5.7% in patients admitted without delirium. Hypoactive delirium was found to be the most frequent subtype of delirium [24].

Identification

Ideally, delirium detection should occur at the time of admission [24]. Each resident with delirium should be evaluated for the multiple risk factors of delirium, especially those that are reversible. When investigating the cause of delirium, it is essential to review the medical history and medication list for all chronic medical illnesses and medications that increase the risk for delirium. Dementia is a leading risk factor for delirium, as are anticholinergic and analgesic medications. An unfamiliar environment or change in staff, such as experienced during a hospital stay, can by itself precipitate delirium. In the hospital setting, up to one-third of the cases of delirium are thought to be either preventable or iatrogenic. For other risk factors for delirium, see Table 4 [26].

Assessment of Delirium

One of the simplest ways to evaluate a resident for delirium is the Confusion Assessment Method (CAM) [27]. It is a four-item evaluation that was developed by Inouye et al. and entails the following characteristics:

1. Acute onset and fluctuating course.
2. Inattention.
3. Disorganized thinking.
4. Altered level of consciousness.

The diagnosis of delirium is made by the presence of both (1) and (2), with *either* (3) or (4). The CAM has been shown to have excellent sensitivity and specificity and has been validated in some care settings [28]. Other methods of diagnosing delirium include a brief assessment for the CAM, which is a 3-min diagnostic assessment (3D-CAM) (and the 4As Test (4AT), which has been validated in clinical settings involving dementia. Some of the more widely used tools to detect delirium severity are the Delirium Rating Scale Revised-98 (DRS-98), the Cam-Severity Scale (CAM-S), and the Memorial Delirium Assessment Scale (MDAS).

As with any change in mental status, an evaluation of the resident/patient must investigate all potentially reversible causes. This should include a complete interval history to determine when there was a change in mental status and the time course of the resident's mental status. Another essential part of the history is medication review. Medications that were recently prescribed had a dosage change or were recently discontinued should be noted. All prescription medications, over-the-counter medications, supplements, and substances with potential for abuse (alcohol, illicit, and prescription drugs) should be reviewed carefully. It is also essential to include any topical medications, such as eye drops, nasal sprays, or suppositories. A *withdrawal syndrome* from prescription drugs (e.g., analgesics, benzodiazepines, or antidepressants), alcohol, or illicit drugs should be considered as a possible cause of delirium. These medications may have been prescribed at the facility or discretely brought into the facility by the resident, a family member, or a friend.

Medication interactions, changes in metabolism with aging (such as decreased renal or liver function), or recently acquired or progressing disease (such as dementia or diabetes) all increase the likelihood that a medication will cause or contribute to delirium. Medications that were previously necessary or recommended may now be causing unwanted effects and thus may need to be discontinued.

A physical exam should include vital signs: temperature, pulse, and blood pressure, as well as pulse oximetry and blood sugar. A careful mental status and neurologic examination should be performed. The remainder of the physical exam should focus on signs and symptoms that may indicate either an acute underlying disease process or a chronic condition that has worsened.

Diagnostic tests should be guided by findings from the history and physical examination. Laboratory tests should include a complete blood count, electrolytes, renal function, and a urinalysis. Other lab tests to consider are thyroid function tests, B12 level, and serum levels of prescribed medications (such as digoxin, lithium, and valproic acid). If indicated, an arterial blood gas or chest X-ray should be done. Other diagnostic testing to consider are neuroimaging and an EKG. Neuroimaging may reveal a subdural hematoma, stroke, brain tumor, or normal pressure hydrocephalus. An acute coronary syndrome and/or arrhythmia may be seen on EKG. On a rare occasion, there may be an indication for either a lumbar puncture to evaluate for infectious or neoplastic processes or an EEG to look for seizure activity [4,

Table 5 Interventions to prevent or ameliorate delirium

Problem	Intervention
Cognitive impairment	Reorientation to time, location, care team Provision of cognitively stimulation activities Caffeine-free warm beverages Music Back massage
Dehydration	Volume repletion (encouragement of oral intake)
Hearing impairment	Disimpaction of cerumen, use of hearing aids and portable amplifiers
Immobility	Encourage early ambulation or active range of motion
Sleep deprivation	Noise reduction measures in patient care areas Minimize sleep deprivation by staff or medication aide
Vision impairment	Use of eyeglasses, magnifying lenses, and adaptive equipment

From: Aging in the Know: www.americangeriatrics.org

21–23]. *In most cases of delirium, the EEG will show nondiagnostic generalized slowing that does not contribute to establishing the cause of delirium nor helpful in its treatment.*

Prevention

Most of all, it is vital to strive to prevent delirium. As noted, studies in the hospital setting have shown that up to one-third of cases of delirium are either potentially preventable or iatrogenic. Interventions used in the hospital that may also help prevent delirium in the PA/LTC setting are listed in Table 5. Despite incorporating systematic screening tools, delirium prevention strategies have not yet been found to be beneficial beyond the acute-care setting [29]. However, pharmacists reviewing medications on a computerized system to identify high risk medications has been supported in the literature [29]. In addition, educating facility care staff led to more delirium cases being recognized and changes in staff attitude [24].

Treatment

Since the causes of delirium are diverse, there is no standard treatment. A safe and calming environment needs to be established for the patient with delirium, while adequate nutrition and hydration are maintained. Patient reassurance, redirection, reality orientation, with the involvement of family and caregivers, can assist in alleviating the delirium. On occasion, treatment of the underlying medical condition causing the delirium will not be sufficient to lessen symptoms promptly to prevent harm to the patient, other patients, staff, and/or the caregiver. In such cases, short-term use of a LOW DOSE of antipsychotic may be necessary. The use of haloperidol is the most clinically established, with only limited studies on using atypical antipsychotics. Benzodiazepines have not shown efficacy except in acute withdrawal from sedatives, hypnotics, or alcohol. *Be aware that antipsychotics and benzodiazepines can cause a paradoxical worsening of anxiety, agitation, and confusion.* In PA settings, patients without objective evidence of delirium who received antipsychotics had worse outcomes and an increased rate of death [30].

COVID-19 and Delirium

With the ongoing COVID-19 pandemic, the geriatric population and those with associated comorbidities are more prone to developing the severe disease.

On retrospective analysis, delirium incidence in the inpatient setting ranges between 11% and 42%, representing a common complication especially in older patients with neuropsychiatric comorbidity, higher serum urea, and elevated lactate-dehydrogenase Poor functional outcomes with long-term sequelae were also reported in this population. On observational analysis, the prevalence of probable delirium is significantly higher in frail compared to non-frail older adults.

Several pathophysiologic pathways have been suggested as promoters of encephalopathy with delirious features, including cytokine storm, endothelial damage, increased oxidative stress, hypoxemia, and direct infection of the central nervous system.

Data on COVID-19 in LTC facilities' residents are scant. Blain et al. reported an atypical presentation of COVID-19 with prodromal symptoms of diarrhea, fall, hypothermia, delirium, and hypotension, followed by respiratory symptoms. Unfortunately, this atypical presentation contributed to a diagnosis delay and rapid dissemination among other patients and health care workers, which increased the risk of mortality in the residents.

The early identification of frailty in COVID-19 patients will facilitate a precise clinical approach, which focuses on both typical and atypical symptoms to diminish the incidence and prevalence of delirium in that patient population.

Depression

Depression is a major illness affecting many elderly who reside in PA/LTC, frequently having an impact on every aspect of their life from mental to physical health. Recent meta-analysis demonstrated an estimated prevalence of depression in nursing facility residents to be around 7%, however, extended review of the literature showed the prevalence of major depressive disorder ranges anywhere from 10% to 29% [31] According to Hoover et al., 54% of nursing home residents older than 65 years had physician-diagnosed depression in their first year of residing in the nursing home [32]. Depression is more likely to occur in patients because of *comorbid medical* (e.g., dementia, stroke, cancer, coronary artery disease, or Parkinson's disease) *and psychiatric conditions* that are frequent in this population. Although depression is very common, it can remain undiagnosed when its symptoms are confused with those of another illness. When depression is untreated, it can worsen any coexisting medical illness and lead to poorer outcomes and increased risk of suicide [1, 4, 33]. Depression in the elderly also result in premature institutionalization. In 2004 the World Health Organization reported that unipolar depressive disorders ranked as a leading cause of the global disease burden and that by 2030 it would be ranked first [34]. Depression is associated with increased disability, greater medical burden, and patients perceiving they have poor health [35, 36].

It is important to be able to differentiate the symptoms of depression from those of delirium and dementia. These disorders often coexist making the diagnosis difficult. Depressive symptoms can be vague, atypical, and nondiagnostic in and of themselves, thus challenging to establish a diagnosis. Both long-term care residents and community-dwelling elders often have undiagnosed and untreated (or undertreated) depression [37].

Symptoms and Risk Factors

The symptoms of depression can be typical or atypical in nature and are commonly overlooked or under recognized. The elderly tend to report less symptoms of depression due to fear of being stigmatized. When they do complain, their somatic symptoms of depression may be incorrectly attributed to physical illness. Finally, even when symptoms of depression are recognized, the false belief that depression is a normal part of aging can keep the depression from being treated [19].

The Classic Symptoms of Depression Include [10]:
- Depressed mood.
- Loss of interest or pleasure (i.e., anhedonia).
- Weight loss or gain, with change in appetite (decreased or increased).
- Change in sleep pattern.
- Psychomotor disturbance.
- Lack of energy or fatigue.
- Guilt.
- Inability to concentrate.
- Suicidal thoughts.

Multiple illnesses can mimic or mask symptoms making it even more difficult for the clinician to recognize depression. Studies have demonstrated a need for *late-life depression* to have a separate classification and diagnostic criteria as it presents differently than depression in younger people [38]. A depressive syndrome that is prevalent in the elderly is "*depression without sadness*" where patients present with lack of vigor, social withdrawal, and apathy [10]. "*Depression-executive dysfunction syndrome*" has also been described in the elderly. It includes psychomotor retardation, loss of interest and task initiation, as well as a language dysfunction characterized by difficulties with visual naming and verbal fluency [38]. When the elderly are depressed, they are also more likely to experience anergia, anhedonia, appetite changes, and sleep dysfunction [39]. Rather than self-report depression or sadness the elderly are more likely to report somatic complaints (i.e., anxiety or hypochondriasis). It is critical to have a low threshold for screening for depression when the organic causes of symptoms are ruled out or when no physical cause of symptoms can be established.

There are several risk factors for late-life depression that encompass social, demographic, psychological, and health domains. One study showed that low economic status, psychosocial stressors, chronic illness, disability, and disrupted relationships all are associated with late-life depression [40]. Another study showed that poor self-rated health, comorbidities, frequent hospitalizations, and lack of friends at the NF are associated with depressive symptoms [12]. Other risk factors included in the health domain that have been found associated with depression are delirium, dementia, or mild cognitive impairment at a younger age, a myocardial infarction or coronary artery disease, and pain or diabetes. Physical disability and hearing loss are other risk factors associated with depression [11, 33].

Differentiating Depression from Dementia

Many patients in long-term care facilities have dementia or some degree of cognitive impairment. It can be difficult to differentiate between cognitive impairment and depression, but it is important to do so as their treatments and potential outcomes are different. *Pseudodementia* is an entity in which cognitive impairment is actually due to a depressive disorder and not dementia [1]. The symptoms of depression and dementia frequently overlap, which can make it difficult for clinicians to differentiate between the two. The Cornell Scale for Depression in Dementia is a tool that uses an interview with the patient and the caregiver (see diagnosis/screening tools below). *Any resident with newly recognized memory or cognitive impairment should also be evaluated for depression,* as they may actually be suffering from pseudodementia rather than dementia. Aggressive treatment of depression in the resident with suspected pseudodementia will lead to a gradual improvement or resolution of the cognitive impairment associated with their depression [41]. Dementia is a known risk factor for depression and there is also evidence that depression may be a precursor to dementia, therefore when depression or dementia is present, the other should be considered [42].

In summary depression is frequently undiagnosed or underdiagnosed in the geriatric patient population. It is postulated that this occurs for many different reasons. The reasons include an overlap between symptoms of depression and those of dementia, a lack of a biologic gold standard test that would diagnose geriatric psychiatric disorders, and preconceptions that depression is a natural part of aging. There is also concern that clinicians have inadequate diagnostic skills and are unable to recognize subtle clinical features of depression in geriatric patients [4, 41].

Diagnosis

It is important to note that a resident may experience a depressed or sad mood and yet not meet the criteria for depression. The key to the diagnosis and treatment of depression is determining whether or not the mood has a significant negative impact on the resident's quality of life. The diagnosis of depression may be guided by the American Psychiatric Association Diagnostic and Statistical Manual of Mental Disorders–version V [10]. *If a resident has significant psychiatric disease, comorbid substance abuse, or depression with psychotic features, it may be helpful to consult a psychiatrist for help with a resident's diagnosis and treatment.*

The DSM-V criteria are currently used to diagnose a major depressive disorder (MDD). In order to make this diagnosis the patient must have *five or more symptoms present for a continuous 2-week period* in which at least one of the symptoms is either *depressed mood or lack of interest or pleasure* [10]. Other symptoms are:

- Significant weight loss or gain.
- Increase or decrease in appetite nearly every day.
- Insomnia or hypersomnia.
- Psychomotor agitation or retardation.
- Fatigue or anergia.
- Feelings of excessive or inappropriate guilt or worthlessness.
- Lack of concentration.
- Recurrent thoughts of death, suicidal ideation, or a suicide attempt.

When using symptoms to diagnose depression, the symptoms should be different from the patient's previous level of functioning and not due to a general medical condition. Standard criteria for depression may not apply to the frail elderly; in these patients, a change in functioning or mood from baseline for more than 2 weeks may indicate an underlying depression. Two other depressive disorders may occur in long-term care: *depressive disorder due to a medical condition* or *other specified depressive disorder.* Other specified depressive disorders include *recurrent brief depression, short duration depressive episode* (lasts 4–13 days), and *depressive episode with insufficient symptoms* to meet criteria for major depressive disorder [10]. These depressive disorders should be considered when a patient is not thought to be suffering from a major depressive episode. It is necessary to ensure that neither a medical condition nor a medication is the cause of the patient's depressive symptoms as treatment would be aimed at the underlying disease (e.g., hypothyroidism).

The evaluation of depression, as with the evaluation of delirium and dementia, should begin with a history, physical exam, and testing guided by the patient's presentation to determine any causative or contributing factors. The investigation should be guided by the goals of care and life expectancy of each patient. For example, in the case of a patient whose life expectancy can be measured in weeks, it may be less important to determine the cause of the depression than it is to treat the depression with therapy that will help relieve symptoms. Careful attention should be given to medication reconciliation and investigating whether the patient recently received any new medications as many medications and some drug–drug interactions may cause or worsen depression. If so, then medication and dose reductions could lessen these effects. Commonly used medications that may cause symptoms of depression include [28]:

- Cardiac medications such as antiarrhythmic or antihypertensive drugs.
- Psychotropic medications such as benzodiazepines or barbiturates.
- Antiseizure medications.
- Steroids.
- GI drugs such as H2 blockers and metoclopramide.
- Opioid analgesics.
- Carbidopa/levodopa.

Laboratory tests that should be considered include: electrolytes, a complete blood count, thyroid function studies, B_{12} and folate levels. If indicated consider medication levels (including, but not limited to antiepileptic drugs, digoxin, lithium, and tricyclic antidepressants). Other investigations may include evaluation for infection (e.g., urinalysis and culture, blood cultures) and an EKG to evaluate for a cardiac ischemia or arrhythmia [4].

Screening Tools

Many different diagnostic and screening tools for depression have been developed and studied. In PA/LTC facilities the Beck Depression Index (BDI), Geriatric Depression Scale (GDS), and the Cornell Scale for Depression in Dementia (CSDD) have been proven useful [43]. A simple screening tool for evaluating depression is SIGECAPS; it is a mnemonic reminder with eight questions (a version of this tool shown in Table 6), which only requires a patient interview. *Five or more positive answers* (indicated in bold) *on SIGECAPS **may** indicate depression.* The GDS-30 is favored by many, consisting of a 30-question interview that evaluates feelings and behaviors of the resident using a "yes/no" format. Scores of 0–10 are considered in the normal range, 11–20 indicates mild depression, and 21–30 severe depression. Use of the GDS-30 is limited because it has a poor predictive value in patients with a MMSE score of 15 or lower. The GDS-15 (see Table 7) is a short form of the GDS-30 that has been reported to be valid in the elderly, but it is thought to still have the same limitation as the GDS-30 in patients with severe cognitive impairment [44]. The CSDD is a 19-item tool used to assess a wide variety of depressive symptoms in patients with cognitive impairment. Its use has been validated in patients with a wide range of cognition, from intact to severely impaired. The CCDD shortcomings are that information needs to be gathered from interviewing the patient *and* interviewer observations, causing it to not only require more time but also a trained clinician to conduct the assessment [44]. The Mood Questionnaire is a modified version of the PHQ-9 and can be completed in a short amount of time, and can either

Table 6 SIGECAPS mnemonic

S	Are you Sad? (**YES**/NO)
I	Do you suffer from Insomnia (**YES**/NO)
G	Do you have feelings of Guilt (**YES**/NO)
E	Do you have a lack of Energy (**YES**/NO)
C	Do you have difficulty Concentrating (**YES**/NO)
A	Have you had changes in your Appetite (**YES**/NO)
P	Do you receive Pleasure from anything in your life (YES/**NO**)
S	Have you had thoughts of Suicide (**YES**/NO)

Table 7 Geriatric depression scale—short form

Choose the best answer for how you have felt over the past week:
1.   Are you basically satisfied with your life? YES/**NO**
2.   Have you dropped many of your activities and interests? **YES**/NO
3.   Do you feel that your life is empty? **YES**/NO
4.   Do you often get bored? **YES**/NO
5.   Are you in good spirits most of the time? YES/**NO**
6.   Are you afraid that something bad is going to happen to you? **YES**/NO
7.   Do you feel happy most of the time? YES/**NO**
8.   Do you often feel helpless? **YES**/NO
9.   Do you prefer to stay at home, rather than going out and doing new thi3259_ngs? **YES**/NO
10.   Do you feel you have more problems with memory than most? **YES**/NO
11.   Do you think it is wonderful to be alive now? YES/**NO**
12.   Do you feel pretty worthless the way you are now? **YES**/NO
13.   Do you feel full of energy? YES/**NO**
14.   Do you feel that your situation is hopeless? **YES**/NO
15.   Do you think that most people are better off than you are? **YES**/NO

Answers in **bold** indicate depression. Although differing sensitivities and specificities have been obtained across studies, for clinical purposes a score >5 points is suggestive of depression and should warrant a follow-up interview. If the patient has a score >10, they almost always have a depression

be answered or conducted by patient interview. The scale of the Mood Questionnaire ranges from 0 to 27 with increasing scores indicating more severe depression. The Mood Questionnaire is easy to use, has a simple format, and good validity in patients with varying degrees of severity in cognitive function [44]. These tools can be selected on a case-by-case basis according to each patient's characteristics and symptoms. SIGECAPS and the GDS include questions that are asked *only of the resident* as opposed to the Cornell Scale that is comprised of questions asked of *both the caregiver and the resident*. SIGECAPS and the GDS are in the public domain and therefore available for use by anyone.

Once a patient has been diagnosed with depression it is important to assess suicide risk. All patients should be questioned about suicidal ideation, a suicide plan, and previous attempts. Caucasian males and elderly men older than 80 have been shown to have the highest risk for completed suicide, followed by males 65–80 years of age. The most important risk factors for suicide are [4]:

- History of a suicide attempt.
- Poor social support.
- Severe depression.
- Psychotic depression.
- Alcoholism.
- Recent loss or bereavement.
- Abuse of sedatives/hypnotics.
- Development of disability.
- Analgesic abuse.

Treatment

Treatment of depression should be aimed at symptom reduction, addressing suicidal thoughts, improving quality of life and function, and preventing relapse with the ultimate goal of remission. However, accomplishing remission can be difficult with one study showing a sustained remission rate of only 30 % after treatment with citalopram [45].

The mainstay of therapy remains psychotherapy and pharmacotherapy. It is important to consider patient characteristics. Psychotherapy may not be helpful in those who have severe cognitive impairment. For patients who have the cognitive ability, cognitive behavioral therapy and learning based therapy have been shown to be useful. Therapy can be provided by a primary care practitioner, social worker, or psychologist [33]. Other non-pharmacologic measures include lessening the institutional appearance of the facility, especially the resident's own space; providing opportunities for meaningful interaction; as well as social, physical, spiritual, and religious activities.

Pharmacotherapy

There are several variables to consider prior to prescribing an antidepressant. These include:

- The antidepressant.
- Potential medication side effects.
- Potential drug–disease interactions.
- Concomitant medical and psychiatric illness.

For example, patients with bipolar disorder are at risk for developing manic episodes when placed on *selective serotonin-reuptake inhibitors* (SSRI).

The classes of medications used to treat depression include SSRIs, serotonin-norepinephrine reuptake inhibitors (SNRIs), tricyclic antidepressants, monoamine oxidase inhibitors (MAOIs), bupropion, and mirtazapine. *SSRIs are typically used as first-line therapy* due to ease of use and low side effect profile. In the elderly the most tolerated SSRIs are sertraline, citalopram, and escitalopram with fluoxetine being least desirable due to its long half-life. *Paroxetine is not preferred in the elderly because it is anticholinergic and sedating* [45]. *The side effects of SSRIs* include nausea, dyspepsia, hyponatremia (due to SIADH), and anorexia. *Serotonin syndrome* is not infrequent and typically occurs when a SSRI is used with other medications that increase serotonin levels in the brain (e.g., SNRIs, buspirone, oxycodone, St. John's wort, linezolid). Serotonin syndrome is characterized by fever, confusion, muscle rigidity, tachycardia, hyperreflexia, and agitation. Muscle rigidity and hyperpyrexia can lead to rhabdomyolysis, which can then cause renal failure. Not only does paroxetine have more side effects, but because of its short half-life, when stopped it can precipitate a *discontinuation syndrome* characterized by increased anxiety, agitation, and tachycardia.

SNRIs (e.g., duloxetine) are useful in patients who have coexistent pain, in particular neuropathic pain. Nausea, agitation, insomnia, and an increase in diastolic blood pressure are side effects often seen with SNRIs. TCAs are useful for treating depression, but are no longer considered first line due to their higher side effect profile and the cardiac risk for arrhythmias or cardiac arrest in the event of overdose and possibly even at therapeutic blood levels. *The most concerning side effects of TCAs are their anticholinergic effects and hypotension.* TCAs are contraindicated in patients with cognitive impairment, recent history (<2 weeks) of myocardial infarction, cardiac conduction abnormalities, orthostatic hypotension, narrow angle glaucoma, urinary retention, and benign prostatic hypertrophy. Nortriptyline and desipramine are more desirable TCAs due to less anticholinergic effects [41].

MAOIs are *typically not used in the elderly* due to possible *drug–drug interactions and dietary modifications that make them difficult to use.* Mirtazapine has both serotonergic and noradrenergic properties and may be useful in patients with insomnia and weight loss owing to its side effects of improved appetite and weight gain and nighttime sedation. Bupropion has noradrenergic effects and its benefits include stimulant properties and low risk for sexual side effects. However, *bupropion lowers the seizure threshold and thus should not be used in patients with a seizure disorder* [46].

Unfortunately, pharmacotherapy in the elderly is often ineffective; thus, many older adults have treatment-resistant depression (defined as failure of two oral antidepressants). Atypical antipsychotics, namely, apriporazole and electroconvulsive therapy are often the next step in treatment. However, these management options are limited by side effects and availability. Newer agents on the horizon for the treatment of depression in the elderly are psilocybin and ketamine, they have yet to undergo statistical validation to prove efficacy within this population.

Attention should be given to the duration of antidepressant treatment as it has implications in the long-term management of depressive episodes. Recurrence is common in the elderly, so it is important to consider a longer duration of treatment. The PROSPECT trial demonstrated that geriatric patients benefit from longer treatment. However, it is also important to assure compliance and follow-up with the patient to assess tolerance to the antidepressant. Other studies have found that geriatric patients had a lower mortality rate after more than 4 years of treatment for depression with antidepressants and psychotherapy as compared to those receiving usual care [47]. *Maintenance therapy* should be *considered for patients with one or more episodes of depression and for those deemed at high risk for recurrence.* For a first episode of depression between 6 and 12 months of antidepressant therapy should be given before reassessment that evaluates continued benefit and potential for relapse. *Patients with three or more lifetime episodes of depression should be considered for lifelong antidepressant therapy* [46]. Special consideration should be made regarding stratification for suicidal risk. Suicide rates are almost twice as high in the elderly as compared to the general population, and alarmingly most older adults who commit suicide have seen a clinician within the previous month.

Psychotherapy

Unfortunately, there are still significant knowledge gaps regarding various therapeutic modalities for depression and their efficacy. Recent research has demonstrated promise in the use of psychotherapy in the elderly. The major available outpatient psychotherapies are as follows: cognitive behavioral therapy, problem solving therapy, life review therapy, interpersonal therapy, and psychodynamic psychotherapy. However, psychotherapy is not commonly used as a treatment for late depression; the major limiting factors being therapist availability, resident access, and health insurance coverage. As we enter the current decade new modalities for therapeutic delivery are being implemented, the most common being telehealth. This intervention is playing a big role in overcoming barriers. However, telehealth has its limitations, because the treatment is limited by the level of executive functioning of the patient and patients may perceive their therapeutic relationship with the practitioner as weaker than traditional delivery methods.

COVID-19

COVID-19 has presented a significant burden on assessment and treatment of mental health in the elderly. Many of the countermeasures implemented as a protective measure against the pandemic have paradoxically worsened mental health indices in institutionalized individuals. The resultant isolation and loneliness experienced by such vulnerable populations had a severe antagonistic effect on well-being in nursing facilities. Studies have shown increased anxiety and depression in residents of Post-Acute and Long-Term Care settings. Telemedicine may serve to alleviate this social burden, but its effect has yet to be validated.

Summary

Dementia, delirium, and depression comprise a diagnostic challenge for the clinician as one, two, or all three conditions may occur in the same individual at the same time or separately over time. An understanding of each of these three conditions will assist the practitioner in providing appropriate clinical evaluation, intervention, and treatment. Evaluation and treatment should be tailored to the goals of care of each resident, guided by the resident's prognosis, level of functioning, comorbidities, and life expectancy. It is essential that monitoring of response to diagnostic and therapeutic interventions be continued, and to consider consultation with specialists or hospitalization if needed. The patient and family should be involved in decision-making in order to accommodate choice, preferences, and goals of care that evolve or change over time.

Pearls for the Practitioner

Dementia
- Dementia is a chronic, irreversible, progressive condition often with insidious onset.
- There is a high prevalence of dementia as a primary diagnosis in the PA/LTC setting.
- Residents with dementia can exhibit challenging or disruptive behavior, as a natural part of their disease process or unmet needs.
- Remember the potentially reversible causes of dementia and the frequent occurrence of a mixed dementia.

Delirium
- Delirium is a potentially life-threatening condition.
- Hyperactive delirium is more easily recognizable than hypoactive delirium.
- Interventions to prevent delirium have been shown to be effective.
- Be aware that many medications and acute medical conditions can precipitate delirium in frail older adults.

Depression
- The prevalence of a depressive disorder or depressive symptoms in the long-term care population has been estimated to be as high as 70%.
- Depression is not an inevitable consequence of aging.
- Depression frequently occurs in the setting of the other medical conditions.
- Several commonly used medications can cause symptoms of depression, even antidepressants.

Websites
- Alzheimer's Association, www.alz.org.
- American Geriatrics Society, www.americangeriatrics.org.
- American Medical Directors Association for their Clinical Practice Guidelines, www.amda.com.

- Hospitalized Elder Life Program for information on delirium, www.elderlife.med. yale.edu.
- Folstein Mini Mental Status Exam (MMSE), the official form has been copyrighted and must be purchased from www.minimental.com.
- St. Louis University Mental Status Exam (SLUMS) is available at: http://medschool.slu.edu/agingsuccessfully/pdfsurveys/slumsexam_05.pdf.
- St. Louis University Geriatrics www.aging/SLU.edu.

References

1. Gagliardi JP. Differentiating among depression, delirium, and dementia in elderly patients. Virtual Mentor. 2008;10(6):383–8.
2. National Nursing Home Survey 2004. Centers for Disease Control; 2009. http://www.cdc. gov/nchs/data/series/sr_13/sr13_167.pdf. Accessed 9 Jan 2010.
3. Rosenblatt A. The art of managing dementia in the elderly. Cleve Clin J Med. 2005;72(Suppl 3):S3–13.
4. Hazzard WR, Blass JP, Halter JB, Ouslander JG, Tinetti ME. Principles of geriatric medicine & gerontology. 5th ed. New York: McGraw-Hill; 2003.
5. Blackwell T, Yaffe K, Laffan A, et al. Associations between sleep-disordered breathing, nocturnal hypoxemia, and subsequent cognitive decline in older community-dwelling men: the osteoporotic fractures in men sleep study. J Am Geriatr Soc. 2015;63(3):453–61.
6. Turner M, Moran N, Kopelman M. Subcortical dementia. Br J Psychiatry. 2002;180:148–51.
7. American Medical Directors Association. Dementia in the long-term care setting clinical practice guideline. Columbia, MD: AMDA; 2009.
8. American Psychiatric Association. Diagnostic and statistical manual of mental disorders. 5th ed. Arlington, VA: American Psychiatric Association; 2013.
9. Donaghy PC, McKeith IG. The clinical characteristics of dementia with Lewy bodies and a consideration of prodromal diagnosis. Alzheimer's Res Ther. 2014;6(4):46.
10. Kim MO, Geschwind MD. Clinical update of Jakob-Creutzfeldt disease. Curr Opin Neurol. 2015;28(3):302–10.
11. Carney RM, Freedland KE. Depression, mortality, and medical morbidity in patients with coronary heart disease. Biol Psychiatry. 2003;54:241–7.
12. Santiago LM, Mattos IE. Depressive symptoms in institutionalized older adults. Rev Saude Publica. 2014;48(2):216–24.
13. Hogan DB. Long-term efficacy and toxicity of cholinesterase inhibitors in the treatment of Alzheimer's disease. Can J Psychiatry. 2014;59(12):618–23.
14. Kurz A, Grimmer T. Efficacy of menantine hydrochloride once-daily in Alzheimer's disease. Expert Opin Pharmacother. 2014;15(13):1955–60.
15. Buhr GW, White HK. Difficult behaviors in long-term care patients with dementia. J Am Med Dir Assoc. 2007;8:E.101–13.
16. Doshi JA, Shaffer T, Briesacher BA. National estimates of medication use in nursing homes: findings from the 1997 Medicare beneficiary survey and the 1996 medical expenditure survey. J Am Geriatr Soc. 2005;53:438–43.
17. Zhang QH, Sheng ZY, Yao YM. Septic encephalopathy: when cytokines interact with acetylcholine in the brain. Mil Med Res. 2014;1:20.
18. Choi SH, Lee H, Chung TS, et al. Neural network functional connectivity during and after an episode of delirium. Am J Psychiatr. 2012;169(5):498–507.
19. Hshieh TT, Inouye SK, Oh ES. Delirium in the elderly. Psychiatr Clin North Am. 2018;41(1):1–17.

20. Conner KQ, Copeland VC, Grote NK, et al. Mental health treatment seeking among older adults with depression: the impact of stigma and race. Am J Geriatr Psychiatry. 2010;18(6):531–43.
21. American Medical Directors Association. Delirium and acute problematic behavior in the long-term care setting clinical practice guideline. Columbia, MD: AMDA; 2008.
22. Inouye SK. Delirium in older persons. N Engl J Med. 2006;354:1157–65.
23. Fick DM, Agostini JV, Inouye SK. Delirium superimposed on dementia: a systematic review. J Am Geriatr Soc. 2002;50:1723–32.
24. Forsberg MM. Delirium update for post-acute care and long-term care settings: a narrative review. J Am Osteopathic Assoc. 2017;117(1):32–8.
25. Ozbolt LB, Paniagua MA, Kaiser RM. Atypical antipsychotics for the treatment of delirious elders. J Am Med Dir Assoc. 2008;9:18–28.
26. Elie M, Cole MG, Primeau FJ, Bellavance F. Delirium risk factors in elderly hospitalized patients. J Gen Intern Med. 1998;13:204–12.
27. Fong TG, Tulebaey SR, Inouye SK. Delirium in elderly adults: diagnosis; prevention and treatment. Nat Rev Neurol. 2009;5:210–20.
28. Marcantonio ER, Ngo LH, O'Connor M, et al. 3D-CAM: derivation and validation of a 3-minute diagnostic interview for CAM-defined delirium: a cross-sectional diagnostic test study. Ann Intern Med. 2014;161(8):354–61.
29. Clegg A, Siddiqi N, Heaven A, Young J, Holt R. Interventions for preventing delirium in older people in institutional long-term care (Review). Cochrane Library; 2017.
30. Jung H, Meucci M, Unruh MA, et al. Antipsychotic use in nursing home residents admitted with hip fracture. J Am Geriatr Soc. 2013;61(1):101–6.
31. Seitz D, Purandare N, Conn D. Prevalence of psychiatric disorders among older adults in long-term care homes: a systematic review. Int Psychogeriatr. 2010;22(7):1025–39.
32. Hoover DR, Siegel M, Lucas J, Kalay E, Gaboda D, Devan DP, Crystal S. Depression in the first year of stay for elderly long-term nursing home residents in the U.S.A. Int Psychogeriatr. 2010;22(7):1161–71.
33. American Medical Directors Association. Depression clinical practice guideline. Columbia, MD: AMDA; 2003.
34. World Health Organization. Depression. http://www.who.int/mental_health/management/depression/wfmh_paper_depression_wmhd_2012.pdf?ua=1.
35. Barry LC, Murphy TE, Gill TM. Depressive symptoms and functional transitions over time in older persons. Am J Geriatr Psychiatry. 2011;19:789–91.
36. Alexopoulos GS, Buckwalter K, Olin J, et al. Comorbidity of late life depression: an opportunity for research on mechanisms and treatment. Biol Psychiatry. 2002;52:543–8.
37. Cepoiu M, McCusker J, Cole MG, et al. Recognition of depression in older inpatients. J Gen Intern Med. 2007;22:559–64.
38. Jeste DV, Blazer DG, First M. Aging-related diagnostic variations: need for diagnostic criteria appropriate for elderly psychiatric patients. Biol Psychiatry. 2005;58:265–71.
39. Rothschild AJ. The diagnosis and treatment of late-life depression. J Clin Psychiatry. 1996;57(Suppl5):5–11.
40. Alexopoulos GS. Depression in the elderly. Lancet. 2005;365(9475):1961–70.
41. Peskind ER. Management of depression in long-term care of patients with Alzheimer's disease. J Am Med Dir Assoc. 2003;1(Supp Nov/Dec):S141–5.
42. Vilalta-Franch J, Lopez-Pousa S, Llinas-Regla J, Calvo-Perxas L, Merino-Aguado J. Depression subtypes and 5-year risk of dementia and Alzheimer disease in patients aged 70 years. Int J Geriatr Psychiatry. 2013;28(4):341–50.
43. Koopmans RTCM, Zuidema SU, Leontjevas R, Gerritsen DL. Review: comprehensive assessment of depression and behavioral problems in long-term care. Int Psychogeriatr. 2010;22(7):1054–62.
44. Azulai A, Walsh CA. Screening for geriatric depression in residential care facilities: a systematic narrative review. J Gerontol Social Work. 2014;

45. Zisook S, Ganadijan K, Moutier C, et al. Sequenced Treatment Alternatives to Relieve Depression (STAR*D): lessons learned. J Clin Psychiatry. 2008;69:1184–5.
46. Rojas-Fernandez C, Mikhail M. Contemporary concepts in the pharmacotherapy of depression in older people. Can Pharm J (Ott). 2012;145(3):128–35.
47. Gallo JJ, Bogner HR, Morales KH, et al. The effect of primary care practice-based depression intervention on mortality in older adults: a randomized trial. Ann Intern Med. 2007;146:689–98.

Ethical and Legal Issues in Post-Acute and Long-Term Care

David A. Smith and Randall D. Huss

Introduction

Ethical dilemmas and legal issues commonly occur in post-acute and long-term care. Health care ethics provides a framework for the application of *values* (patient, caregiver, and societal) to the process of clinical/medical decision-making. This process requires the weighing of values, facts, and prognostication in order to produce a just and supportable decision. However, clinicians/practitioners often encounter competing values, e.g., the right of self-determination of an individual versus the interests of society as a whole, and thus must make decisions based on the facts, as well as the likelihood and consequences of various potential outcomes.

D. A. Smith (✉)
Geriatric Consultants of Central Texas, Brownwood, TX, USA

R. D. Huss
Department of Family Medicine and Geriatrics, Mercy Clinic, Rolla, MO, USA

© The Author(s), under exclusive license to Springer Nature Switzerland AG 2023
P. Winn et al. (eds.), *Post-Acute and Long-Term Care Medicine*, Current Clinical Practice, https://doi.org/10.1007/978-3-031-28628-5_15

The *law* is a society's compilation of rules that are intended to be uniformly applied (equal protection under the law), mandatory (ignorance of the law is no excuse), and modifiable only through the legislative process (the rule of law). Fortunately, the tenets of health care ethics continue to be considered in the establishment of laws that interface with the practice of medicine. Challenging situations often arise for practitioners when applying the principles of health care ethics within the constraints of existing State and Federal law. All state and federal surveys of long-term care facilities follow regulations that are dictated by law. Clinicians are admonished to know the laws of the jurisdiction in which they practice and to seek legal counsel for clarification when needed. The contents of this chapter are educational only and not formal legal advice.

Principles of Health Care Ethics

The five principles of health care ethics include *autonomy, beneficence, justice, non-maleficence,* and *fidelity*. These principles do not stand alone or in a hierarchy, but must be considered in the context of each other. Frequently these ethical principles compete. However, a decision based upon one of the ethical principles usually predominates.

Autonomy is the principle attesting to an individual's right to sovereignty over oneself. It encompasses the right to self-determination and privacy. The law recognizes the right to privacy in statutes that codify the privacy of medical records such as the Health Insurance Portability and Accountability Act (HIPAA), informed consent, and the individual's right to decline life-sustaining treatment. Mental incapacity may alter the implementation of the principle of autonomy.

Beneficence is the ethical principle that holds a practitioner responsible to do good to others. Good Samaritan laws are designed to protect individuals when they act by this principle. Similarly, laws that require health care professionals to report suspected elder abuse is an example of this principle. Laws related to guardianship and other forms of surrogate decision-making for those either adjudicated *incompetent in a court of law* or clinically determined not to have mental capacity derive from the principle of beneficence. Beneficence also holds that any procedure or intervention proposed for a patient by a health care professional must be capable of providing a benefit to the patient, and that by its application, does not provide greater burden than benefit. Ethically, there is no obligation for a health care professional to provide or even offer an intervention incapable of providing a benefit or whose burden is greater than any benefit to a patient (*futile* care). This stands as an ethical check (to do good to others) versus unbridled autonomy. An example where this may apply in PA/LTC are decisions in patients with advanced dementia who fail oral feeding, and the provision of tube feeding is raised and/or suggested by staff or family in an attempt to provide adequate nutrition and hydration.

Non-maleficence, a corollary to beneficence, holds that it is the responsibility of the practitioner to do no harm, to not provide interventions whose burdens or potential harm would outweigh benefit. Avoiding unnecessary surgery and optimizing patient safety are examples. Laws regarding medical malpractice are based on this principle and claims for punitive damages stem from what plaintiffs perceive as a breach of this principle.

Justice is the ethical principle espousing the responsibility of medical professionals to treat patients equitably (fairly) and to consider not only one's patient, but also the good of society. An example of this principle is when a physician assists with terminating the driving privileges of an unsafe driver. This principle also entails the equitable allocation of society's limited healthcare dollars and resources (*distributive justice*).

Finally, *fidelity, a corollary to the principle of justice*, involves the medical practitioner's responsibility to keep the terms of the "doctor/patient contract." Truthfulness and substantial compliance with informed consent are components of fidelity as is *non-abandonment*. Practitioners should not summarily cease to act for the benefit of one's patient even when that patient has not lived up to their side of the doctor/patient contract (e.g., noncompliance) or exerted their autonomy and chosen a course of medical action with which the physician disagrees. In such circumstances the physician should attempt to provide the best possible outcome in the context of the patient's treatment choices. Alternatively, practitioners may exit the doctor/patient contract by providing emergency care as needed, while affording the patient sufficient time to become established with another health care professional.

Historically, physicians often made decisions for patients based on the principle of beneficence without an appreciation of patient autonomy, a practice known as *paternalism*. Society's response was a consumer movement, which included the *Patient's Bill of Rights*. While needed, it may have inadvertently resulted in patient autonomy to supersede other ethical principles. We must recognize that the principles of autonomy, beneficence, non-maleficence and justice all be considered to guide ethical decision-making. For example, autonomy and the right to privacy could be subordinate to the principles of beneficence and justice in the case of an individual with a contagious illness posing a public health threat who refuses to follow guidelines to prevent the transmission of the disease to others. Conversely, beneficence and justice (the State's interest in protecting life) would be subordinate to autonomy when a capacitated adult Jehovah's Witness declines a lifesaving blood transfusion. However, if a patient were a child below the age of consent, the State's interest in protecting life would prevail.

The vast majority of applications of these ethical principles are not played out in the legal arena, but rather in everyday patient/practitioner medical decision-making. The practice of medicine within the long-term care continuum commonly involves issues related to diminished mental capacity and mental illness, treatments with narrow risk/benefit ratios, end-of-life care, elder abuse and exploitation, and utilization of limited and expensive medical resources. Practice in post-acute and long-term care challenges every practitioner to abide by these principles and to competently apply them with skill and confidence. Input from the interdisciplinary team and from the patient/family is essential to applying these principles and to choosing an appropriate course of action. As such, every practitioner must be able to effectively communicate and to apply and balance these principles to the specifics of the patient's clinical scenario and to them succinctly record his/her reasoning in the medical record.

Resident Rights

When an individual enters any facility or program within the long-term care continuum they do not lose their fundamental *constitutional rights*. Providers have an obligation to inform residents of their rights and to encourage and assist them in exercising these rights. It is illegal for a facility, program, or any employee to infringe upon a person's human rights by threatening, coercing, intimidating, or retaliating against a resident who is exercising their rights. A facility or program should educate residents on how to use the complaint process if they feel their human rights are being violated. Specific responsibilities of PALTC institutions are further described in the Abuse, Neglect, and Exploitation section of this chapter. A synopsis of Resident rights are listed in state and federal regulations, which are summarized in Table 1. For full text see [1].

A resident's rights may only be restricted when it is necessary to protect the resident or another individual (resident, staff or family) from potential harm, or to protect the rights of another resident, e.g., infringement on another's privacy. Facility rules must be fully disclosed before admission, such as scheduled smoking breaks or a nonsmoking policy. These can only be enforced if the resident or their surrogate have agreed to these rules as a condition of admission. Furthermore, problem behaviors may be addressed by practitioners through behavior modification programming, behavioral contracting with the resident, or as a condition of continued residence in the facility if done as part of a therapeutic plan of care and in keeping with nursing facility regulations. A resident with mental incapacity still retains all of the rights outlined in Table 1. However, if a resident lacks capacity, their rights would be advocated by their legally designated surrogate decision-maker. For instance, a mentally incapacitated resident with diabetes mellitus who wants to spend their money on candy and soda may be care planned to receive budgeted amounts of spending money from their facility account and to be encouraged to choose more healthy snacks, given that the resident's surrogate decision-maker is in agreement. *Facilities and practitioners should be aware that litigation alleging infringement on a resident's human rights may not be covered under malpractice insurance.*

Table 1 Synopsis of CMS' statement of resident rights

Your rights and protections as a nursing home resident
What are my rights in a nursing home?
As a nursing home resident, you have certain rights and protections under federal and state law that help ensure you get the care and services you need. You have the right to be informed, make your own decisions, and have your personal information private
The nursing home must tell you about these rights and explain them in writing in a language you understand. They must also explain in writing how you should act and what you're responsible for while you're in the nursing home. This must be done before or at the time you're admitted, as well as during your stay. You must acknowledge in writing that you got this information
At a minimum, federal law specifies that nursing homes must protect and promote the following rights of each resident. You have the right to:
Be treated with respect
Make your own schedule
Participate in activities
Be free from discrimination based on race, color, national origin, disability, age, or religion
Be free from abuse and neglect
Be free from restraints, physical or chemical
Make complaints without fear of punishment: the nursing home must address the issue promptly
Get proper medical care: To be fully informed of your total health status, involved in choice of doctor, participate in decisions that affect your care, take part in developing your care plan, have access to your medical records, to express any complaints you have about your care or treatment, to create advanced directives in accordance with state law, and to refuse participation in experimental treatment
Have your representative notified: If you are involved in an accident, your physical, mental or psychosocial status worsens, you have a life-threatening condition, you have medical complications, your treatment needs to change significantly, or the nursing home decides to transfer or discharge you
Get information on services and fees: To be told in writing about all nursing home services and fees before admission and if these change. Before admission, the nursing home must tell you orally and in writing and display written information on how to apply for and use Medicare/Medicaid benefits
Manage your money: Or choose someone you trust, have access to your money and financial records
Get proper privacy, property, and living arrangements: To keep and use your personal belongings, have private visits, make or get private phone calls, have privacy in sending or receiving mail or emails, be protected from theft, share a room with your spouse if both agree, be notified before changes in roommate or room (taking your preferences into account), and to review the nursing home's health and fire safety inspections
Spend time with visitors: At any time not interfering with care or privacy of others, and to see any person for help with health, social, legal, or other services
Get social services: For counseling, solving problems with other residents, help in contacting legal or financial professionals, and discharge planning
Leave the nursing home: For visits or leave of absence (consistent with health insurance rules) or to move out

(continued)

Table 1 (continued)

Your rights and protections as a nursing home resident
Have protection against unfair transfer or discharges: unless it's necessary for the welfare, health, or safety of you or others, nursing home care is no longer necessary or the nursing home has not been paid or closes. You have the right of appeal
Form or participate in resident groups: including resident councils and the home must provide space and act upon grievances/recommendations of the group

Centers for Medicare and Medicaid Services

Elder Abuse, Neglect, and Exploitation

Residents within the long-term care continuum represent a population vulnerable to abuse, neglect, and exploitation by a family member, another resident, a member of the health care team, or even the facility. Abuse, neglect, and exploitation may be deliberate or arise due to inadequate staff knowledge and training.

Abuse is an *act of commission* intended to do harm. Abuse can be physical, financial, sexual, or emotional in nature. Many episodes of physical and emotional abuse are sporadic and occur as an unguarded response to an elderly, demented, or mentally ill person's behavior directed toward a facility caregiver. Resistive, combative, and assaultive behaviors by the resident may trigger retaliation if the caregiver fails to understand the behavior is inherent to the disease process. Caregivers are more likely to be abusive if they lack knowledge of alternative behavioral approaches or become unduly focused on the need to complete caregiving tasks. Unresolved stress, depression, and cultural acceptance of punishment increase the risk that a caregiver be abusive. Abusive caregivers are also more likely to have been abused in the past or present.

Neglect is an *act of omission*, the failure to meet one's obligation to anticipate and meet the needs of a vulnerable or elderly person. Elders who have been unrecognized as mentally incapacitated, may be neglectful of themselves, refusing assistance, living in squalor, and not attending to their health, hygiene, or safety (a common occurrence in cases of Adult Protective Services). Neglect may be purposeful or retaliatory. When an elder shows no gratitude or is critical of the care they receive, neglect may occur. Frequently, neglect is the result of inadequate understanding and anticipation by the caregiver of a vulnerable person's needs. Poor knowledge and training on the specifics of care giving, inadequate care planning to delineate anticipated needs, lack of "job ownership," unprofessional attitudes, and low motivation of caregivers are all potential risk factors for neglect. Elders with challenging needs due to morbid obesity or who are slow with assisted feeding have been shown to be at increased risk for neglect. Neglect can occur when caregivers fail to recognize that an individual's disability is progressing and subsequently have increased care needs. Changes in the plan of care should occur when a change of resident condition is recognized. Neglect may also occur at the institutional level due to understaffing, or as a result of inadequate supervision, orientation, or training. Lack of staff cohesion, high staff turnover, and inadequate resources can also lead to institutional neglect.

Exploitation refers to *acts of misappropriation of a vulnerable person's money or property*. This is not necessarily for the purpose of enriching the perpetrator. For example, two daughters may have their mother's best interest in mind as they decided to sell the home of their mentally or physically incapacitated mother while she is in the nursing facility recuperating from surgery following a hip fracture, having determined she will no longer be safe and be at high risk for repeated falls if she continues to live alone. However, exploitation can be overt fraud or theft. Misappropriating an elder's pension and Social Security checks for their own use, and illegal transfers of property without proper consent are examples of exploitation commonly perpetrated by families. Pilfering a resident's personal property or medication is another type of exploitation commonly committed by facility staff. Occasionally, even guardians and those designated as Power of Attorney may exploit the person they are obligated to protect. Although the Courts require a yearly report from guardians in order to discourage exploitation, no such oversight is required of persons with other types of surrogate decision-making authority. Practitioners should be alert to evidence of exploitation and report such concerns to the appropriate authority. The state government agency responsible for nursing home surveys is typically the authority to investigate abuse of a nursing home resident by staff or a family member. State Adult Protective Services or the State Ombudsman can also be contacted to investigate abuse, neglect, or exploitation.

Abuse, neglect, and exploitation perpetrated by a family member, unpaid caregiver, or other private individual are usually resolved without bringing criminal charges. In contrast, abuse, neglect, and exploitation of a resident by an institution or a certified/licensed caregiver within the long-term care continuum are usually handled by the formal survey process, and increasingly by licensure review and even criminalization. The CMS State Operations Manual (SOM) requires nursing facilities to be proactive to:

- Have policies and procedures on abuse prevention.
- Screen potential employees to be hired.
- Provide initial and ongoing staff training on elder abuse.
- Identify potential abuse events to include setting expectations among staff for reporting.
- Investigate alleged abuse events and incidents that might constitute abuse.
- Protect residents from retaliation or distress during investigations of abuse.
- Report incidents, alleged abuse events, investigations, and facility actions in response to investigations as required by state and federal authority.

Racial Disparity in Quality of Care/Patient Outcomes

Examples of poorer medical outcomes in patients of color compared to Caucasians include: higher use of restraints, more frequent pressure injuries, decreased provision of recommended immunizations, inadequate control of pain, and poor quality of life. Also, there is an increased burden of illness in persons of color: higher rates

Table 2 Factors associated with racial disparity

• Geographic/demographic
– Discriminatory community housing practices detrimental to geographic/demographic diversity
– Discriminatory community financial lending practices
– Discriminatory community educational practices contributing to disparity in wealth
– Trend to locate assisted living and skilled nursing facilities in higher income areas
• Financial
– Inadequate support of Medicare/Medicaid funding of PA LTC coupled with racial wealth disparity
– Funding dynamics that concentrate residents of color in lower resourced facilities
– Racial discrimination in staff hiring, salaries, career advancement
– Financially punitive survey practices levying civil monetary penalties on lower resourced facilities caring disproportionally for residents of color
• Attitudinal
– Racist attitudes causing inequity in access to care and delivery of treatment
– Facility language, menu, activities, and milieu insensitive to or contrary to the preferences and needs of residents of color
– Attitudes explaining or contextualizing disparities as due to biological or genetic factors
– Historically justified mistrust of caregivers and institutions held by patients of color
– Transfer and placement decisions by discharge planners, social workers, administrators, attending physicians that are racially biased
– Racist verbal assaults directed toward residents and staff persons of color by other staff or other mentally capacitated residents

of heart attack, hospitalization, and mortality. The current COVID 19 pandemic in the USA attests to such systemic inequity. A complex array of contributing factors include geography, demography, financial policy (proprietary and government), employment policy, and personal attitudes/discrimination. Many, if not most of these factors are not under the direct control of administrators and medical practitioners. Table 2 is a partial listing of structural/institutional, cultural and personal factors that contribute to racial disparities in healthcare outcomes in nursing facilities (adapted from [2]).

Mental Capacity, Competence, and Surrogate Decision-Making

All adults are considered mentally competent by law unless adjudicated otherwise. A court adjudicates *competency* or *incompetency*. Physicians and other providers, as recognized by individual state law, may make a determination of an individual's mental *capacity* or *incapacity*. Either may be *partial* or *total* or be specific to a particular circumstance. *Capacity is often decision-specific.* To be determined to have decisional capacity for a proposed procedure or treatment, a person must be able to understand its benefits, risks, and alternatives (including no treatment); be able to reason among alternatives; and be able to communicate their decision (i.e., be able to give *informed consent*). Incapacity may be *permanent* as in advanced dementia, or *temporary* as in delirium or intoxication. While often used interchangeably, competency is a legal determination by a court of law while mental capacity is a clinical one.

There are several distinct types of competencies under the law. A person is competent to stand trial for a crime if they know the difference between right and wrong and are able to participate in their own defense. Different criteria exist for competency to make or change a will; this is referred to as *testamentary capacity*. When making or changing a will, a person is considered to have testamentary capacity if they know the nature/extent of their property; know the natural objects of their bounty (heirs); the disposition that their will is making; and understand the implications of their bequeathal; and be free of undue influence or coercion.

Practitioners are rarely asked to provide an opinion on mental capacity as it relates to competence to stand trial, though in cases of resident-to-resident physical or sexual assault this may occur. Most often practitioners are asked to evaluate mental capacity as it relates to testamentary capacity. Asking open ended questions that relate to criteria for testamentary capacity, as well as performing a standard test of cognition, can help determine capacity.

Mental capacity assessment is often needed in long-term care practice to determine a person's ability to make decisions in their own best interest of a personal, medical, and financial nature. Often an adult child is perfunctorily listed as the *"Responsible Party"* on the nursing facility demographic face sheet and delegated to make decisions without any formal authority, with no attempt made to determine whether the resident is partially or fully able to make their own decisions. This practice runs contrary to the ethical principle of autonomy and exemplifies *agism*. Indeed, cases have occurred where a mentally capacitated individual has been kept in nursing home care against their will, through the combined efforts of the facility, attending physician, and family.

Conversely, there are nursing or assisted living facilities, which list the resident as the "Responsible Party" even though the resident is moderately or severely demented, psychotic, or neuropsychiatrically impaired, and clearly do not have decisional capacity. This usually occurs when the resident has no close family or proxy legal representative. When an elder is found to be mentally incapacitated and is facing a situation requiring an informed decision, the practitioner must consider all the surrogate decision-making options. In such situations, look for documents such as living wills or advance care directives, or any individuals who can provide "substituted judgment" for what the individual would have decided if he or she were able to express an informed decision.

In many States, statutes have been adopted that list a hierarchy of family decision-makers, which usually begin with the spouse, then the oldest adult child, and so forth. This then obviates the need for a more involved legal process (i.e., guardianship). In such cases, practitioners make a determination of a resident's temporary or permanent mental incapacity in the medical record, and then proceed to contact the family member highest on the hierarchy list who is both capable and willing to be the surrogate decision-maker. Should a practitioner subsequently believe that this individual is not acting in the best interest of the patient, then he/she should challenge the person's surrogate decision-making by submitting a report to either Adult Protective Services or perhaps to the court dependent as the resident's area of jurisdiction.

Other types of surrogate decision-making include a *Power of Attorney* and *Conservatorships*. The latter typically deals only with financial matters while a Powers of Attorney may be designated as to decision-making related to "person" or "estate" or both.

- A ***General Power of Attorney*** is a legal document by which a mentally capacitated (presumed competent) person chooses another to make decisions on their behalf commencing from the time the document is executed and *endures until either death or a future time of mental incapacity*. These documents may entrust broad powers or be limited in scope, e.g., only grant authority to complete a real estate transaction.
- A ***Springing Power of Attorney*** is completed by a mentally capacitated person to give "their chosen surrogate" decision-making powers *at some future time when the person may become mentally incapacitated.*
- A ***Durable Power of Attorney*** *goes into effect at execution* (if agreed to by the capacitated person) and continues to grant surrogate decision-making power to the chosen person *beyond the occurrence of mental incapacity* of the person who established the durable power of attorney.

Practitioners should remain alert to the circumstance under which a family and lawyer draw up a Power of Attorney and encourage a mentally incapacitated person to sign it. Remember that only *a person who has mental capacity can execute a Power of Attorney*. Once a person is mentally incapacitated, a Power of Attorney cannot be legally completed. Then another form of surrogate decision-making such as a *guardianship* must be established.

Guardianship. This may be either *temporary* or *permanent*. A physician will often be asked to provide the court an opinion as to a person's mental incapacity (in part or total) stating the reason for incapacity and elaborating on any medical condition and medications that affect that person's mental status and capacity. Typically this is done using a standardized legal form to be submitted to the court. Upon making a ruling of incompetence, the court judge will name a guardian for surrogate decision-making. The guardianship may have limitations. For example, a guardian may not have authority to sign consent for admission to inpatient psychiatric care, sign a Do Not Resuscitate (DNR), or authorize the withdrawal of life sustaining treatment. These latter medical decisions may require separate petition to the court for action. In most States a surrogate decision-maker cannot give permission for the nursing facility to hide antipsychotic medication in food, give it by force, or by injection on a routine basis. Even a severely demented or mentally ill person who has objected to taking medication cannot be forced or tricked to do so. This usually would not apply to the treatment of a psychiatric emergency in which the behavior puts the patient at imminent danger to self or others. In some states, the need for psychiatric treatment may be sufficient to establish a forced medication order while in others the standard of danger or imminent danger to self or others must be met.

Guardians should attempt to represent resident/patient choices that follow existing advanced directives. If no such directives exist then the guardian should make a best effort to make decisions on behalf of their ward that are consistent with known values, culture, and life history of the ward. When partial capacity exists, the wishes of the ward should be respected for those decisions made within the confines of their capacity. When totally incapacitated, the guardian and caregivers should still attempt to ascertain the resident/patient opinions on different choices, especially when the probable outcomes of such choices are inconsequential. Wherever possible, *assent* should be solicited even when *consent* cannot. Ultimately, guardians or caregivers exercising substituted judgment must make decisions in the "best interest" of the resident.

Evaluation of Capacity

An elder's capacity may be challenged when they make a decision with which others do not agree and should not be prejudiced by either the examiner's or the caregiver's preferred choice in a decision. Lifelong poor judgment does not necessarily indicate mental incapacity. People have *a* right to make mistakes, and some exercise this right again and again. However, poor judgment that results from disease of the brain and that represents a decline from prior intellectual/cognitive functioning may indicate mental incapacity.

A capacity evaluation should include a formal mental status examination (Table 3). This includes testing of judgment, orientation (time, person, place, situation), memory (recent and remote), the ability to think in the abstract, and to do

Table 3 Elements of a mental capacity evaluation (*J O M A C*)

• *J*udgment
• *O*rientation (time, person, place)
• *M*emory (recent, remote)
• *A*bility to think in the abstract
• *A*bility to calculate
• *A*bility to explain the nature of the needed decision at hand
• *A*bility to explain personal implications of choices, understand risks/benefits
• *A*bility to explain the rationale for choices
• *A*bility to explain how their decision best matches their personal goals
• *A*bility to persist in a decision unless new facts or circumstances arise
• *A*bility to negotiate (unless the issue at hand is a core value)
• *E*valuate for undue influence or coercion
• *C*onsider the effect of mental illness on decision-making

calculations. Formal brief mental status testing with the *Mini Mental Status Examination* (MMSE) or the *Saint Louis University Mental Status Exam* (SLUMS) can be helpful.

Judgment can be tested with hypothetical scenarios such as requesting a solution to the problem, "What would you do if you were the first person in a crowded movie theater to discover that it was on fire?" Answers not recognizing the need to avoid causing a panic would indicate faulty judgment. If the need for a specific and important decision has required an evaluation, the clinician should explore the individual's ability to explain the nature of the decision to be made, their thoughts on the various possible choices, and assessment of risks and benefits. A person with capacity should also be able to articulate how they have come to a decision, what factors were important to them, and what values and preferences they applied to come to the decision. Be aware that poor hearing or eyesight can interfere with the individual's understanding of the issues at hand. Overall, this process is similar to the tenants of *informed consent*.

Good *judgment* involves the *ability to negotiate* in their best interest, and be congruent to their fundamental human or religious values. For example, an individual may decline a blood transfusion as a Jehovah's Witness. A person with a compelling need to be admitted to long-term care facility yet refuses to discuss the matter and insists that her daughter can meet her needs, though the daughter has categorically told her she cannot, would demonstrate questionable mental capacity. If the potential consequences are not too high, such a dilemma may best be handled by allowing the mother to experience the consequences of her decision. *Self-neglect* by a person should be recognized and would support a determination of mental incapacity.

The *ability to think in the abstract* can be evaluated by asking the individual to explain the idiomatic meaning of a proverb with which the individual is familiar. A concrete (non-abstract) answer may indicate low IQ, low educational level or an organic impairment of the brain.

Ability to calculate can be tested by requesting the individual to subtract 7 serial from 100. A value comparison of certain assets may be helpful, e.g., "Which is worth more? Your farm or your antique car?"

An "enmeshed" family can place undue coercion on an elder family member. Practitioners should be aware that in certain cultures the opinion of a family leader or a family consensus is the accepted norm for decision-making.

Mental illness, (e.g., depression and psychosis), can be an underlying cause of mental incapacity. However, decisions that conform to the individual's historical value system, culture, and life history, prior to the onset of mental illness, may be considered valid. A patient afflicted with paranoid schizophrenia who, while scowling at the examiner, refuses evaluation and treatment of a breast mass "because it's probably nothing," probably lacks capacity to make this decision. Or a patient with suicidal depression who declines electroconvulsive therapy because "it won't do any good" or because "I don't deserve to feel better" is likely incapacitated, while a similar patient who declines because "I'm scared I'll have memory loss, you told me ECT can cause that" is likely capacitated.

A diagnosis of dementia does not necessarily imply mental incapacity. The degree of mental capacity will depend on the severity of cognitive loss, the domains affected, the kind and complexity of the issue, and the potential consequences of the decision. A study by Marson et al. had shown that most participants with Alzheimer's disease with MMSE of 19 or greater had capacity to make and communicate choices, as well as the potential consequences and rational for their choices [3]. However, practitioners should not use the MMSE score as the sole criterion when determining capacity. A Standardized evaluation such as the *MacArthur Capacity Assessment Test* is not designed to determine if an elder has capacity at a certain score [4].

End-of-Life Issues

Residents in long-term care facilities often have a limited life expectancy, commonly 2–3 years. As such, end-of-life issues commonly arise. It is a federal mandate that upon admission to a hospital, a long-term care facility, home health or hospice, to inquire whether a patient has an *advance directive*. In an emergency, persons without a known advance directive are presumed to have elected to pursue life-saving and life-sustaining treatment. In some States, persons with an advance directive that includes a DNR, would be presumed the person to have verbally withdrawn their DNR if they had called for an ambulance. Advance directives should be reviewed upon admission to the hospital or a long-term care facility.

An Advance Directive for health care may take the form of a *Living Will*. Both a Springing and Durable Power of Attorney are also advance directives that include designation of a proxy decision-maker. The Living Will outlines the general and specific wishes of a capacitated individual (or previously capacitated person) as to various health care interventions to be (or not be) provided irrespective of future loss of mental capacity. Most living wills lack sufficient directives to address specific clinical circumstance, and often result in doubt and controversy. However, a living will can provide guidance to the family and thus lessen discord and relieve guilt. Note that a Living Will may state a person's desire to receive aggressive treatment such as cardiopulmonary resuscitation (CPR), respiratory intubation, or insertion of a feeding tube.

Issues to consider when completing a Living Will include
- Whether the person agrees or declines to give a Power of Attorney the authority to consent to research.
- Whether they wish to be an organ donor.
- Whether they wish to accept or decline psychotropic drug treatment and/or electroconvulsive treatment.
- Whether they wish to be allowed to have an emotional, physical, or sexual relationship with another person if the latter express assent.

- Whether they wish to continue to have a physical relationship with their spouse if he/she assents. Be aware that some state surveyors and caregivers (both formal and informal) believe that once mentally incapacitated, a person may no longer be able to consent to intimacy with their spouse.

The wishes expressed in a Living Will do not oblige the practitioner to provide *futile care*. The American Medical Association defines futile care as medical treatment that would provide little or no benefit. Offering futile care (e.g., CPR in an unwitnessed cardiopulmonary arrest in the nursing home or feeding tube placement in a patient with end stage dementia) as if it were a reasonable treatment option breaches the ethical principles of beneficence, non-maleficence, and fidelity. It would be prudent to educate families on futile medical treatments.

There is no ethical difference between withholding or withdrawing a treatment. For instance, placing a person on a respirator when in acute respiratory failure does not oblige the practitioner to continue artificial ventilation when it is evident that the patient has intractable adult respiratory distress syndrome. Similarly, a feeding tube begun in an acute situation where the prognosis for recovery is uncertain, may be legally and ethically removed at a later time when a poor prognosis becomes clear and meaningful recovery unlikely. At end-of-life controversial issues may arise such as *active euthanasia* and *physician-assisted suicide*. Both the AMA and AMDA have issued policy statements and white papers on these issues [5–7].

Ethical and Legal Aspects of Research in Long-Term Care

Given the unresolved issues in long-term care, the value of research cannot be understated. Studies rarely focus on this population because potential subjects often have confounding diseases and conditions and are at risk to drop out of a study due to unexpected death or intervening illness. They are also considered a "vulnerable population" that require a high ethical and legal standard for informed consent to participate in research. In the past lack of a high standard has resulted in victimization of patients and research subjects on the basis of race (e.g., Tuskegee study of untreated syphilis, and Henrieta Lack unauthorized use of HeLa cells). Tragically, this has caused mistrust in racial communities such that they are underrepresented in current research. The high prevalence of cognitive impairment also makes the LTC population vulnerable to abuse in recruitment for research. Protections and processes for the ethical and legal recruitment of incapacitated persons do allow for a legally recognized surrogate decision-maker to consent on behalf of the incapacitated person to be a research subject. However, an elder who in any way demonstrates lack of assent to the research should be either not enrolled or withdrawn.

Liability in Long-Term Care

An awareness of liability issues in LTC is crucial to practitioners to the delivery of care and care transitions. Most practitioners agree that when medical errors occur as a result of either negligence or purposeful misdeeds that the injured party should be informed, and if indicated, compensated. Common liability issues in long-term care are listed in Table 4 [8]. Many LTC providers concur that inevitable poor medical outcomes, inevitable decline in function or cognition, and unavoidable accidents/ injuries are frequently litigated unfairly. A negative view of long-term care by the public and the press may result in the facility and practitioners open to criticism and liability.

In order for a *medical malpractice* **action to have merit, plaintiffs must show**
- Defendant(s) had a *duty* to the patient.
- A *breach of* an existing *standard of care* occurred.
- The breach was a *substantial proximate cause* of harm suffered by the plaintiff.
- Harm, injuries, (e.g., *damages*) and their value.

Given that many nursing facility and assisted living residents have a limited life expectancy and are not employable, economic damages are often limited. But, *non-economic damages*, (e.g., pain and suffering or family/spouse loss of counsel and consortium) may increase damage. In addition, *punitive damages* can occur that are designed as financial punishment for bad practices by a defendant.

Duty exists when a practitioner or facility has an ongoing relationship with the patient. Practitioners are duty bound to act in accordance with their *professional standards*, while facilities have a duty to act within existing state and federal regulations. Some institutional policies and procedures may exceed professional standards or regulations. A practitioner is expected to exercise the degree of care and skill that would be expected of a reasonably prudent practitioner of that same discipline under the same or similar circumstances.

Table 4 Common liability issues in long-term care	
	• Dehydration
	• Elopement
	• Emotional distress
	• Falls/fractures
	• Improper use of restraints (clinical and physical)
	• Medication errors
	• Pressure ulcers/injuries
	• Sexual assault
	• Single event injuries
	• Weight loss

Standards of care were once thought to be unique to a local geographic area but are now viewed as national in scope. Regulations, clinical practice guidelines, and evidence-based practice as well as the testimony of expert witnesses, are often used to establish the standard of care. A breach of a standard of care may be either a matter of omission or commission. Once a malpractice action is initiated, failure to protect the integrity of the medical record and alterations of the medical record can be damaging to the defense. Not all breaches of a standard of care will contribute to causation of harm. It should be recognized that there could be more than one *proximate cause* for an injury or poor outcome.

Practitioners should be aware of circumstances that can place them at increased risk of facility litigation. These can include:

- Inadequate documentation, criticisms, or bickering in the medical record.
- Failure to follow policies and procedures without documentation of a supportable reason.
- Documentation of care in a manner not concordant with that care.
- Failure to notify the physician and family of changes in condition.
- Outdated and unnecessary policies and procedures.
- Care plans not updated to reflect the current condition of the resident and the care being given.
- Failure to follow the care plan.
- Unrealistic goals in the care plan.

Summary

Ethical and legal issues abound in the everyday practice of post-acute and long-term care medicine. Practitioners must acquire understanding of medical ethics and the law in one's jurisdiction and be able to discuss these issues with the interdisciplinary team, family, and patients in a manner that will foster collaboration and consensus. A skilled and confident practitioner can guide patients, families, and caregivers through shared medical decision-making. Guidance that will provide clarity, comfort, and consistency to the plan of care within the goals and personal values of the person receiving that care.

Pearls for the Practitioner
- The principles of health care ethics are *autonomy, beneficence, justice, nonmaleficence,* and *fidelity.* For ethical decision-making, each principle must be considered in the context of the others.
- No person loses his/her human rights upon entering a long-term care facility.
- Federal and State regulations require facilities to proactively prevent and address abuse, neglect, and exploitation.

- Practitioners in long-term care need to acquire skills to assess mental capacity in order to determine a person's ability to make personal, medical, and financial decisions in their own best interest.
- End of life issues are common in post-acute and long-term care, and thus practitioners must acquire skills in engaging patients and surrogate decision-makers and be cognizant of applicable laws.
- While litigation is common in long-term care, for a malpractice action to be successfully pursued, all four elements of duty, breach of the standard of care, causation, and harm (damages) must be proven.

References

1. https://downloads.cms.gov/medicare/Your_Resident. Accessed 5 Aug 21.
2. Sloane P, Yearby R, Konetzka RT, et al. Addressing systemic racism in nursing homes: a time for action. J Am Med Dir Assoc. 2021;22:886–92.
3. Marson DC, Ingram KK, Cody HA, et al. Assessing the competency of patients with Alzheimer's disease under different legal standards. Arch Neurol. 1995;52:949–54.
4. Grisso T, Applebaum PS, Hill-Fotouhi C. The MacCat-T: clinical tool to assess patient's capacity to make treatment decisions. Psychiatr Serv. 1997;48:1415–9.
5. www.ama-assn.org/ama/pub/physician-resources/medical-ethics. Accessed 5 Aug 21.
6. www.amda.com/governance/papers.cfm. Accessed 5 Aug 21.
7. www.amda.com/governance/resolutions/m03.cfm. Accessed 5 Aug 21.
8. Huss R, Smith DA, Horowitz A. Lessons from litigation: minimizing liability and regulatory enforcement risk in PALTC. In: AMDA annual conference 2021, virtual.

Working with Families and Person-Centered Care

David Brechtelsbauer

Introduction

Despite efforts to precisely define PCC [1], its definition remains diverse. In many PA/LTC communities "culture change" is often interchanged with PCC. The Centers for Medicare and Medicaid Services (CMS) uses the following to define *"Person-centered Care": "means to focus on the resident as the locus of control and support the resident in making their own choices and having control over their daily lives"* [2]. Use of the word "person" is preferred by advocates of PCC to reinforce the fact that people residing in these communities are unique individuals while CMS uses the designation "resident."

Person-Centered Care: Impact on Patient/Resident Assessment and Care Planning

Studies are emerging that assess the impacts of PCC on persons and their families. Studies have generally focused on two long-term care populations, those who are cognitively intact who can advocate for themselves, and those who have dementia where family members need to provide relevant information about the person's history for the development and implement a comprehensive person-centered care plan. Benefits have been noted on psychological wellbeing and Quality of Life (QoL). Person-centered dementia care decreased behavioral symptoms and decreased use of psychotropic medications. Family satisfaction has also improved [3].

D. Brechtelsbauer (✉)
University of South Dakota Sanford SOM, Sioux Falls, SD, USA

© The Author(s), under exclusive license to Springer Nature
Switzerland AG 2023
P. Winn et al. (eds.), *Post-Acute and Long-Term Care Medicine*, Current Clinical
Practice, https://doi.org/10.1007/978-3-031-28628-5_16

Traditionally many families are valuable allies when a loved one is admitted to or living in a PA/LTC community. Family members can provide emotional support, manage their loved one's finances, assist with the resident's ADLs, and participate at care plan meetings. PCC has changed the family role to "partners" in care who can provide valuable input to the care planning process by clarifying the residents past medical and social history, life journey, any post-traumatic events, family customs and traditions, likes and dislikes, usual daily routine, and personal values and preferences. As to medical decision-making, the family may be able to recount how the resident's priorities have determined past medical decisions. The transition from a community residence or an acute hospitalization to a PA/LTC community can be stressful for family caregivers. They may feel guilty for deciding that the resident transition to a nursing home instead of continuing to care for a spouse or parent at home. Family members who may have promised not to put their loved one in a nursing home are particularly conflicted. It is necessary for the attending practitioner to address this issue [4]. There are other practicalities that face family caregivers. The realities of possibly being separated by long distances and having employment and nuclear family obligations can limit an adult child's opportunity to actively participate in caregiving. While those who are able to be involved often feel awkward with the *role reversal* created when they find themselves *parenting their parent*. Frequently the parent can be distressed and resentful toward children who are now making decisions for them.

Attitudes

It is pivotal that IDT work with families to examine their own attitude toward families and the issues that commonly arise. Prejudicial assessments, blind spots in problem solving, and ineffective interventions can result when a health care provider (HCP) is unaware of her/his own beliefs and values contrasted to how families are defined and how they function. This may unconsciously impact communication style and decision making. While health care providers are encouraged to set aside personal biases, *feelings* about traditional verses nontraditional family structure, gender roles, locus of decision-making, and filial obligation all can impact a health care professional's attitudes and effectiveness when dealing with families.

Some of the discomfort when dealing with family issues probably relates to the lack of attention to effective communication, particularly with persons other than the patient. In many professional training programs, the emphasis placed on the doctor–patient relationship and confidentiality is often an attitudinal barrier that must be recognized and addressed in order to effectively interact with families. Practitioners who feel they are exclusively responsible to the patient may respond by avoiding encounters with families, a response that only worsens an issue or situation. Changing from an exclusive focus on the patient to that of *the family system* can be helpful. This can promote a collaborative relationship between the IDT and the family to the benefit of the patient/resident and the facility. Other families, due to personal preference or barriers created by living far away or holding down two jobs, will want to be informed, but not be able to share in the care of the patient/resident. Unfortunately, a few families have no desire to be involved. It is essential to determine the level of interest desired by each family, and to periodically determine if the desired level of involvement has changed to another family member.

A major attitudinal issue is reflected in the use of the word *"dysfunctional"* when describing a family. Too often this word signals a professional caregiver feeling hopeless or powerless to intervene in a difficult family situation. Whenever a care team member utters this word, that person needs to be encouraged to examine what he/she understands the word to mean and why use of "dysfunctional" is spoken in the situation at hand. At times dysfunctional may be an accurate description, but dwelling on that aspect of the problem will interfere with problem solving. *Cross-cultural issues* can also raise attitudinal issues and create disparity in one's thinking. Increasing diversity in the general population (as well as in health care workers and patients/residents) requires reexamination of systems of care and communication skills.

Knowledge

A physician's knowledge of the dynamics of the health system can be invaluable to families and to patients/residents as families vary in their level of experiential knowledge of the health care system. The public at large generally have little understanding as to the workings of PA/LTC. Family members may harbor negative feelings toward nursing home care. Sharing knowledge of the health care system in a non-condescending manner is an important first step in building credibility, rapport, and trust with the patient/resident and family. Studies have shown that moving into a PA/LTC community (which for many PA/LTC professionals is considered routine and straightforward), is often a major stressor for the resident and their family.

Upon resident admission it is helpful to discuss the facility and State policy regarding restraints as the family likely had observed bedside rails used in the acute care setting and thought this was a good idea. Learning of the "no restraints" regulations in PA/LTC can cause confusion and resentment for the resident and family. Explaining the risks of restraints and the indignity restraints will cause to their loved one may help resolve this contentious issue.

Education of the person and family about PCC can begin with the question, "If I used the phrase 'person-centered care', would that mean anything to you?" If the answer is "no," it provides the opportunity to describe the tenets of PCC. If the answer is "yes," ask them to share what they know. This will allow practitioners to address misperceptions. Compassionately guiding the family through the transition from hospital (or other setting) to the PA/LTC community will enable a positive beginning to the physician–patient and physician–family relationships. In turn, it will help foster a collaborative and positive demeanor and relationship between the *professional (formal)* and *family (informal) caregivers* that will help the family understand its role and the role of the facility's interdisciplinary team (IDT).

Subsequent issues that are likely to confront the family and that will need prompt and proactive efforts by facility practitioners and the IDT include:

- Informing the family of an incident (fall, medication error, skin tear, etc.)
- Notifying the family of an acute change of status (fall with injury, acute illness, exacerbation of a chronic illness).
- Advising the family of a problematic behavior and its consequences.
- Apprising the family of progressive frailty and that consideration be given to a focus on palliative care or hospice.

Chronic illness, particularly chronic diseases that impair a person's function to the extent that necessitates moving from home to a residential care setting are stressful for the person and the person's family. Accordingly, it's vital to inquire about *caregiver stress and distress*. Ask the family caregiver, *"And how are you doing with all this?"* Encourage family caregivers to take time for themselves and to seek help if overburdened. Urge participation in a caregiver support group.

Advance Care Planning (ACP) can be stressful to families. Discussion of goals of care and scope of treatment regularly occur. ACP has shown mixed efficacy. As such, a series of guidelines have been developed to support a more coherent process [5]. Recently a consensus definition of ACP has been proposed [6]:

1. Advance care planning is a process that supports adults at any age or stage of health in understanding and sharing their personal values, life goals, and preferences regarding future medical care.
2. The goal of advance care planning is to help ensure that people receive medical care that is consistent with their values, goals, and preferences during serious and chronic illness.
3. For many people, this process may include choosing and preparing another trusted person or persons to make medical decisions in the event the person can no longer make his or her own decisions.

A goals of care (GOC) discussion on medical interventions (or not) for those residents with advanced dementia has shown some efficacy in supporting family members in end-of-life conversations. The intervention involved a GOC video decision aid plus a structured discussion with nurses, social workers, therapists, and nutritionist who then create a care plan [7]. Some knowledge of *clinical psychology* and *family systems* is fundamental to effective "working with families." Full discussion of this is beyond the scope of this chapter. Excellent texts are available [8, 9].

Skills

Skills in "working with families" can be *learned* and will *improve with practice.* If one finds oneself struggling to respond to texts, phone calls, or emails from families, avoiding family contact, or when unable to attend family meetings or care conferences, it is helpful to find a person who is skilled and effective in this area. Practicing these skills under the watchful eye of a mentor, being open to feedback and willing to try a new approach will lead to improvement. It is important to recognize situations that may be medically complex and emotionally challenging for patient/residents and families as well as clinicians and staff. In such situations it is imperative to choose one's words carefully [10]. An unfortunate phrase is "There is nothing more to do." To the patient/resident this can sound like abandonment. An **alternative phrase** would be *"There is nothing more we can do to cure your illness."* Such a statement opens the door to discuss symptom management, psychosocial and spiritual support, and other measures that promote comfort and dignity for the person and caring and support for the family.

A similar problematic question posed to patient/residents is, "Would you like us to do everything?" Clinicians usually are thinking about aggressive ICU level of care. Families will often answer "yes" to such a question, while clinicians are rather thinking about efforts to relieve pain and suffering, not about a transfer back to the hospital. A *better phrase* is, *"I recognize your mother is in distress, and of course that is upsetting for you. I don't think sending her to the hospital for more tests and treatments would resolve her distress, let me explain what we can do here, working with nurses and other staff members who know your mother well. I think we can get her pain (or any distressing symptom) under better control."* You may want to add the phrase "I will write orders for *aggressive* symptom management." There are times when a patient/resident may need to be admitted to hospital for symptom control, but many symptoms can be successfully managed by the practitioner and skilled nursing facility IDT without hospitalization. The physician's awareness of the level of expertise and confidence (or not) of the staff needs to be assessed to ensure the needs of the patient can be met.

Selection of a Family Spokesperson

In most circumstances communication is more effective when a family spokesperson can be designated to respond to messages from the facility IDT and to then share that information with other family members. The spokesperson can also communicate family concerns back to the attending physician and the IDT. While the physician and IDT may have a preference as to which family member should be the spokesperson, the choice should rest with the family. The family's choice is often revealing as it typically reflects how the family unit has functioned in the past. The team needs to inquire as to the spokesperson's preferred method of communication—phone call, text, email, or in-person. Be sure that the spokesperson's phone numbers (cell, home, work) and email address are correct and easily retrievable. By the same token, the spokesperson should be provided with contact information for the facility attending physician, medical director, director of nursing, administrator, social worker, and the nurse most familiar with the person/patient whom the spokesperson represents. The administrator should be available to answer questions on nursing home regulations and policies. As the family spokesperson will not always be available so a backup family member should be determined.

Responding to a Phone Call from an Unhappy Family Member

A useful phrase to initially use when returning phone calls is, "Hello Mrs. Jones. This is Dr. Smith. I understand you are *concerned about your mother.*" Mrs. Jones is not likely to disagree with this greeting. If you don't know what is going on, call the facility staff member most likely to provide relevant information *before* returning the phone call. If the situation is complex or it appears the caller is emotionally distraught, consider making a face-to-face or telemedicine visit with the resident in order to collect more information if this can be accomplished without causing too much of a delay before returning the call. The need for prompt communication needs to be balanced with the need for preparation and obtaining accurate information on the resident situation.

The next useful comment is to *very briefly* state your understanding of the issue— "I think at least some of your concerns relate to your mother's bruises, but please explain to me what you noticed." Then do what too many HCPs find difficult: *listen to the whole story before interrupting or attempting to explain.* Families often are as concerned that they are not being heard or that they are considered by staff as the problem. Important things to listen for are family perceptions and interpretations that you did not anticipate, and whether the caller is an eager or reluctant family spokesperson. Sometimes the spokesperson has been put up to calling by another family member and the caller's own feelings and perceptions are not congruent with feelings and perceptions of the other family member. While working through a family spokesperson is generally recommended, in this case the practitioner may want to ask the spokesperson if it would be better to speak directly with the person who has the concern.

After listening, reflect back to the family on what you have heard with enough detail for the family member to be convinced that you have heard and understand what the family has said. Depending on the issues involved, you may be able to provide education, reassurance, and an action plan that will satisfy the caller. If the caller is not satisfied and the situation is not an emergency, the *best response is,* "I'm going to have to look further into your concerns in order to better understand what's going on. I will visit your loved one early tomorrow. What is the best way to reach you tomorrow morning?"

Effective communication by phone includes creating a succinct record of what was said. This is an extremely important skill. Consider the following example of a phone call from a family member who's loved one had been transferred from the PA/LTC community to the hospital the day before. The phone call is "real" and was transcribed verbatim (names have been changed) in order to enter it into the medical record.

"This is Donna Smith. I am Richard Martin's daughter. Richard was taken yesterday from Sunset Manor to the hospital, at first with thoughts of a stroke or whatever. I guess we just really, really frustrated. Nobody, Dr. Collins or I know he has students or whatever that come in and are under him [the caller is referring to resident physicians], my mom has not heard anything from him as far as treatment, what is the plan, what are they going to do? If it was a stroke, what were the blood test results? We need to know. He has been laying up there for a full day with nothing to eat, we don't know if he can eat. He can't speak. It is pretty frustrating and I believe probably somebody needs to get on the ball and find out what is going on and let the family know. My number is xxx-xxxx, and my mother's number is xxx-xxxx. Her name is Darla Martin and she is retired. She is on her way up to the hospital right now. Again, we want some answers and we want to know what is going on. Thank you."

When this call is returned, an apology needs to be promptly stated. What is informative in this case scenario is the concerned tone of the message when it was reviewed by *listening to the voice mail,* in contrast to the hostile tone one quickly detects upon reading the transcription. A major lesson is not to read too much into a transcribed message. In situations where there seems to be hostility it's best to respond by phone in order to hear the tone of voice and its inflection. When face-to-face the clinician can better observe and respond to nonverbal cues.

Email and texting have become popular for family communication with clinicians. Both allow for synchronous communication and efficient record keeping. Like the above example, emails and texts generally cannot accurately convey the emotional state of the family member sending the email or text, nor can it convey the compassion of the responding health care professional. When the content of an email or text conveys urgency, it is generally better to pick up the phone and call than to respond via return email or text. It is important to carefully proofread your email response before sending it, and be careful to send it to the right person. Inadvertently clicking on "reply all" can create problems!

Convening and Conducting a Family Meeting (Refer to Table 1)

Effective phone, email, and text communication and face-to-face meetings with the family spokesperson can often resolve family concerns. Other situations, either because of complex medical or ethical issues, or complex family dynamics, require a more formal process to achieve resolution. Expertise in convening and

Table 1 Family meetings

• Guidelines have been developed by various professional organizations
• Usually occur at the time of a health crisis and in an acute setting
• Often involve the need to deal with an issue that needs to be decided upon on an urgent basis
• Often involves a conflict between the professional care team (physician, nurse, and social worker are core, others as needed) and the patient/family
• Sometimes involves understanding and managing a conflict within the family system
• Ideally involves all family members
• Goals of care discussion focuses on one issue
• Moderated by an IDT member caring for the patient
• Overall goal is to resolve conflict and come to an acceptable action plan

participating in family meetings is an important skill for professionals, particularly physicians, advance practice nurses, and social workers in the PA/LTC setting [8].

- *Preparation for a family meeting* needs to be more thorough and thoughtful than that for a phone call. The convener of the meeting needs to learn as much as possible about the patient/resident and the situation to be addressed at the family meeting. Ideally all family members will be in attendance. Consulting with the PA/LTC community's social worker can provide insight into family structure and dynamics. Staff participants should be aware of the capabilities and culture of the community. If the issue is a controversy about a medical issue, it is important for the practitioner to examine the patient/resident *prior* to the meeting and review the medical record. Obtaining insights from other community professionals can be helpful. If the issue involves a conflict that relates to a federal regulation or a facility policy the administrator should be present.
- *Once preparation is complete, set a date, time, and place for the meeting.* Relevant staff and practitioners need to clear their schedules to allow for uninterrupted participation. Avoid having too many staff members attend in order to not to appear as ganging up on the family. However, all family members should attend. Out of town family members should be encouraged to participate by conference call or speakerphone. If family members want to attend by a virtual platform, the platform must be HIPAA compliant.
- The convener should *begin with introductions* and then *state the "rules" for the meeting.*

Many physicians, with training and experience, are comfortable in the convener role, but the role can be assumed by any team member. Most social work training programs provide training and experience in moderating family meetings.

- The first rule is *every person will be invited to share his/her perception of the issue at hand.*

The person speaking should not be interrupted. If another person interrupts the moderator can make a note of the concern without comment, and say the concern will be discussed during the time for that person's time to speak. Generally speaking, *the patient/resident, if present,* or the *least empowered person should speak first.* The selection of the least empowered person may be based on being the person present via speaker phone, or the person with the least education. In an effort to put family members at ease, assure everyone that *all comments are useful* to help understand the concerns that precipitated the need for the family meeting. If the moderator is aware of a family member who is either intimidating to other family members, or has strong feelings about what should be done, call on that person last. The family meeting may be daunting and seem like a time-consuming process, especially with large families. Often however, once a few family members have spoken, others will just express agreement or will only have a brief comment.

- *After the family has spoken,* the moderator should summarize what has been said and obtain assent that the summary is basically correct. *Then each staff professional is called upon to state, without interruption, her/his perception of the issue.* Avoid offering solutions at this point. After the professional team has spoken, the moderator should offer a brief summary of what has been said.

- *Next,* the person with the most credibility (this is often, but not always, the practitioner) can *provide education and suggest realistic goals and expectations.* Open discussion, problem solving, and hopefully agreement on next steps will follow. It is useful to explicitly define what will be measured to monitor the results of the intervention(s). Ask, *"If this plan works, how will we know?"* Also, agree on how the results will be communicated to the family, the IDT, and particularly to front-line caregivers who are to be involved in executing the plan. Most of the time this process will lead to a plan that is acceptable to the family and the IDT. If things go poorly it may only be possible to say, "We only agree that we disagree."
- At this point the team and the family can be *assigned tasks* (obtaining a second opinion, obtaining a copy of the advance directive, check to find out if some of the "facts" stated in the meeting are instead opinions) that may impact the situation and provide additional useful information for a follow-up meeting (if needed). *Suggest that the family may want to meet together before returning to the follow-up meeting.* If there is little hope that the next meeting will go any better than the first, select another moderator. In an extremely difficult or tense situation a skilled family therapist should participate. Other options could include referral to an ethics committee or even formal arbitration.
- While periodic family meetings often save time (and improve outcomes and patient/resident, family and IDT satisfaction), there can be disincentives. Equitable reimbursement for the work involved in preparing and holding family meetings is usually unavailable. If the patient/resident is *meaningfully* present at the family meeting the physician can bill for and be reimbursed for patient education, counseling, and coordination of care using appropriate nursing facility subsequent care codes. Facilities will recognize the value of family meetings, both in terms of resident/family satisfaction and risk management, and thus should be willing to pay a professional moderator a reasonable fee.

The Covid-19 pandemic has catalyzed a quantum leap in sophistication and acceptance of telemedicine platforms, as well as the acceptance of virtual meetings. Such scenarios can be extremely helpful when families are geographically remote and when clinicians are busy at other clinical sites. Sometimes the inpatient and outpatient teams can both attend the meeting with surprising positive results [11].

Convening and Conducting a Person-Centered Care Plan Meeting (CPM) (Refer to Table 2)

Care plan meetings are very different than family meetings. Federal statute and its associated regulations impact almost every aspect of the PA/LTC care planning process. The *State Operations Manual Appendix PP—Guidance to Surveyors for Long*

Table 2 Care plan meetings (CPMs)

• Federally mandated resident assessment instrument (RAI) must be used
• RAI has three basic components:
1. MDS 3.0. Provides for a comprehensive and standardized assessment
2. Care area assessment (CAA) process-aids in decision-making
3. RAI utilization guidelines-instructions for when and how to use the RAI
• Does not involve urgent decision-making; short windows to complete some tasks
• Generally collaborative in tone, disagreements resolve by consensus
• CPM IDT: Attending physician, RN and CNA with responsibility for patient, dietary staff member, resident and resident's representative per CMS regulations
• Goals of care discussion involves health and functional status, quality of life, preferences for assistance needed to manage activities of daily living (ADLs)
• Moderated by a registered nurse (MDS nurse)
• Meeting facilitated by the federally prescribed resident assessment instrument (RAI) health and functional status are reviewed as well as the resident's quality of life
• Goal of CPM is to develop, review and revise the patient-centered, personalized care plan

Term Care Facilities contains all the Federal regulations (F-tags) with "interpretative guidelines" to State and Federal surveyors. Appendix PP is in the public domain [3]. The following is the Federal Regulation regarding the resident comprehensive care plans. The facility should strive to have the person/resident or representative attend care plan meetings.

    F657—Comprehensive Care Plans

    "A Comprehensive Care Plan must be developed by an interdisciplinary team, that includes but is not limited to

(A) *The attending physician*

(B) *A registered nurse with responsibility for the resident*

(C) *A nurse aide with responsibility for the resident*

(D) *A member of food and nutrition services staff*

(E) *To the extent practicable, the participation of the resident and the resident's representative(s). An explanation must be included in a resident's medical record if participation of the resident and their resident representative is determined not practicable for the development of the resident's care plan.*

(F) *Other appropriate staff or professionals in disciplines as determined by the resident's needs or as requested by the resident."*

Empowering the Patient/Resident and the Resident's Representative

In care plan meetings all health care providers need to be familiar with the person's current cognitive status and to encourage the person's representative to be present. If the person is able to clearly express his/her preferences and goals, able to make informed choices, and has control of daily life, the person's input should be honored. The representative may just observe, but also be called to corroborate and clarify their loved one's responses. If the person/patient is not able to participate then the person's representative will need to provide relevant information. The representative needs to be reminded to respond to whatever is being discussed exactly as the *person* would respond if they were able. Note that when developing the *admission* person-centered care plan the information being sent from the hospital usually contains many details about the hospital course but little useful information about the patient as a person. There are a number of strategies to address this dilemma. Over 70% of hospitals with 50+ beds have inpatient palliative care programs [12]. With a new facility admission there is a good likelihood that the patient/resident could have had a palliative care consult that would have included a discussion of goals of care and the creation or review and updating of any Advance Directive for healthcare. Contacting the person's community-based primary care physician can also provide valuable information and insight as to the patient's past medical and family history. The involvement of the family over the years may also be helpful. Addressing the patient's **family system** and creating a **family genogram** can be helpful. Creating a family genogram is a skill taught in most nursing and social work training programs, but less familiar to most medical professionals. Let us consider the Jones family genogram (Fig. 1).

By convention, male family members are represented as squares and female members as circles. A horizontal line connecting two people indicates a marriage, a double slash through the line a divorce or separation. An "X" inside a square or circle indicates that person is deceased. An arrow designates the patient. Each family generation has a separate level in the genogram [9].

This genogram displays four generations of the Jones family. "Grandma" Jones' husband and father both died at home. It is likely Ethel was the at-home caregiver for her husband and perhaps for her father. No wonder Ethel is upset that her family could not make arrangements for her to be able to die at home. Looking at Ethel's children and their spouses, it appears that the daughter Janice would be the best person to serve as Ethel's representative.

Family's dynamics and relations can change over time so the genogram in the chart may need to be updated periodically. Referring to the genogram before returning a phone call or text, or participating in a family or care plan meeting can quickly refresh one's memory of family structure and dynamics, making the call, text, or meeting more productive and efficient.

During the Care Plan Meeting

After the initial care plan is developed, subsequent care plan meetings should start with determining the impact of the previous care plan interventions and the impact it had on the resident's quality of life. The resident may report that the intervention was more burdensome than the problem it was trying to solve or mitigate. Given

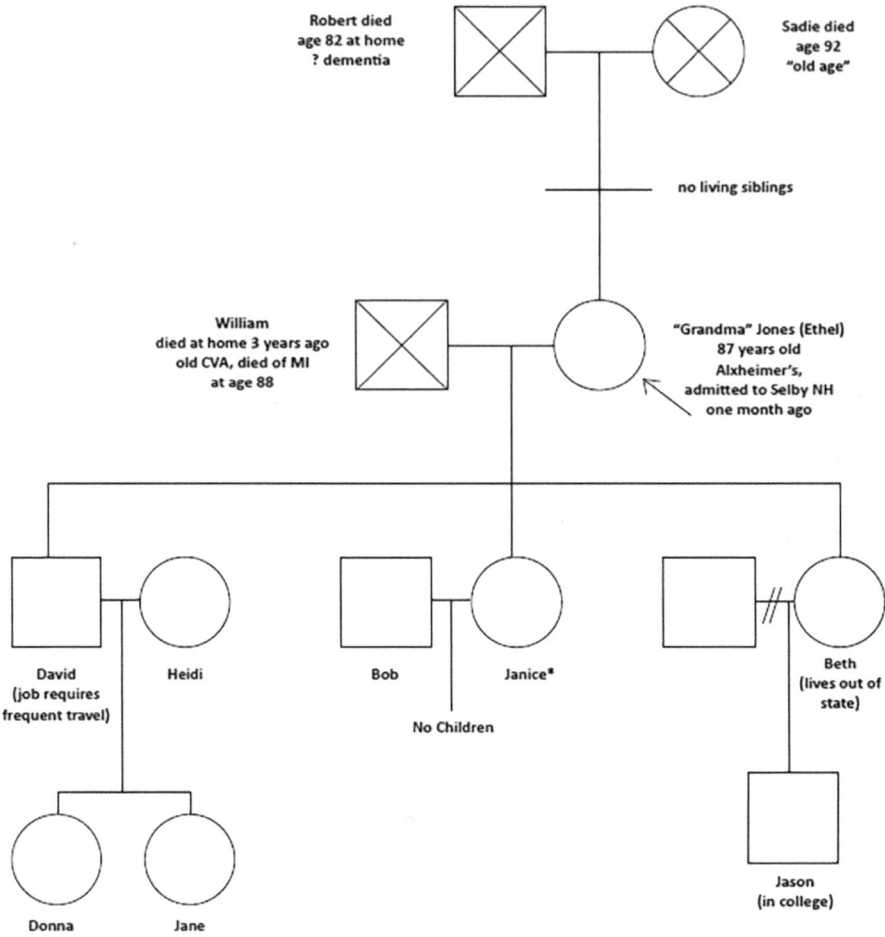

Robert died
age 82 at home
? dementia

Sadie died
age 92
"old age"

no living siblings

William
died at home 3 years ago
old CVA, died of MI
at age 88

"Grandma" Jones (Ethel)
87 years old
Alxheimer's,
admitted to Selby NH
one month ago

David
(job requires
frequent travel)

Heidi

Bob

Janice*

No Children

Beth
(lives out of
state)

Donna   Jane

Jason
(in college)

*visited her mother almost every day since her dad died, continues to visit at nursing home

Fig. 1 Jones Family Genogram

that patient-centered care recognizes the patient/resident as the center of focus by the care plan IDT, members of the IDT must avoid use of medical jargon and abbreviations, and periodically check for understanding when the discussion addresses complex issues. The patient/resident's or family member's input is critical in deciding how to proceed. If the suggested intervention is declined and could result in an adverse outcome then a discussion of how to mitigate risk is appropriate. This may cause anxiety among staff. A useful resource is listed under Suggested Reading/Viewing.

The Resident Assessment Instrument for implementing a care plan does not specify care plan structure or format. Various advocacy groups have created care plan templates. If the PA/LTC community utilizes an electronic medical record they likely already have a built-in template for documenting the care plan. The patient/resident and/or the family member should receive a copy of the care plan.

When There Are Cultural Differences

Cultural differences can sometimes interfere with family communication. In an age when political correctness can block efforts to address a problem, cultural values and consideration may further create confusion and misunderstanding.

- To help manage misunderstanding, reflect on your personal and professional culture. What assumptions might others make based on knowing you are an African-American physician or a Filipino nurse? If thoughts about a cultural group would be true or false, how would they apply to you?
- Next, consider the cultural background of the patient/resident and her/his family. What do you know, or think you know, about their culture and values? No one expects a health care provider to have an intimate knowledge of each patient/resident's culture, but some basic knowledge is useful. Professional colleagues from the same culture of the patient/resident may be helpful. Other resources can quickly be found on line. Just as you may recognize yourself as an African-American physician, but meet none of the stereotypes, you cannot assume the patient/resident and his/her family will be well characterized by generalizations about their culture. A useful way to address this is to ask, "I have learned that it is common in Bulgaria for adult children to care for their elderly parent. How true is that for your family?"

Sometimes, despite being knowledgeable and respectful of the family and the family's cultural/ethnicity background, communication can still be challenging. In this case, it is usually helpful to find a mutually acceptable facilitator. The person selected is often a community or religious leader from the same cultural group who can bridge the gap between the prevailing and/or professional culture and the minority and/or lay culture. *When a translator is necessary,* effective communication requires behaviors that may not be intuitive. It is important to talk directly to the person and not to the translator. "How are you feeling today?" is more likely to engender engagement and a meaningful response than "Ask her how she is feeling today." Talking directly to the person makes the translator's job easier. Professional translators are preferred over use of family members, although financial and logistical barriers may require the use of untrained family members. Companies offering telephone and computer-based translators can be found by searching "translation providers" on the Internet. Prices and available languages vary.

Summary

Post-Acute and Long-Term Care communities, as well as other venues in health care, are embracing the precepts of *person-centered care*. Implementation of this approach to care has been endorsed by CMS and advocacy organizations, notably by the Pioneer Network. Comprehensive assessments and subsequent care planning are vital elements of the PCC process. This approach emphasizes that practitioners and other members of the PA/LTC community's IDT elicit the values and preferences of the person living in the community, and incorporate those values and preferences when creating, reviewing, and revising a patient-centered care plan. Practitioners must put aside the role of principal decision-maker in deference to the person living in the community, and the person's representative for health care decision-making. This requires practitioners to thoroughly understand the Federal statutes and regulations related to the care planning process, and how it differs from traditional family meetings. Development of a family genogram can be a helpful tool in understanding family structure and function.

Pearls for the Practitioner
- Recognize and acknowledge that chronic illness and having a family member move into a PA/LTC community are major stressors for both the person and the family.
- In almost every situation it is import to listen before offering solutions.
- Determine the level of involvement the family desires; whenever possible support that involvement.
- Practice until you can comfortably and skillfully:

  - Return a phone call from a family member.
  - Respond to an email or text message from a family member.
  - Participate successfully in a family meeting.
  - Participate successfully in a person-centered care planning meeting.
  - Successfully communicate when utilizing a translator.

Suggested Reading/Viewing
- Honoring preferences when the choice involves risk: A process for shared decision making and care planning.—pdf can be downloaded from the Pioneer Network web site.
- Family Meetings on Behalf of Patients with Serious Illness—12-min video of a family meeting with commentary—available on the New England Journal of Medicine web site <nejm.org>.
- https://www.mypcnow.org/fast-facts/ Fast Facts are concise (2 page), peer-reviewed and evidence-based summaries on key palliative care topics. Fast Facts 16 and 222–227 provide guidance for holding Family Meetings.

References

1. The American Geriatrics Society Expert Panel on Person-Centered Care. Person-centered care: a definition and essential elements. J Am Geriatr Soc. 2016;64(1):15–8.
2. Appendix PP State Operations Manual (Revised 11/22/2017) (PDF).
3. Li J, Porock D. Resident outcomes of person-centered care in long-term care: a narrative review of interventional research. Int J Nurs Stud. 2014;51:1395–415.
4. Lane ML, Hirst SP, Hawranik P. What do family members really want when older adults transition to a nursing home? J Gerontol Nurs. 2017;43(11):9–14.
5. McMahan RD, Tellez I, Sudore RLL. Deconstructing the complexities of advance care planning outcomes: what do we know and where do we go? A scoping review. J Am Geriatr Soc. 2021;69:234–44.
6. Sudor RL, Lum HD, You JJ, et al. Defining advance care planning for adults: a consensus definition for a multidisciplinary Delphi panel. J Pain Symptom Manag. 2017;53(5):821–832.e1.
7. Hanson LC, Zimmerman S, Song M, et al. Effect of the goals of care intervention for advanced dementia: a randomized trial. JAMA Intern Med. 2017;177(1):24–31.
8. Bloom MV, Smith DA. Brief mental health interventions for the family physician. New York: Springer; 2012. p. 260–82.
9. McGoldrick M, Gerson R, Petry S. Genograms: assessment and treatment. 4th ed. New York: W.W. Norton & Company; 2020.
10. Pantilat SZ. Communicating with seriously ill patients: better words to say. JAMA. 2009;301:1279–81.
11. Lee TH. Zoom family meeting. N Engl J Med. 2021;384:1586–7.
12. Center to Advance Palliative Care and the National Palliative Care Research Center. America's care of serious illness: a state-by-state report care on access to palliative care in our nation's hospitals. New York: Center to Advance Palliative Care; 2019.

Documentation and Coding

Peter Winn and Leonard Gelman

Introduction

The provision of care to residents in long-term care facilities entails different requirements in documentation and coding for physician and practitioner services than those in the clinic and hospital setting. Both the **documentation of care** provided and determination of the correct **evaluation and management (E/M) code** are essential to ensure appropriate reimbursement for the level of services rendered. A glossary of terms is reviewed in Table 1.

P. Winn (✉)
Department of Family and Preventive Medicine, University of Oklahoma, College of Medicine, Oklahoma City, OK, USA

L. Gelman
Community Care, Ballston Spa, NY, USA

© The Author(s), under exclusive license to Springer Nature Switzerland AG 2023
P. Winn et al. (eds.), *Post-Acute and Long-Term Care Medicine*, Current Clinical Practice, https://doi.org/10.1007/978-3-031-28628-5_17

327

Table 1 Glossary of terms

Admission—When a patient enters a NF or SNF and there are no open clinical or financial records pertaining to the current stay
Readmission—There is no clarity from CMS concerning the definition of this term, and it may be used in two ways, the more logical of which, based on the CMS wording in the Medicare Carrier Manual, is number two below
1. When a patient returns to a NF or SNF after leaving with a bed hold status; the clinical and financial records have remained open and the patient is considered to be continuing the current stay that began prior to leaving with the bed hold status; all services are billed using the subsequent care codes (99307–99310)
2. When a patient returns to a NF or SNF after leaving with a discharged status; the clinical and financial records from the prior stay have been closed and the patient is considered to be starting a new stay; an initial visit is again required and this is billed using the initial care codes (99304–99306)
Discharge—When a patient leaves a NF or SNF to go to another venue of care (home, hospital, assisted living, group home, etc.) and the clinical and financial records pertaining to the current stay are closed, even if there is a possibility or probability that the patient will return to the same NF or SNF
Bed Hold—When a patient leaves a NF or SNF to go to another venue of care (usually, hospital) and the clinical and financial records pertaining to the current stay remain open in expectation of the patient's return
MDS—Acronym for Minimum Data Set, the comprehensive multidisciplinary evaluation performed for a patient on admission and periodically thereafter as long as the patient remains a resident in the NF or SNF; the MDS is electronically to State and Federal agencies
Initial Visit—"the initial comprehensive assessment visit during which the physician completes a thorough assessment, develops a plan of care and writes or verifies admitting orders for the nursing facility resident"
CMS—Acronym for The Centers for Medicare and Medicaid Services
Nursing Facility (NF)—An institution (or a distinct part of an institution), which is primarily engaged in providing skilled nursing care and related services for residents who require medical or nursing care, or rehabilitation services for the rehabilitation of injured, disabled, or sick persons. *Patients (residents) in a NF do not receive Medicare Part A benefits*
Skilled Nursing Facility (SNF)—An institution (or a distinct part of an institution), which is primarily engaged in providing skilled nursing care and related services for residents who require medical or nursing care, or rehabilitation services for the rehabilitation of injured, disabled, or sick persons. *Patients (residents) in a SNF are receiving skilled services that are being paid for by the resident's Medicare Part A benefits*

Documenting the Visit

While the centers for medicare and medicaid services (CMS) issues documentation guidelines for the evaluation and management (E/M) services the American Medical Association (AMA) is responsible for both the establishment and updating of the Current Procedural Terminology (CPT) codes. AMDA-The Society for Post-Acute and Long-Term Care Medicine, has issued a *Guide to Post-Acute and Long-Term Care Coding, Reimbursement, and Documentation* based upon the AMA's CPT guidelines [1]. It summarizes documentation requirements and provides coding vignettes for several facility visit codes, in addition to those related to chronic care management, advance care planning, and behavioral health integrated services. Updated CPT E/M codes became effective January 1, 2023. Note that many E/M service codes are now based on medical decision making **or** time [2].

There are **seven components** that constitute a practitioner's patient visit. In most instances the **first three are the** *Key Components* that determine the level of E/M services.

- Extensiveness of **history** (Chief Complaint (CC), HPI, Review of Systems (ROS), and Past Family and Social History (PFSH)).
- Extensiveness of the **physical examination.**
- **Complexity of medical decision making.**
- Patient counseling.
- Coordination of care.
- Severity of the presenting problem and.
- Suggested time or duration needed to render the service.

Each of the three key components have four levels of extensiveness and complexity.

History

There are four levels of **history**. *Note that a chief complaint is needed for each encounter.*

- *Problem focused*: *Brief* history of present illness (HPI) or problem.
- *Expanded problem focused*: *Brief* HPI; and a *problem pertinent* system review.
- *Detailed*: Extended HPI; *problem pertinent* review of systems; and pertinent past, family, and/or social history directly related to the patient's problems.
- *Comprehensive*: *Extended* HPI; review of systems that is directly related to the problem(s) identified in the HPI in addition to a review of all additional body systems; and a *complete* past, family, and social history.

Physical Examination

There are four levels of physical examination
- *Problem focused*: A *limited* examination of the affected body area or organ system.
- *Expanded problem focused*: A *limited* examination of the affected body area or organ system and other symptomatic or related body area(s) or organ system(s).
- *Detailed*: An *extended* examination of the affected body area(s) and other symptomatic related body area(s) or organ system(s).

- *Comprehensive*: A general *multisystem* examination *or* a complete examination of a single organ system and other symptomatic or related body area(s) or organ system(s).

Medical Decision Making

There are several factors that can increase the **complexity** of medical decision making. These include:

- Number and complexity of problem(s) addressed at the encounter.
- Number of management options that are considered and selected.
- Amount and complexity of medical data and other relevant information that has been reviewed and analyzed.
- Risk of significant complications, and/or morbidity and/or mortality, in addition to comorbidities and their respective severity and how these can impact patient management options.

There are four levels of complexity of medical decision making
- *Straightforward*: *Minimal* number of diagnoses or management options; *minimal* or no data to be reviewed; *minimal* risk of complications, morbidity, and mortality.
- *Low complexity*: *Limited* number of diagnoses or management options; *limited* amount or complexity of data to be reviewed; *low* risk of complications, morbidity, and mortality.
- *Moderate complexity*: *Multiple* diagnoses or management options; *moderate* amount of complexity of data to be reviewed; *moderate* risk of complications, morbidity, and mortality.
- *High complexity*: *Extensive* diagnoses or management options; *extensive* amount or complexity of data to be reviewed; *high* risk of complications, morbidity, and mortality.

Visit Time

As of January 1, 2023, the time allocated to an E/M visit code (see Tables 2 and 3) can now be used to determine the level of service. **Remember that the documentation of each encounter must be of sufficient detail to support the E/M code**. Visit time can be used to determine the level of an E/M service if counselling and coordination of care are greater than 50% of the total time spent with a patient or resident. The prolonged service E/M codes are described later in the chapter.

Table 2 Initial SNF or NF visit codes

99304	99305	99306

• 99304 (REQUIRES THREE OF THREE E&M COMPONENTS)
  – DETAILED OR COMPREHENSIVE HX
  – DETAILED OR COMPREHENSIVE EXAM
  – MEDICAL DECISION MAKING:
    • STRAIGHTFORWARD LOW
  – 25 min must be met or exceeded
• USED FOR:
  – INITIAL ADMISSION/READMISSION
  – Usually, the problem(s) requiring admission are of low severity		

99305
- • 99305 (REQUIRES THREE OF THREE E&M COMPONENTS)
  - COMPREHENSIVE HX
  - COMPREHENSIVE EXAM
  - MEDICAL DECISION MAKING:
    - • Moderate
  - 35 min must be met or exceeded
- • USED FOR
  - INITIAL ADMISSION/READMISSION
  - Usually, the problem(s) requiring admission are of moderate severity

99306
- • 99306 (REQUIRES THREE OF THREE E&M COMPONENTS)
  - COMPREHENSIVE HX
  - COMPREHENSIVE EXAM
  - MEDICAL DECISION MAKING:
    - • HIGH
  - 45 min must be met or exceeded
- • USED FOR:
  - INITIAL ADMISSION/READMISSION
  - Usually, the problem(s) requiring admission are of high severity

Note: for services 60 min or longer, use prolonged services code 993X0

Table 3 Subsequent SNF or NF visit codes: 99307–99310

99307
- • 99307 (REQUIRES TWO OF THREE E&M COMPONENTS)
  - PROBLEM FOCUSED HX
  - PROBLEM FOCUSED EXAM
  - MEDICAL DECISION MAKING:
    - • STRAIGHTFORWARD
  - 10 min must be met or exceeded
- • USED FOR
  - PATIENT STABLE, RECOVERING, OR IMPROVING
  - "ROUTINE/REGULATORY" VISIT

(continued)

Table 3 (continued)

99308
- • 99308 (REQUIRES TWO OF THREE E&M COMPONENTS)
  - – EXPANDED PROBLEM FOCUSED HX
  - – EXPANDED PROBLEM FOCUSED EXAM
  - – MEDICAL DECISION MAKING:
    - • Low
  - – 15 min must be met or exceeded
- • USED FOR:
  - – PATIENT RESPONDING INADEQUATELY TO RX OR DEVELOPED MINOR
  COMPLICATION
  - – "ROUTINE/REGULATORY" VISIT

99309
- • 99309 (REQUIRES TWO OF THREE E&M COMPONENTS)
  - – DETAILED HX
  - – DETAILED EXAM
  - – MEDICAL DECISION MAKING:
    - • Moderate
  - – 30 min must be met or exceeded
- • USED FOR
  - – PATIENT DEVELOPED SIGNIFICANT COMPLICATION OR SIGNIFICANT NEW
  PROBLEM
  - – "ROUTINE/REGULATORY" VISIT

99310
- • 99310 (REQUIRES TWO OF THREE E&M COMPONENTS)
  - – COMPREHENSIVE HX
  - – COMPREHENSIVE EXAM
  - – MEDICAL DECISION MAKING:
    - • HIGH
  - – 45 min must be met or exceeded
- • USED FOR
  - – The patient may be unstable or may have developed a significant new problem
  requiring immediate physician attention

Note: for services 60 min or longer, use prolonged service codes 993X0

Coding and Billing for Skilled Nursing and Non-Skilled Nursing Facility Visits

The E/M service code selected is based upon fulfilling the requirements of the individual CPT code. Each patient visit must always meet the requirement as to **medical necessity**. Having provided the service and properly documented the care, selection of the appropriate CPT code is usually straightforward.

For practitioner services in nursing facilities there are four categories of service codes

- • _**Initial** Nursing Facility Care_ (services provided on admission to the SNF or NF for the _initial comprehensive assessment)_: 99304, 99305, 99306. The patient's attending physician of record must append the modifier "AI" to the bill when performing initial visits.

- ***Subsequent*** *Nursing Facility Care* (services provided *subsequent to* **or** *prior* to the initial comprehensive assessment): 99307, 99308, 99309, 99310.
- *Services provided for* ***discharge***: 99315 or 99316 (based on time 30 min or less, more than 30 min).
- *Services provided for the* ***annual health evaluation***: 99318 (This code has been **deleted** as of January 1, 2023).

Note that all these codes apply to both new and established patients.

The appropriate *Initial Nursing Facility Care* code is determined by the extensiveness and complexity of the components of the E/M service provided; with the most comprehensive service being billed at level 99306 (see Table 2). *Use of the initial codes require that* **all three E/M components** *be performed* (*history, physical, medical decision making*). These codes are used for the initial admission (or readmission, if the patient has previously resided in the nursing facility and had been discharged, i.e., no bed hold). Note that the *initial codes* are related to the **place of service** to which a patient is being admitted. For clarification, note that if a patient from your practice is being admitted to a NF/SNF, it is *not* a subsequent patient visit, but an *initial visit to that facility* and should be coded as an initial visit.

The *Subsequent Nursing Facility* care codes are reviewed in Table 3. The appropriate subsequent care code is determined by the complexity of the components of the E/M service provided, with the most complex and comprehensive services being coded at the 99310 level that is associated with a high risk of complications, morbidity and/or mortality. *When billing for* **subsequent care**, *only* **two of the three** *E/M components need be* **performed**, though optimal medical care would entail that all three components be performed and documented.

The codes for *services provided upon discharge* from a SNF or NF are 99315 and 99316 (see Table 4). For these discharge services, the differentiation of the appropriate code is determined by the total time spent performing all of the tasks and services required for the patient's discharge (final exam, instructions for continuing care, preparation of discharge records, prescriptions, referral forms and communication with practitioners who are to provide follow-up care for the patient after discharge). *It is important to remember that these discharge visit codes, as all the other visit codes, require a face-to-face visit.* If the visit is performed on a day different than the actual day of discharge, the date of service for billing should be the actual date of the visit. The discharge code can be used for a visit when a

Table 4 SNF or NF discharge visit codes: 99315 or 99316

- 99315—30 MIN OR LESS DURATION OF TIME
- 99316—MORE THAN 30 MIN DURATION OF TIME
- USED FOR:
  - FINAL EXAM
  - INSTRUCTIONS FOR CONTINUING CARE
  - PREPARATION OF DISCHARGE RECORDS
  - PRESCRIPTIONS
  - REFERRAL FORMS
  - COMMUNICATIONS WITH AFTER-DISCHARGE PROVIDERS

resident has died; however it is only billable if the physician fulfills the requirement of a face-to-face visit and pronounces the death of the patient!

CMS requires that any E/M code for a **SNF visit** be modified with the **Place of Service Code modifier "31"** and that for a **NF visit** with the **Place of Service Code modifier "32."**

Other Coding Issues in Nursing Facilities

Consultations

A specialist/consultant or a primary care physician may perform consultations **in** a nursing or skilled nursing facility. A billable consultation requires a request/order from the attending physician of record who is overseeing the care of the patient. As of 2010, the initial consultation visit is billed using the nursing facility initial assessment E/M codes (99304–99306). The patient's principal physician of record must append the modifier "AI" to the bill when performing initial visit to differentiate the attending initial visit from a consultant's initial visit for which no modifier is needed. The principal "physician of record" is identified by Medicare as the physician who oversees the patient's overall care at the facility. Follow-up visits by the consultant are billed using the subsequent nursing facility visit codes (99307–99310).

Hospice Care

When a patient is receiving care under the Medicare Hospice Benefit, there are additional guidelines for billing for provided services that depends on whether the physician has a relationship with the hospice and whether that care is related to the terminal illness or not (see Table 5). However, physicians should ask their Medicare Administrative Contractor (formerly called Medicare Fiscal Intermediary or Carrier) to verify whom to bill for physician services related to the terminal diagnosis (i.e., whether the hospice or Medicare Part B). Usually if the patient's attending

Table 5 Billing for services on patients receiving the medicare hospice benefit

- For care *not* related to terminal illness
  - Bill Medicare Part B—Modifier GW
- For care *related* to terminal illness (check with your Medicare Administrative Contractor)
  - If the physician is not associated with the hospice
    - Bill Medicare Part B—Modifier GV
  - If the physician is associated with/employed by the hospice
    - Bill hospice unless services are covered by a contract or agreement with hospice

Table 6 Group practice

• Same group—same specialty
– Bill and be paid as though they were single physician
– One E/M code per day
– Can combine same day visits and submit appropriate code
– Unrelated problems: can submit different bills; documentation critical
• Same group—different specialty
– Bill and be paid without regard to membership in group

physician is also the medical director of the hospice from which the patient is receiving hospice services, then that physician should bill the hospice for services rendered. If not the hospice medical director, then the attending physician should bill Medicare Part B. Also, for a consultant who performs a follow-up *office visit* related to the *patient's hospice diagnosis*, then the physician should bill the hospice on an agreed negotiated reimbursement. Often this is not done and the visit erroneously billed to Medicare Part B.

Physicians in Group Practice

In certain circumstances, providers of a group practice of the same specialty may bill for services provided to a patient on the same day (see Table 6 on Group Practice).

Multi-Site Same Day Visits

The only instances in which Medicare will pay for two different services provided by the **same** physician for the **same** patient on the **same** day at **different sites of service** is for hospital discharge (99238, 99239) and the nursing facility admission (99304, 99305, 33906). Documentation must meet the E/M requirements for each site of service. It is not acceptable that the nursing facility admission H and P state "see hospital discharge H and P."

Split or Shared Visits

Previously Medicare did *not* recognize split or shared E/M visits at the nursing facility and thus would not reimburse for them. However, starting in 2022 CMS now permits such visits for new and establish patients, for initial and subsequent visits, for critical care services, prolonged E/M visits, and SNF E/M visits (**except** those visits that are required to be done by the attending physician).

"Incident To" Services

"Incident to" services provided in the nursing facility are *not* recognized by Medicare and will not be reimbursed. However, **if** the physician has established an office in the nursing facility (a discrete space that the physician rents and uses for patient care visits), "incident to" services provided in that discrete office space are billable and thus reimbursable. In this case, the "incident to" services should be billed utilizing the **office** E/M codes.

Prolonged Face-to-Face Service Codes (99417, 993X0)

The E/M codes for prolonged service with direct patient contact (99354–99357) have been **deleted** as of January 1, 2023. For prolonged evaluation and management services on the date of an outpatient service or a private home or residence, use code 99417. While for prolonged E/M services on the date of a face-to-face **nursing home service**, use code 993X0.

Prolonged Non-Face-to-Face Service Codes (99358, 99359)

These service codes are used when a prolonged service is provided on a date **other** than the date of the face-to-face visit (E/M encounter) that occurred with the patient and/or family/caregiver. Use of these codes must be related to the face-to-face patient care visit that previously occurred, regardless of the place of service.

These codes are used for prolonged physician services *without* direct patient contact such as speaking to family members or extraordinary chart/medical record review. Time spent must be documented and include what was reviewed. These codes are *not* an add-on code and must be performed on a **different day** *and* be directly related to the previous face-to-face visit, are to be performed on a single day and time, *not* accumulated over several days; and cannot overlap with chronic care management codes, *may not be reimbursable*. Using these prolonged service codes does not guarantee reimbursement. For clarification on their use and reimbursement contact the CMS Physician Fee Schedule web page, the CMS Division of Practitioner Services, or your local Medicare Administrative Contractor.

Code 99358 is used to report the first 60 min of the prolonged visit code on a given date regardless of place of service and only used once per date. Code 99359 is used to report each additional 30 min beyond the first 60 min and to report the final 15–30 min of the prolonged given service date. An initial service time **less** than 30 min is not reportable nor re-imbursed.

Chronic Care Management Services

Some practitioners have queried whether Medicare would allow billing (and thus receive reimbursement) for CCM services for patients who reside in nursing and assisted living facilities. If a CCM service is billed and payment received it does not necessarily indicate such services are covered. Erroneous payment, once detected, could potentially put practitioners at risk of fraud. Accordingly, be in contact for those sources previously suggested for clarification in the previous section.

Annual Nursing Facility Resident Assessment (AWVs): (G0438, G0439)

Are Medicare Annual Wellness Visits (AWV) able to be performed and reimbursed for residents in nursing facilities? For residents in assisted living facilities? AWVs entail a "personalized preventive plan of service." As such could this assessment be performed at the nursing or assisted living facility? Or at a physician's community-based clinic? It is suggested you contact CMS or the local Medicare Administrative Contractor for clarification. If allowable, remember that you must meet all the required components of the initial AWV and subsequent AWV.

Telehealth Services

During the COVID-19 pandemic CMS authorized the use of telehealth for nursing facility and domiciliary (assisted living) facilities for both newly admitted and established patients. For nursing facility residents, telehealth visits were limited to once every 14 days. There is a concern that emergency use authorization under COVID-19 will be rescinded once the COVID-19 pandemic Public Health Emergency (PHE) is declared to have ended. CMS is proposing that nursing facility **initial service (99304–99306)** will be removed from the allowable telehealth list 151 days after the PHE ends, stating that all regulatory visits must be done in person, given that the initial visit is considered a regulatory visit.

Visits by Qualified Nonphysician Practitioners

Nonphysician practitioners (NPP) include nurse practitioners (NP), physician assistants (PA), and clinical nurse specialists (CNS). All E/M visits must be performed within their State scope of practice and licensure requirements. Any federal and state requirements for physician collaboration and physician supervision must be met. Refer to Table 7 for the Federal regulations related to which services may be

Table 7 Nonphysician practitioner services

	Order to admit	Admission treatment orders	Initial comprehensive visit	Other required visits	Other medically necessary visits	Other medically necessary orders	Certification, recertification
SNF							
PA, NP, and CNS employed by facility	N	N	N	Y (alternate)	Y	Y	N
PA, NP, and CNS not a facility employee	N	N	N	Y (alternate)	Y	Y	Y
NF							
NP, CNS, and PA employed by facility	N	N	N	N	Y	Y	Y
NP, CNS, and PA not a facility employee	Y	Y	Y	Y	Y	Y	Y

provided by various NPPs as related to their employment status and care setting. Note that these requirements may vary from one state to another and can change over time.

Services Provided in the NF or SNF That Are Not Reimbursable by Medicare

Care plan oversight, telephone calls, and medical team conferences (interdisciplinary team meetings) are not reimbursable and prolonged services without a face-to-face visit may not be reimbursable. Contact your local Medicare Administrative Contractor for clarification.

Coding and Billing for Assisted Living Facilities

Levels of E/M services for assisted living facilities are determined by the **same first three key components**. See Table 8. These billing codes are used for assisted living facilities, group homes, custodial care facilities, and residential substance abuse facilities. It is important to use the correct **place of service code** for each of these venues (**13, 14, 33,** and **55,** respectively). Note that as of January 1, 2023 the service

Table 8 Private home/residence and assisted living visit codes (as of January 1, 2023)

Initial care	Subsequent care
• 99341–15′	• 99347–20′
• 99342–30′	• 99348–30′
• 99343—Deleted′	• 99349–40′
• 99344–60′	• 99350–60′
• 99345–75′	• 75′ or longer use add on 99417
• 90′ or longer use add on 99417	

E/M codes 99324–99328 and **99334–99337 have been deleted**. Accordingly, the **home visit E/M codes** are now to be used for assisted living visits: 99341, 99342, 99344, and 99345 for new patient visits and 99347–99350 for established patient visits.

Coding and Billing for Home Visits

Visit services provided in the patient's home are billed using the same set of codes as listed in Table 8 and follow the same parameters for E/M intensity, and also guided by the same duration time of service with **place of service code 12**.

Summary

Proper documentation and coding of patient visits, irrespective of place of service, is a skill that practitioners must attain and maintain. Documentation must be thorough, appropriate to the condition(s) being assessed and truthful. The extensiveness of the history, physical examination, and medial decision making must support the chosen visit code. Time for the visit can now guide the choice of a given code. Over-coding (and thus over-billing) can be considered fraud, which can result in a dire situation for practitioners that could include payback to Medicare, financial penalties, and criminal changes. When unsure whether to use a specific visit code, contact the CMS Division of Practitioner Services or your local Medicare Administrative Contractor.

Pearls for the Practitioner
- Medical necessity and fulfilling the requirements of the individual CPT code are necessary for choosing the level of an E/M code.
- Appropriate and thorough documentation in the medical record must support the chosen level of service E/M code.
- The extensiveness of the history, physical examination, and the complexity of medical decision making must be linked to the presenting complaint(s) or clinical situation.
- The three key components of any E/M code are history, physical examination, and medical decision making.

- For billing purposes, it is essential to use the appropriate place of service and modifier codes.
- Contact your local Medicare Administrative Contractor (MAC) for queries on billing and coding.
- The home visit codes **are now** to be used for those visits performed at an assisted living facility, a residential care facility, a group home, custodial care facility, or a residential substance abuse facility.
- Be cognizant that an E/M code and documentation requirements may change over time and the responsibility rests with practitioners to keep informed of any changes. (Updated January 1, 2023).
- CMS has published a memorandum (04/07/2022) ending several waivers related to the COVID-19 Emergency Declaration Waivers for SNFs/NFs (Ref: QSO-22-15-NH&NLTS&LSC).
- The authors of this edition recognize Drs. Alva 'Buzz' Baker and Leonard Gelman who wrote the first and second editions on Documentation and Coding from which content for this third edition was updated and expanded upon.

Web Resources
- Centers for Medicare and Medicaid Services Manual Update on Prolonged Service Codes from April 2008. http://www.cms.hhs.gov/transmittals/downloads/R1490CP.pdf.
- AMA Website CPT Code/Relative Value Search Engine based on Current CPT codes and Medicare payment information. https://catalog.ama-assn.org/Catalog/cpt/cpt_search.jsp.
- Find-A-Code, a commercially available website that helps find ICD and CPT codes. http://www.findacode.com.
- CMS Revisions to Consultation Services Payment Policy, information for physicians. http://www.cms.hhs.gov/MLNMattersArticles/downloads/MM6740.pdf.
- *Guide to Post-Acute and Long-Term Coding, Reimbursement and Documentation* can be obtained. http://www.paltc.org.

Acknowledgements Information in this section was partially extracted from a presentation on: "Billing and Coding in PALTC and Beyond!" Presented by Charles Crecelius MD, PhD, FACP, CMD and Robert Zorowitz MD, MBA, CMD at the PALCT 22 Annual Conference in Baltimore, MD given by AMDA—The Society for Post-Acute and Long-Term Care Medicine in March 2022.

References

1. American Medical Association. Current procedural terminology CPT, professional edition. Chicago: American Medical Association; 2022.
2. AMA CPT Evaluation and Management (E/M) Codes and Guideline Changes effective January 1, 2023. https://www.ama-assn.org/system/files/2023-e-m-descriptors-guidelines.pdf. Accessed 16 Dec 2022.

Medication Management in Long-Term Care

Keith A. Swanson, Raghuveer Vedala, and Peter Winn

Introduction

Two-thirds of Americans over the age of 65 have multiple chronic conditions (i.e., multi-morbidities) that affect both quality of life and longevity. The most common chronic diseases and the leading causes of death in older adults are heart disease, cancer, stroke, respiratory disease, dementia, and diabetes mellitus. Census projections estimate that by 2030, 20% of the US population will be 65 years of age and older. As pharmacotherapy is an essential part of care in older adults, optimization of their drug regimen (where benefit outweighs risk) is an important public health issue [1]. Chronic disease, limited physiologic reserves, changes in pharmacokinetics and pharmacodynamics, and impaired immune and inflammatory systems all predispose elders to serious adverse drug events (ADEs) such as falls, hip fractures, weight loss, cognitive and functional decline.

K. A. Swanson (✉)
Department of Pharmacy: Clinical and Administrative Sciences, OU College of Pharmacy, Oklahoma City, OK, USA

R. Vedala · P. Winn
Department of Family and Preventive Medicine, University of Oklahoma Health Sciences Center, Oklahoma City, OK, USA

© The Author(s), under exclusive license to Springer Nature Switzerland AG 2023
P. Winn et al. (eds.), *Post-Acute and Long-Term Care Medicine*, Current Clinical Practice, https://doi.org/10.1007/978-3-031-28628-5_18

Since 27% of patients in a long-term care facility (LTC) routinely take nine or more medications a day, it is not surprising that over 65% will have an ADE occur during a 4-year period, with one in seven of these ADEs resulting in a hospital transfer [2]. Thus, the prevention and recognition of medication-related events is a principal *health care quality* and *safety* issue at LTC facilities, hospitals, and community settings. Understanding the basics of drug pharmacokinetics and pharmacodynamics is essential to quality and safe prescribing.

Physiologic Changes in the Elderly

Both the physiologic changes that occur with normal aging, and pathophysiologic changes due to disease can affect the pharmacokinetics and disposition of many drugs that includes their absorption, distribution, metabolism, and elimination that must be considered when prescribing any medication.

Absorption

Medications enter the systemic circulation via oral, rectal, inhalation, percutaneous, subcutaneous, intravenous, and intramuscular routes. The effect of aging on decreased gastric and intestinal motility have not shown to have a consistent effect on drug absorption. Gastric hypochlorhydria seen with normal aging can decrease the absorption of some medications such as ketoconazole. The widespread use of acid suppressive therapies [proton pump inhibitors (PPIs) and H2 antagonists] results in hypochlorhydria with consequences on drug and vitamin B-12 absorption (decreased) being more prevalent [3, 4]. Physiologic changes of reduced gastric motility, slowed gastric emptying, and reduced peristalsis can alter drug absorption [5].

Comorbid conditions can also alter the absorption of some medications. Congestive heart failure causing bowel wall edema can decrease the absorption of diuretics such as furosemide and thus reduce its clinical efficacy. The transdermal absorption of medication can be significantly decreased [6]. Epidermal thinning and other skin changes common to aging can significantly decrease the absorption of fentanyl from patches although reduced clearance may increase analgesic effect and risk. Other skin changes that decrease drug absorption include:

- Diminished peripheral blood flow and impaired microcirculation (especially in patients with cardiovascular and peripheral vascular disease).
- Increased keratinization.
- Decreased hydration and surface lipid content affect both water-soluble and fat-soluble topical medications.
- Increased intramuscular connective tissue.

Distribution

Once absorbed, drug distribution within body compartments depends upon its lipid and water solubility and the extent to which it is bound to plasma proteins. The volume of distribution (*V*d) is the pharmacokinetic variable that relates the drug dose administered to its concentration in body fluids. Aging decreases the body's lean-to-fat ratio and total body water is reduced by 10–15% by age 80 [7]. Subsequently, this results in a decreased *V*d for water-soluble drugs and those drugs distributed to lean body tissues (e.g., muscle). Therefore, it is recommended to *reduce loading doses* by 10–20% for water-soluble medication. Conversely, the age-related increase in body fat content *increases* the *V*d for lipid-soluble medication such as benzodiazepines, amiodarone, and some hormones (e.g., thyroid), thereby reducing clearance and increasing its metabolic half-life.

Albumin and alpha-1-acid glycoprotein are the most common plasma proteins to which many drugs are bound. Although the concentrations of these plasma proteins do not normally decline significantly with normal aging, nutritional deficiencies, or catabolic states may cause a clinically important decline. Drugs that are highly protein-bound, such as carbamazepine, phenytoin, valproic acid, and warfarin will have *higher free serum concentrations* in the elderly with a decreased level of plasma carrier proteins [8]. To avoid the adverse effects associated with drug toxicity, dose adjustments may need to be based on the *free* medication concentration, not on the total blood concentration (e.g., free phenytoin).

Metabolism

Liver mass and liver blood flow decrease significantly with aging, reducing clearance and increasing the half-life and bioavailability of drugs that undergo extensive first-pass liver metabolism such as propranolol and labetolol [7]. On the other hand, the bioavailability of some ACE inhibitors, (e.g., enalapril) and opioids (e.g., codeine) are reduced as they require hepatic activation [9]. The activity of the cytochrome P450 oxidase system decreases with age, as well as **Phase I reactions** (reduction, oxidation, hydroxylation, and demethylation). Table 1 summarizes isoenzymes of the P450 cytochrome system and commonly prescribed drugs whose metabolism is affected by them. Of note, grapefruit juice is a known inhibitor of the cytochrome P450 3A4 pathway. Such inhibitors can decrease clearance, increase half-life, and thus increase toxicity of some drugs [10]. **Phase II reactions** (drug glucuronidation, sulfation, and acetylation) are minimally influenced by aging.

Table 1 Potential metabolic effects of P450 cytochrome isoenzymes enzymes

P450 enzyme	Common substrate medications	Common inhibitor/ inducer[a] medications	Problematic drug–drug interactions	Clinical problem
CYP 3A4	Simvastatin Atorvastatin Amiodarone Azithromycin Erythromycin Warfarin Quetiapine Solefenain Losartan Amlodipine Prednisone Omeprazole Sertraline Sitagliptin Oxycontin Vardenafil Mirtazapine Indinavir Saquinavir ritonavir Cyclosporine Tacrolimus	Amiodarone (moderate) Erythromycin (moderate) Ciprofloxacin (moderate) Amlodipine (weak) Rifampin Atripla®	Fat soluble statin + Amiodarone Fat soluble statin + Cipro	Increased statin level, which can cause a myopathy
			Azithromycin + Amiodarone Amiodarone + Ciprofloxacin	Leads to QT prolongation, and arrhythmia
			Warfarin + Amiodarone	High INR can lead to bleeding
			Statin + Atripla	Decreases statin levels
			Warfarin + Rifampin	Decreases INR and efficacy
			Rifampin + Atripla®	Decreased HAART efficacy
CYP 2D6	Fluoxetine Paroxetine Aripiprazole Metoprolol, timolol, carvedilol Sertraline Oxycontin Mirtazapine	Fluoxetine (strong) Sertraline (weak) Amiodarone (weak)	Metoprolol + Fluoxetine	Bradycardia, AV block
CYP 2C9	Losartan Glipizide Phenytoin Warfarin	Fluoxetine (weak) Amiodarone (weak)	Warfarin + Fluoxetine	High INR can lead to bleeding
			Glipizide + Amniodarone	Hypoglycemia
CYP 2C19	Clopidogrel Fluoxetine Omeprazole Sertraline Warfarin	Fluoxetine (moderate) Omeprazole (moderate)	Omeprazole + Warfarin	High INR can lead to bleeding

(Adapted from [10])

[a]enzyme inhibitors or inducers may respectively reduce or enhance the molecular metabolic pathway and thus increase or decrease substrate concentrations

INR international normalized ratio, HAART highly active antiretroviral therapy

Renal Elimination and Clearance

Decreased renal elimination of drugs is the most significant pharmacokinetic change seen in older adults. In one study of 10,000 long-term care residents, 40% had significant renal insufficiency [11]. Renal mass decreases an average of 20% from the fourth to the eighth decade of life with a concomitant reduction in renal blood flow, glomerular filtration rate, and tubular secretion. Thus drugs that are dependent upon renal clearance require a dosage reduction [12].

With decreased muscle mass, reduced physical activity, decreased protein intake, and altered tubular secretion of creatinine, serum creatinine by itself is not an accurate measure of renal function. Calculators based on equations such as the *Cockcroft–Gault Equation* that take into account a patient's serum creatinine, sex, age, and estimated lean body weight, provide a more accurate approximation of creatinine clearance [13]. Another formula that estimates glomerular filtration rate, the *Modification of Diet in Renal Disease (MDRD) equation*, has also become a standard for determine renal function used by some clinical laboratories, although it hasn't totally replaced the *Cockcroft–Gault Equation* [14].

Pharmacodynamics

Pharmacodynamics is the interaction between a drug and its effector organ(s) (i.e., receptor) that results in either a therapeutic or adverse effect or both. In addition, the elderly can exhibit increased sensitivity to the therapeutic as well as the toxic effects of many medications due to comorbid illness such as Alzheimer's, Parkinson's, strokes, congestive heart failure, and frailty that reduce the ability of the body to maintain homeostasis. Age-related pharmacodynamic changes that commonly occur in the elderly [3, 9] include:

Increased response
- Increased sensitivity to the CNS effects of benzodiazepines and alcohol.
- Greater analgesic response to opioids.
- Increased sensitivity to anticoagulants (warfarin, heparin).
- Increased risk of delirium from anticholinergic medication.
- Increased risk of bladder outlet obstruction from anticholinergics.
- Increased risk of extrapyramidal side effects and tardive dyskinesia from antipsychotics.

Decreased response
- Reduced sensitivity to beta-adrenergic agonists and antagonists.

Medication Selection in the Elderly

In LTCFs, the primary responsibility for prescribing, dosing, ordering, procuring, administering, monitoring, and when appropriate, altering or discontinuing medication therapy involves the **triad** of prescriber, nursing personnel, and pharmacy provider/consultant. Each has a specific role and responsibility to ensure that patients receive the most appropriate medical therapy (maximize benefit and minimize the risk). Collaborative practice and respectful communication between these health care providers is thus essential.

Preventing Adverse Drug Events

Several years ago, a consensus panel of experts established a list of medications commonly called the "Beers' List" that should be prescribed with caution in older adults. The **current** American Geriatrics Society Beers' Criteria for **Potentially Inappropriate** Medication [15] has evolved into evidence-based recommendations listing medications that have increased risk-to-benefit ratio that are best avoided or cautiously prescribed in the elderly due to the high likelihood of *potential* adverse effects. This tool has been subsequently adapted and applied by State surveyors of LTCFs. The AGS Beers Criteria include a list of medications with significant anticholinergic effects such as antihistamines (e.g., diphenhydramine) and antiemetics (e.g., promethazine), and other medications with a propensity to worsen mental status, (i.e., delirium/encephalopathy), and cause falls, urinary retention, orthostatic hypotension, dehydration, and movement disturbances such as extrapyramidal symptoms (EPS) and tardive dyskinesia. Benzodiazepines increase the risk of altered mental status, sedation, and falls. Limiting the use of medications on the AGS Beers' Criteria is not necessarily contraindicated when a patient is receiving hospice care [15].

Another screening tool to promote optimization of medication use is the *STOPP* criteria (*S*creening *T*ool of *O*lder *P*erson's *P*rescriptions). This may be more user-friendly than the AGS Beers Criteria. A systematic review found this tool to be a more sensitive measure of potentially inappropriate prescribing patterns in community-dwelling and acute and long-term care facilities in Europe, Asia, and North America. The STOPP criteria were developed as many clinicians considered that certain drugs designated as inappropriate by the AGS Beers' Criteria were debatable, and rather could be safely prescribed in certain specific clinical situations [16].

Tools such as the AGS Beers Criteria and STOPP criteria do not substitute for thorough clinical assessment and good judgment, as clinicians must first and foremost consider whether medications are possibly the cause of signs and symptoms presenting in older adults. By optimizing and minimizing medication use, unnecessary and potentially harmful adverse side effects and *prescribing cascades* (use of a medication to treat the side effects of another) can be lessened or avoided [17, 18]. The STOPP criteria are summarized in Table 2 with examples of potential adverse drug outcomes [16].

Table 2 STOPP criteria for potentially inappropriate prescribing

Medication by physiological system	Prescribing pitfall	Potential adverse outcome
Cardiovascular system		
Digoxin	>125 µg per day with impaired renal function	Digoxin toxicity from decreased renal clearance
Thiazide diuretics	With history of gout	Gout attack, nephropathy
β-Blockers	With COPD	COPD exacerbation
Diltiazem or verapamil	Class III or IV heart failure	CHF exacerbation
Calcium channel blockers	Chronic constipation	Worsening constipation, impaction
Dipyridamole	As monotherapy for cardiovascular secondary prevention	Orthostatic hypotension
Warfarin	Use in first episode of uncomplicated pulmonary embolus for >12 months	Increased risk of bleeding
Warfarin, clopidogrel, or aspirin	Use with concurrent bleeding disorder	Development of hidden or covert bleeding
Aspirin	With history of PUD without histamine H2 antagonist or PPI	Gastrointestinal bleeding
	≥150 mg/day	
	With no history of coronary, cerebral, or peripheral vascular symptoms or Occlusive event	
Central nervous system		
TCAs	With dementia	CNS adverse effects
	With cardiac conductive abnormalities	Cardiac arrhythmia
	With constipation	Impaction, worsening constipation
	With prostatism or history of urinary retention	Urinary retention
Long-term, long-acting benzodiazepines	Any use	Falls, confusion, lethargy, overdose
Long-term neuroleptics	In those with parkinsonism or dementia	CNS and extrapyramidal adverse effects, cardiovascular events
Phenothiazines	Use in patients with epilepsy	Increased risk of seizure
SSRI antidepressants	Use in patients with history of hyponatremia	Increased risk of altered mental status
First-generation antihistamines	Prolonged use	Falls, CNS adverse effects
Gastrointestinal system		
Diphenoxylate, loperamide or codeine phosphate	For treatment of diarrhea of unknown cause	Delay in treatment of bacterial/other causes of diarrhea
	For severe infective gastroenteritis, i.e., bloody diarrhea, high fever, or severe systemic toxicity	Bacteremia, sepsis, death

(continued)

Table 2 (continued)

Medication by physiological system	Prescribing pitfall	Potential adverse outcome
Proton pump inhibitors	For peptic ulcer disease at full therapeutic dosage for >8 weeks	Aspiration pneumonia, B12 deficiency, magnesium deficiency
Respiratory system		
Nebulized ipratropium	Use in glaucoma	Worsens symptoms
Theophylline	As monotherapy for COPD	Poorly controlled COPD, theophylline toxicity
Systemic corticosteroids	Instead of inhaled corticosteroids for maintenance therapy in moderate–severe COPD	Any corticosteroid side effect, especially hyperglycemia, osteoporosis, cataracts, confusion
Musculoskeletal system		
NSAIDs	With history of PUD or gastrointestinal bleeding, unless with concurrent histamine H2 receptor antagonist, PPI, or misoprostol (Cytotec)	Gastrointestinal bleeding
	With moderate to severe HTN	Poorly controlled HTN
	With heart failure	Exacerbation of HF
	With warfarin (Coumadin)	Bleeding
	With chronic renal failure	Worsening renal function
	For relief of mild–moderate joint pain in osteoarthritis	Bleeding, exacerbation of renal function, heart failure, hypertension
Long-term corticosteroid	As monotherapy for rheumatoid or osteoarthritis	Corticosteroid adverse effects (see above)
Long-term NSAID or colchicine	For chronic treatment of gout where there is no contraindication to allopurinol	NSAID or colchicine adverse effects
Urogenital system		
Bladder antimuscarinic drugs	With dementia	CNS adverse effects
Antimuscarinic drugs	With chronic prostatism	Urinary retention
Endocrine system		
β-Blockers	In those with DM	Unrecognized hypoglycemia
Drugs that adversely affect persons who are at risk to fall		
Benzodiazepines		Fall with or without injury
Neuroleptic drugs		
Vasodilator drugs	With postural hypotension	
Long-acting benzodiazepine		
Long-term opiates	In those with recurrent falls	
Analgesic drugs		

Table 2 (continued)

Medication by physiological system	Prescribing pitfall	Potential adverse outcome
Long-term potent opioids	Use as first-line therapy for mild-moderate pain, e.g., morphine or fentanyl patch	CNS adverse effects, falls with or without injury, hypotension
Long-term opioids	In those with dementia unless used for palliative care	
Regular scheduled opioids	For more than 2 weeks in those with chronic constipation without concurrent use of laxatives	Impaction, worsening constipation, bowel perforation, and ischemia

Adapted from reference [16]

The AGS Beers Criteria and the STOPP and START screening tools (the latter to be discussed later) aim to both reduce polypharmacy and the incidence of adverse drug events. However, these tools are more applicable to the general adult older population and not specifically frail *individuals with a limited life expectancy*. A recent addition to these tools is the **STOPPFrail** list, which was developed to help guide *deprescribing* for persons in the last year of life [19]. For example, frail elderly patients with limited life expectancy most likely will not survive long enough to reap the benefits of medication suggested by the START criteria. Furthermore, the STOPP criteria do not exclude medications that should be stopped due to their limited benefit in those with a limited life expectancy (e.g., statins). The STOPFrail list consists of 27 criteria relating to medication that may be considered unnecessary or inappropriate in frail elderly and thus encourage practitioners to deprescribe. In general, this list of medication appropriate for discontinuation is recommended under the following conditions:

- End-stage irreversible disease.
- Poor 1-year survival prognosis.
- Severe functional or severe cognitive impairment (or both).
- Symptom control is the priority (palliation) rather than prevention of disease progression.
- Medications that are persistently refused, forgotten, or have intolerable side effects despite adequate patient education and optimized dosing safeguards.

In a randomized controlled trial using STOPPFrail, individuals did not suffer undue harm or negative outcomes when potentially unnecessary medications were discontinued versus those who continued usual drug therapy [19, 20].

Though studies that assess suboptimal prescribing often focus on *overuse* and *misuse* of medication, it is equally important to ensure against the *underuse* of medication or the *omission* of a clinically indicated drug for treatment or prevention of disease, if compatible with a patient's goals of care and goals of life. Such occurrences (that is underuse or omission) are reported in up to 50% of community dwelling elders. Examples of drug omissions in LTCFs include the lack of GI protection with proton pump inhibitors (PPIs) for patients taking a NSAID or prednisone, no ACE inhibitor therapy in diabetics, no vitamin D supplementation for those at risk for osteoporosis, and lack of venous thromboembolism (VTE) prophylaxis.

The START (*Screening Tool to Alert Doctors to Right Treatment*) (see Table 3), is a tool to help identify potentially beneficial medications that may have been omitted from a LTCF resident's treatment regimen. The START tool is similar to the STOPP criteria in that both have been validated in the elderly, derived from evidence-based prescribing practice, and arranged by physiological systems; but

Table 3 START: *Screening Tool to Alert doctors to Right Treatments*

These medications should be considered for people ≥65 years of age based on other clinical conditions and no contraindication to the recommendation

Cardiovascular conditions

- Initiate anticoagulation to reduce stroke/thrombosis risk in chronic atrial fibrillation—direct acting anticoagulant (ex. apixaban, others), warfarin, aspirin (when DOAC or warfarin is contraindicated)
- Aspirin or clopidogrel in documented history of atherosclerotic coronary, cerebral, or peripheral vascular disease in patients with sinus rhythm
- Antihypertensive therapy when systolic blood pressure is consistently >160 mmHg
- Lipid lowering therapy (statin) with documented history of coronary, cerebral, or peripheral vascular disease, where the patient's functional status remains independent for ADLs and life expectancy is greater than 5 years
- Initiate or optimize treatment for chronic heart failure according to current guidelines when not contraindicated by current clinical conditions or status [which may include: ACEi indicates angiotensin-converting enzyme inhibitor(ACEi), angiotensin receptor blocker (ARB), angiotensin receptor-neprilysin inhibitor (ARNi), hydralazine, isosorbide dinitrate, mineralocorticoid receptor antagonist (MRA), sodium-glucose cotransporter 2 inhibitor (SGLT2i), or diuretics]
- Initiate or optimize treatment according to current guidelines for acute myocardial infarction (e.g., ACEi) or chronic stable angina (e.g., beta-blocker)

Respiratory system

- Initiate or optimize treatment for moderate to severe symptoms of COPD and/or frequent emergency room visits or hospitalization (which may include: inhaled beta2 agonist, anticholinergics, inhaled corticosteroids, others)
- Initiate or optimize treatment for moderate to severe symptoms of asthma (which may include: inhaled corticosteroids, inhaled beta2 agonist, others)
- Initiate or optimize oxygen therapy for documented chronic respiratory failure

Central nervous system

- Initiate or optimize treatment for Parkinson's disease with functional impairment and disability (which may include: L-DOPA, COMT inhibitors, MAO-B inhibitors, dopamine receptor agonists, others)
- Initiate or optimize treatment for moderate to severe depressive symptoms with or without anxiety [which may include: selective serotonin reuptake inhibitors (SSRIs), serotonin and norepinephrine reuptake inhibitors (SNRIs), norepinephrine and dopamine reuptake inhibitors (NDRIs), mixed serotonin effect agents, serotonin and α2-adrenergic antagonists, others]
- Initiate or optimize treatment for cognitive impairment/dementia in individuals where the patient's functional status remains independent for ADLs and life expectancy is greater than 5 years and treatment is appropriate according to the individual's goals of care [which may include: acetylcholinesterase inhibitor (AChI) or *n*-methyl-D-aspartate antagonists (NMDA)]

Table 3 (continued)

Gastrointestinal system
• Initiate or optimize treatment for moderate to severe gastroesophageal reflux disease (GERD) especially with history of erosive esophagitis and/or strictures [which may include: daily doses of proton pump inhibitor (PPI) or high dose histamine-2 receptor antagonist (H2RA)]
• Initiate or optimize treatment for prevention of peptic ulcers due to nonsteroidal anti-inflammatory drugs (NSAIDs) when use is absolutely necessary strictures [which may include: daily doses of proton pump inhibitor (PPI) or high dose histamine-2 receptor antagonist (H2RA)]
• Initiate or optimize fiber supplementation for chronic, symptomatic diverticular disease with constipation
Musculoskeletal system
• Initiate or optimize treatment for active moderate to severe rheumatoid arthritis strictures [which may include: disease-modifying anti-rheumatic drugs (DMARDs), immune modulating agents such as monoclonal antibodies against TNF-α, leukocyte adhesion and migration inhibitors, interleukin inhibitors, JAK inhibitors, others]
• Initiate or optimize treatment for osteoporosis or individuals requiring maintenance corticosteroids (therapy may include: bisphosphonates, calcium, and vitamin D, others)
Endocrine system
• Initiate or optimize treatment for diabetes and or metabolic syndrome (therapy may include: metformin, others)
• Initiate or optimize therapy to reduce risk of nephropathy associated with diabetes (therapy may include ACEI or ARB)
• Initiate or optimize therapy to reduce major cardiovascular risk in individuals with diabetes [therapy may include: antiplatelet agents, lipid-lowering agents (e.g., statins), others]

(Adapted from Ref. [16])

unlike STOPP, START identifies *possible prescribing omissions* in older adults as opposed to medication overuse by STOPP. These tools can enable practitioners to better evaluate an older person's "prescription" drug regimen in the context of current clinical diagnoses [16].

Issues in Medication Management

Anticholinergic Burden

Medications that block cholinergic neurons are considered potentially harmful in older individual due to adverse effects that include dry mouth, constipation, urinary retention, precipitation of glaucoma, and altered mental status or cognition. Highly anticholinergic medications have also been associated with increased risk of hospitalization and mortality, dementia, and pneumonia. Several tools have been developed to determine the cumulative risk for anticholinergic effects, such as the Anticholinergic Cognitive Burden List (ACB), the Anticholinergic Drug Scale

(ADS), and the Anticholinergic Risk Scale (ARS). These tools categorize medications as Highly Anticholinergic (Score = 3), Moderately Anticholinergic (Score = 2), and Mildly Anticholinergic (Score = 1). The use of multiple drugs with anticholinergic activity will result in a cumulative *anticholinergic burden* that in turn increase the risk of delirium, worsening dementia, hospitalization, and mortality [21–23].

"Deprescribing" and Gradual Dose Reduction (GDR)

Known as **deprescribing**, many initiatives have been undertaken to identify the risks and *benefits* to reducing medication burden via systematic evaluation and discontinuation of potentially unnecessary medication. Prescribers are often hesitant to deprescribe due to concerns that this may cause patient decompensation in clinical and functional status. Cautious and gradual discontinuation of medication through a process termed by CMS as Gradual Dose Reduction (GDR), often causes little if any detrimental effects in older and/or frail adults [24]. In 2021, AMDA-The Society for Post-Acute Care and Long-Term Care Medicine launched an initiative titled "Drive to Deprescribe" (D2D). This program addresses the issue of polypharmacy and inappropriate medication use in post-acute and long-term care (PALTC) with the goal to reduce (unnecessary) medication use by 25% [24]. Federal nursing facility regulation require that gradual dose reductions (GDR) be attempted at least quarterly for all *sedative/hypnotics* and *psychotropics* that are prescribed on a scheduled basis and continued beyond the manufacturer's recommended duration of use. *Current practice extends GDR to all medication.* Any medication should be determined as whether necessary in order to lessen the risk of a potentially harmful outcome.

However, a consultant pharmacist's recommendation for a GDR can be declined on clinical grounds if

1. Continued use of the medication is in accordance with the current standard of practice and a GDR would likely impair the patient's function or cause psychiatric or instability by either exacerbating an underlying medical condition or psychiatric disorder.

or

2. Patient's target symptoms for which the medication had been prescribed either returned or worsened after the most recent GDR, and further GDR attempts would likely impair the patient's function or psychiatric stability.

Practitioners should note that current State Operations Manual (SOM) guidelines to surveyors state that medication should be prescribed *only* when necessary and in the lowest effective dose and that each resident's drug regimen be free from *unnecessary* drugs *(F-Tag 757)*. Once symptoms have resolved or stabilized, these guidelines recommend that attempts be made to either discontinue the medication or reduce the dose through GDR. Previous efforts to reduce unnecessary medication focused solely on antipsychotics, benzodiazepines, and centrally acting drugs. The current guidelines encourage GDR be attempted for *all medications* unless the patient's current condition would be adversely affected. Refer to **Appendix A** for more detailed information on what defines an unnecessary medication and the intent of the federal regulation.

Transitions in Care and Medication Errors

Transitions in care portend significant risk for patients with changes in location, level of care, and/or providers. Such transitions can result in *unrecognized* medication errors and adverse patient outcomes. Medication-related adverse events are common after discharge from the hospital [25]. For this reason, one of the National Patient Safety goals of the Joint Commission on Accreditation of Hospital Organizations (JCAHO) continues to be *medication reconciliation* and the transmission of accurate up-to-date medication information between care settings.

Risk factors for medication-related adverse events during a care transition include:

- Polypharmacy (>4 medications)
- Inadequate monitoring of high-risk medications such as insulin, warfarin
- Chronic complex illness: stroke, cancer, diabetes, COPD, heart disease
- Hurried transfers during nonstandard times of day/night/weekend
- Inadequate patient support post-discharge from one care setting to another

Hand-off communication must include comprehensive and up-to-date records to accompany the patient through any care transition and ensure a timely evaluation of the patient upon admission to their new residence. This can help alleviate medication errors, diagnose new problems, and prevent the occurrence of deteriorating conditions. Use of a universally accessible electronic health care records (EHR) across all care settings is essential to meet this goal [26].

Use of Psychoactive Medication

Older adults are especially vulnerable to adverse effects from psychoactive medication especially the atypical antipsychotics that can cause delirium, extrapyramidal symptoms, postural hypotension, falls (with/without fractures), and cardiac arrhythmias. Although these medications have been used *off-label* to manage behavioral and psychological symptoms of dementia (BPSD), safety concerns have been raised and well documented [17, 27]. Other adverse outcomes include hospitalization [28] and acute kidney injury [18].

In 2014, the American Geriatrics Society (AGS) recommended *Choosing Wisely®* guidelines that staff and physicians should initiate non-pharmacologic strategies as first-line treatment for aggression and disruptive behaviors associated with dementia. Identifying and addressing the underlying cause of the behavior (the antecedent) may preclude the use of psychoactive medication. If these approaches fail and the clinician decides that there is a need to prescribe an antipsychotic medication, patients and their families should be informed on the drug's potential adverse effects. *Many facilities now require the family to sign informed consent prior to their use.* Proactive monitoring of blood pressure, as well as serum lipid, glucose, and creatinine levels should be part of the treatment plan for any patient prescribed an antipsychotic medication. Additionally, recent meta-analysis studies have shown (though of low quality) that antipsychotics may be successfully discontinued in older adults with dementia and other neuropsychiatric symptoms who have been on antipsychotics for 3 months. The discontinuation of these medications had little or no rebound effect on behavioral and psychological symptoms [29].

Overprescribing of Antibiotics

The over-prescribing of antibiotics continues to be a concern in the older aged population, specifically those who reside in a nursing home setting. **Antibiotic stewardship** is an integral component of quality assurance and performance improvement in LTCFs. Antibiotic overuse has been linked to multiple risks including antibiotic drug–drug interactions, colonization with multiresistant organisms, and creation of "super-bugs" in which no antibiotic will be effective. Preventive use of antibiotics is an ongoing concern in long-term care facilities [30]. Research questions the evidence for prescribing antibiotics to prevent recurrent urinary tract infections, to treating acute bronchitis (often viral) to prevent bacterial pneumonia, to treat acute sinusitis to prevent bacterial superinfection, to ongoing antibiotic treatment in persons with COPD to prevent exacerbations or hospitalizations, to prevent soft tissue skin infections in a patient with frequent cellulitis (often over-diagnosed), and for treatment at the time of dental procedures to prevent endocarditis in patients with heart disease or to prevent joint infection in those patients with artificial joints.

Overprescribing of Proton Pump Inhibitors

Proton pump inhibitors (PPIs) are gastric acid suppressive medications that are used to treat gastrointestinal disorders such as Gastroesophageal Reflux Disease (GERD) and Peptic Ulcer Disease (PUD). Since their approval for use in the United States over 30 years ago, they have expanded to worldwide use, are deemed low risk medications in most countries, and often obtained without a prescription. However more recent studies regarding PPIs have reported adverse effects when prescribed long term. PPIs have been linked to an increased risk of *Clostridium difficile* infection, increased infection risk in cirrhotic patients, acute interstitial nephritis, prevention of clopidegrol conversion to its active metabolite, increased risk of hip fracture, increased risk of chronic kidney disease, increased risk of community acquired pneumonia, decreased iron, B12, and magnesium absorption leading to deficiencies, and *rebound* gastric acid hypersecretion after discontinuation of use.

Given these multiple risk factors, cautious prescribing and regular monitoring of PPI use is essential in older adults who may be at higher risk of those adverse reactions mentioned above. **Deprescribing** should be considered and entails decreasing dosage, switching to as needed use, or stopping altogether and starting a different medication for symptom management. Histamine 2 receptor blockers are an appropriate alternative, and have been associated with less *C difficile*, and fracture risk [31, 32]. Patients should be educated on non-pharmacologic lifestyle modifications to reduce the need for acid suppressive therapy. These include weight loss, elevated head of bed, limiting bedtime meals, and avoiding high-fat greasy meals.

Selection of Diabetic Medication

Several studies have suggested that older adults with diabetes and high comorbidity have diminished cardiovascular benefit from intensive blood glucose control (Hgb A1C less than 6.5–7%), and an increased risk for hypoglycemia. These patients would *benefit more from improved control of other risk factors* including serum lipids, dietary consumption of sodium, and blood pressure [33, 34]. Current treatment options for diabetes have increased with multiple medications now available. Each has its own mode of action and risk. Renal status should always be considered when prescribing. Some of these medications have been shown to have cardiovascular benefits as well. Table 4 provides a summary of these medications as to route of administration, risk of hypoglycemia, weight loss or gain, cardiovascular effect, renal effect, and side effect risk and contraindications [35]. For more detailed information on the management of diabetes in PALTC refer to the chapter on "Common Clinical Conditions in Long-Term Care."

Table 4 Commonly used diabetic medication in older adults

Common diabetic medications in older patients

Class/drug	Route	Hypoglycemia	Weight	CV effect	Renal effect	Contraindications/side effects
Metformin	Oral	NO	Loss	Potential benefit	Contraindicated if GFP <30	• GI side common • Potential for B12 deficiency • Lactic acidosis
Thiazolidinediones	Oral	NO	Gain	Increased risk of CHF (Black cox warning: Rosiglitazone and Pioglitazone)	Not recommender in renal impairment—can cause fluid retention	• Fluid retention/edema-CHF • Benefit in NASH • Risk of bone fracture • Bladder cancer (Pioglitazone) • ↑LDL (Rosiglitazone)
Sulfonylurea	Oral	YES	Gain	Neutral	Avoid glyburide in renal impaired	• Glipizide preferred in older population
GLP 1 analogs	Subq	NO	Loss	Benefit (Liraglutide and semaglutide)	Caution if GFR <30	• Risk of thyroid C cell tumors (Liraglutide, Exenatide, Dulaglutide, Albiglutide) • GI side effects (delayed gastric emptying → n/v, diarrhea)—care in elderly/frail/malnourished • Injection site reactions • ↑Risk of pancreatitis
SGLT-2 inhibitors	Oral	NO	Loss	Benefit (Canagiflozin, Empagiflozin)	Cangiflozin (Cl in GFR <45) Dapigaflozin [caution in GFR <60, Cl GFR <30 Empagiflozin (Cl GFR <30)]	• Risk of amputation (Canagiflozin) • DKA risk (all agents, rare in type 2 DM) • GU infection (bacterial/fungal) • Risk of volume depletion/hypotension • ↑LDL

Common diabetic medications in older patients

Class/drug	Route	Hypoglycemia	Weight	CV effect	Renal effect	Contraindications/side effects
DPP-4 inhibitors	Oral	NO	Neutral	CHF risk (Saxogliptin, Alogliptin)	Dose adjustment required if renal impaired	• Risk of pancreatitis • Joint pain • Well tolerated in elderly
Insulin	Subq	YES	Gain	Neutral	Lower doses for renal impaired	• Injection site reactions • Hypoglycemia

Adapted from: https://professional.diabetes.org/sites/professional.diabetes.org/files/media/mendez_how_to_use_the_type_2_diabetes_treatment_algo-rithm.pdf

Choice and Use of Analgesics

Guidelines published by the American Geriatric Society (AGS) caution against the use of *nonselective NSAIDs* (especially those with a long half-life such as naproxen and piroxicam) and *COX-2 selective inhibitors* due to their potential cardiac (fluid and sodium retention), gastrointestinal (inflammation, bleeding), CNS (altered mental status, psychosis), and renal effects (altered blood flow) [36]. Both these classes of medication have significant drug interactions with ACE inhibitors (potential for hyperkalemia), diuretics (diminished diuresis due to changes in renal blood flow), methotrexate (decreased clearance), anticoagulants (potentiated effects), and lithium (decreased renal clearance and increase risk of lithium toxicity). Additionally, there is concern that concomitant use of a NSAID (especially ibuprofen) or a COX-2 inhibitor with a once daily cardio-preventive dose of aspirin *will negate aspirin's cardio-preventive effect* [37].

An FDA Advisory Panel has recommended sweeping safety restrictions on the use of acetaminophen alone and in combination with opioids such as hydrocodone/acetaminophen and oxycodone/acetaminophen due to reports of increased cases of liver damage and acute liver failure associated with acetaminophen overuse. This risk increases with current and chronic use of alcohol. The panel advised that combination opioid/acetaminophen analgesics increase the possibility of accidental overdose and acute liver failure, especially when taken with over-the-counter formulations of acetaminophen. The panel also recommended that the maximal *amount per unit dose of acetaminophen be a lowered to 325* mg tablet in lieu of the current 500 and 650 mg tablets currently available over the counter. And that the maximum daily dosage for osteoarthritis be *less* than 4 g per day [38], i.e., 2–3 g per day. Useful medication guidelines for many drugs can be downloaded from the FDA website. These guidelines provide specific information for patients and caregivers and may help prevent ADEs [39]. Current national initiatives focus on reducing the overuse of opioid analgesics due to the risk of accidental overdose and death. The diversion of controlled substances continues to be major concern. This can also occur in LTC facilities! Every patient visit should include a review of current analgesic utilization (both scheduled and as needed) with a goal to discontinue any unused, unnecessary, or ineffective drugs.

Medication Treatment Goals for Hypertension

The elderly are at high risk for cardiovascular events, thus blood pressure should be monitored and hypertension treated. Recommendations from the Joint National Commission 8 (JNC-8) published in 2014 set BP goals for persons over the age of 60 years at <150/90. This goal has been controversial as many clinicians advocate a lower blood pressure goal of 140/90 in persons under the age of 80 and a higher goal of 150/90 for those over the age of 80. There also has been a change in the recommended BP goals for patients with chronic kidney disease (CKD) and diabetes *from* <130/80 *to* <140/90. The Joint National Commission also recommended that clinicians investigate for secondary causes/contributors to hypertension (see Table 5),

Table 5 Secondary causes of hypertension

Cause	How to identify
Medication	Medication reconciliation: check for nonsteroidal anti-inflammatory (NSAIDS), steroids, venlafaxine, estrogen-containing preparations (found in herbals, over-the-counter meds)
Alcohol abuse	AUDIT-C
Obstructive SA	Epworth sleepiness scale, sleep study, snoring history
Lifestyle	High sodium diet, increased body mass index (BMI), lack of exercise
Primary renal	Basic metabolic profile (BMP), urine sediment, urine for microalbumin/creatinine
Renovascular	Clinical atherosclerosis: PVD, CAD, CVD Acute onset/exacerbation of hypertension; +abdominal bruit, deterioration of renal function after angiotensin-converting enzyme inhibitor (ACEI) or angiotensin receptor blocker (ARB)
Aldosteronism	Electrolytes (low potassium)

Adapted from reference [40]

assess for end organ damage, and better monitor for side effects of antihypertensive medication (including postural hypotension) [40].

Newer recommendations from ACC/AHA in 2017 call for stricter control of blood pressure [41]. These recommendations define elderly as individuals >65 years of age and recommend starting pharmacotherapy with BPs >130/80. It is important to note that the American College of Physicians (ACP) and the American Academy of Family Physicians (AAFP) did not support the ACC/AHA recommendations and continue to recommend the original JNC-8 guidelines with BP goals for individuals over 60 years of age at <150/90. Additionally, in 2018 the European Society of Cardiology (ECS) and European Society of Hypertension (ESH) stratified patients further to a "very old" category, defining those 80 years of age. In these patients, they recommended starting pharmacotherapy at BPs >160/90. A lower BP target of 130–139/70–79 could be considered in those over 65 years old, but not the very old (>85).

Although the ACC/AHA and the ECS/ESH guidelines differ in definitions and thresholds, both agree that treatment of high blood pressure in the elderly is pivotal to reduce atherosclerotic cardiovascular risk, and recommend caution and close monitoring.

If clinically appropriate, it is particularly important in geriatric patients to optimize antihypertensive therapy with lifestyle modifications, including the implementation of the Dietary Approaches to Stop Hypertension (DASH) diet with a sodium restriction of 1500 mg/day (4 g or two-thirds of a teaspoon of table salt) [42]. *Restrictive diets are not recommended in the frail elderly because of the potential to cause weight loss.* If, however, dietary intervention is insufficient to control blood pressure, a low-dose thiazide diuretic and long-acting calcium channel blocker can be prescribed unless comorbidities merit the choice of other drugs. See chapter: "Common Clinical Conditions in Long-Term Care" for further discussion on the treatment of hypertension.

Beta-Blocker Use in Post-Myocardial Infarction

Beta-blocker use is important in the early course of an acute MI and in secondary prevention to reduce cardiac morbidity, mortality, and MI recurrence. Age greater than 75 has been associated with the *underuse* of beta-blockers. This is concerning given that mortality rate has been reported to be 43% less among beta-blocker recipients than non-recipients [43].

Choice of Anticoagulants in Non-Valvular Atrial Fibrillation

Anticoagulation is recommended in patients with atrial fibrillation due to increased risk of stroke. The CHA_2DS_2-VASc calculator incorporates multiple risk factors and its use is recommended by the American Heart Association to predict the yearly stroke risk in patients with chronic *non-valvular* atrial fibrillation [44]. Patients with a score of 1 (male) or greater than 1 (female) are at high risk for embolic stroke and anticoagulation should seriously be considered if not contraindicated.

Warfarin was previously recommended as first-line agent with INR goal of 2–3 in patients with atrial fibrillation older than 75, and those ages 65–75 with risk factors of stroke (i.e., hypertension, diabetes mellitus, CHF, previous history of stroke, transient ischemic attack, or peripheral vascular disease). However more recent studies, and concensus panels now recommend the use of direct acting oral anticoagulants (DOACs) specifically apixaban other oral anticoagulants [45].

Treatment of Subclinical Hypothyroidism

The prevalence of subclinical hypothyroidism increases with age, being higher in females than males, and lower in Black persons than White persons. It has a prevalence up to 18% in elderly persons and progresses to overt hypothyroidism at a rate of 5–18% per year. Causes of subclinical hypothyroidism are similar to those of overt hypothyroidism: autoimmune disease, thyroid injury, thyroid infiltrative disorders such as sarcoidosis or amyloidosis, drugs impairing thyroid function such as amiodarone, lithium, sulfonamides, and sulfonylureas, and inadequate replacement therapy for overt hypothyroidism. The most common cause is chronic autoimmune (Hashimoto's) thyroiditis.

Subclinical hypothyroidism is associated with an increased cardiovascular risk (CHF, CAD), elevated low-density lipoprotein (LDL), blood pressure dysregulation, impaired endothelial function, increased risk of nonalcoholic fatty liver disease, alterations in cerebral blood flow, and impairment of memory. Despite this, treatment of subclinical hypothyroidism is not always indicated.

It is universally accepted that TSH levels ≥10 mU/L should be treated in all ages. However, in elderly persons (ages >65–70) it is suggested to avoid treatment when TSH levels <7. For TSH levels between 7 and 9.9, treatment is only recommended if patients have *symptoms suggestive of hypothyroidism*. Studies have shown that there is *no benefit* to the treatment of older persons *with asymptomatic* subclinical hypothyroidism (TSH 7–9.9), as treatment can increase the risk of *iatrogenic* thyrotoxicosis. Thyroid peroxidase antibody testing may help decision making regarding treatment, since Hashimoto's thyroiditis is the most common cause. Treatment is recommended to start with a low dose of levothyroxine 25–50 mcg daily and rechecking response with a TSH level in 4–6 weeks. This approach avoids overtreatment and is most appropriate in older adults [46].

Choosing Wisely® and Medication Management

The American Board of Internal Medicine Foundation developed and promoted the Choosing Wisely campaign to discourage medication and medical interventions shown to have little or no clinical benefit to patients and that could potentially cause harm. As such, many subspecialties, including AMDA-The Society for Post-Acute and Long-Term Care Medicine have developed several medication-related recommendations. These are listed in **Appendix B** and are available for review at the Choosing Wisely® website where the rationale for each recommendation is discussed. Also, in response to the 2014 GAO report on adverse events in SNF patients, AMDA-The Society for PA and LTC Medicine spearheaded the "Quality Prescribing Initiative" in 2015 in collaboration with CMS and other long-term care provider organizations.

Pharmacogenomics

Pharmacogenomics continues to be an evolving field that investigates how the clinical response to a drug can vary dependent on a person's genetic makeup [47]. The genetic makeup can determine a drug's pharmacodynamics and pharmacokinetics. Pharmacogenomics may help *individualize* pharmacologic therapy, reducing adverse drug reactions while optimizing a drug's benefit. Commercial testing for genetic variants of the hepatic cytochrome P-450 isoforms is now available. Although not currently broadly applied to clinical practice, pharmacogenetic testing can be useful to guide medication prescribing in specific situations. The Pharmacogenetics Research Network was established in 2000 by the National Institutes of Health [5] in order to: investigate the relationship between genetic variation and variable drug responses; create a base of knowledge available to the public, which provides reliable information about genetic makeup and medication responsiveness; and to facilitate collaboration among investigators.

The FDA now provides pharmacogenetic information and recommendations within the approved labeling for approximately 200 medications where pharmacogenomics can play an important role in medication selection and dosing. An example is the variable expression of the production of CYP2D6 isoenzymes with over 160 versions of the CYP2D6 gene. Natural genetic variation may result in excessive production of a variant enzyme, for example, causing overconversion of codeine to its active metabolite morphine, that then results in an excessive response to a normal dose of codeine. Conversely, an individual may have an underactive form of the enzyme to convert enough codeine to sufficient morphine resulting in ineffective analgesia. Situations such as this may reflect the efficacy and/or toxicity of medication [48]. A central web-based repository of known genetic variants that determine drug responses is available at http://www.pharmgkb.org. It is updated regularly and links the results of patient pharmacogenetic tests to specific recommendations on therapeutic dosing for many drugs.

Summary

Timely and aggressive pharmacologic intervention for a newly diagnosed or worsening medical condition is essential. However, the intended positive outcome of any medication must be balanced against the risk of an adverse drug event and a subtherapeutic response. Efforts to optimize appropriate, effective, and safe medication use in the elderly have become a priority for health care systems, clinicians, and state and federal agencies. Tools such as the AGS Beers' Criteria, STOPP, STOPPFrail, and START criteria can aide practitioners to recognize both potentially inappropriate and appropriate medication use. *Quality prescribing* has the potential for primary and secondary prevention and an improved quality of life. It is incumbent upon practitioners to collaborate with pharmacists, nursing personnel, caregivers, and patients and patients' family members. Practitioners must regularly assess for both negative and positive medication-related outcomes and decide whether to continue pharmacologic treatment based upon patient goals and preferences for care, prognosis, and *time needed to treat in order to obtain the desired therapeutic benefit* [49].

Pearls for the Practitioner
- Polypharmacy (sometimes called "multiple medication use") is characterized by excessive or unnecessary use of medications (often at doses higher than necessary) or drug combinations that put older adults at excessive risk due to drug–drug, drug–disease, or drug–nutrient interactions.
- Request patients and their caregivers to bring in all medications, including over-the-counter and herbal medications, to each office visit or upon admission from home to an assisted living or nursing facility.

- Regularly review the LTCF resident's *m*edication *a*dministration *r*ecord (i.e., MAR) looking for unnecessary medication use (i.e., no apparent indication, either a subtherapeutic or an excessive dose, prolonged duration of action, drug interactions, inappropriate dosage forms, and excessive cost) and adjust accordingly.
- Consider a potential adverse drug event in the differential diagnosis of any change in the clinical or functional status of an elderly person.
- *Gradual up-titration* is appropriate when starting a new medication in the elderly, particularly when prescribing thyroid hormone replacement especially in a those with underlying ischemic heart disease.
- The AGS Beers' Criteria, STOPP and STOPPFrail criteria can help practitioners avoid prescribing *potentially* inappropriate medication, especially those with anticholinergic properties or hypotensive effects.
- Dietary and behavioral interventions rather than pharmacotherapy may be more useful and safer, less costly, and have other salutary effects when treating chronic conditions.
- Anticipate decreased renal clearance and hepatic oxidative metabolism; accordingly individualize drug doses when initiating or modifying drug therapy.
- Consider pharmacogenetic testing when clinically necessary and where applicable; such as when a personal or family history of medication intolerance and adverse effects may indicate the presence of genetic variations in CYP-P450 iso-enzymes, that can then guide use of an alternative medication and its dosing. Though its cost may be prohibitive to the health care system.

Websites
- GFR Calculator Using Cockcroft–Gault, MDRD equations. https://www.mdcalc.com/. Site accessed: 19 July 2022.
- AMDA-The Society for Post-Acute Care and Long-Term Care Medicine. 2021. https://paltc.org/drive2deprescribe. Site accessed: 19 July 2022.
- AGS Clinical Practice Guidelines for Pharmacological Management of Persistent Pain in Older Persons. Available at: https://www.aafp.org/pubs/afp/issues/1998/1001/p1213.html. Accessed on 19 July 2022.
- US Food and Drug Administration Medication Guides. http://www.fda.gov/Drugs/DrugSafety/ucm085729.htm. Accessed on 19 July 2022.
- In Brief: Your Guide to Lowering Your Blood Pressure with DASH. The DASH Eating Plan. Available on: http://www.nhlbi.nih.gov/files/docs/public/heart/dash_brief.pdf. Accessed on 19 July 2022.
- Choosing Wisely: An initiative of the American Board of Internal Medicine Foundation.www.choosingwisely.org. Accessed on 19 July 2022.

- Clinical Practice Guidelines of the American Association of Clinical Endocrinologists for management of patients with hypothyroidism and suspected hypothyroidism. 2012 Updates www.aace.com/pub/pdf/guidelines/hypo_hyper.pdf. Accessed on 19 July 2022.
- NIH National Institute of General Medical Sciences. Pharmacogenomics Primer. https://nigms.nih.gov/education/fact-sheets/Pages/pharmacogenomics.aspx. Accessed on 19 July 2022.
- Pharm GKB. The Pharmacogenomics Knowledgebase. Pharmacogenomics. Knowledge, Implementation. Pharm GB is a comprehensive resource that curates knowledge about the impact of genetic variation on drug response for clinicians and researchers. http://www.pharmgkb.org. Accessed on 19 July 2022.

Appendix A: Unnecessary Drugs in the NF/SNF

F-tag #	Regulation	Guidance to surveyors
F757	*Unnecessary drugs* 1. *General.* Each resident's drug regimen must be free from unnecessary drugs. An unnecessary drug is any drug when used: (1) In excessive dose (including duplicate therapy); or (2) For excessive duration; or (3) Without adequate monitoring; or (4) Without adequate indications for its use; or (5) In the presence of adverse consequences which indicate the dose should be reduced or discontinued; or (6) Any combinations of the reasons above	*Intent: Unnecessary drugs* The intent of this requirement is that each resident's entire drug/medication regimen be managed and monitored to achieve the following goals: The medication regimen helps promote or maintain the resident's highest practicable mental, physical, and psychosocial well-being, as identified by the resident and/or representative(s) in collaboration with the attending physician and facility staff Each resident receives only those medications, in doses and for the duration clinically indicated to treat the resident's assessed condition(s) Non-pharmacological interventions (such as behavioral interventions) are considered and used when indicated, instead of, or in addition to medication Clinically significant adverse consequences are minimized; and The potential contribution of the medication regimen to an unanticipated decline or newly emerging or worsening symptom is recognized and evaluated, and the regimen is modified when appropriate *NOTE*: This guidance applies to all categories of medications including antipsychotic medications

Source: Code of Federal Regulations 483.25(l)

Appendix B: Choosing Wisely® and Medication Management in PA/LTC

Organization	Recommendation
AMDA-Society for PA/LTC Medicine	Do *not* use sliding scale insulin for long-term diabetes management for individuals residing in the nursing home Do *not* routinely prescribe lipid-lowing medication in individuals with limited life expectancy Do *not* initiate hypertensive treatment in individuals >60 years of age for SBP <150 mmHg or DBP <90 mmHg Do *not* prescribe antipsychotic medications for behavioral and psychological symptoms of dementia (BPSD) in individuals with dementia without an assessment for an underlying cause of the behavior
American Geriatrics Society	Do *not* prescribe a medication without conducting a drug regimen review Do *not* prescribe cholinesterase inhibitors for dementia without periodic assessment for perceived cognitive benefits and adverse GI effects *Avoid* using prescription appetite stimulants or high calorie supplements for treatment of anorexia or cachexia in order adults
Annual Assembly of Hospice and Palliative Care	Do *not* use ABH gel (Ativan, Benadryl, Haldol) for nausea due to absent or insufficient transdermal absorption of active ingredients
American Psychiatric Association	Do *not* routinely prescribe antipsychotic medication as a first-line intervention for insomnia in adults Do *not* routinely use antipsychotics as first choice to treat BPSD (see above) Do *not* routinely prescribe two or more antipsychotic medications concurrently
American Society of Consultant Pharmacists	Do *not* start new medications to treat new or emerging symptoms caused by existing therapies Do *not* use highly anticholinergic medications when safer alternatives are available Do *not* use anticholinergic medications concomitantly with acetylcholinesterase inhibitors in patients with dementia Do *not* use two or more anticoagulants or antiplatelet agents in older individuals at high risk of bleeding Do *not* use three or more CNS-active medications due to high risk of falls and fractures Do *not* combine opioids with benzodiazepines or gabapentin due to increased risk of serious adverse outcomes including excessive sedation, overdose events, or death Do *not* use tramadol without considering risks sedation, serotonin syndrome, hyponatremia, hypoglycemia, and seizures due to serotonergic excess especially when used in patients with renal insufficiency or with other agents such as SSRIs or CYP2D6 inhibitors
American Society of Nephrology	Do *not* administer erythropoiesis-stimulating agents (ESAs) to chronic renal disease patients with hemoglobin levels ≥10 g/dL (without symptoms of anemia) *Avoid* NSAIDs in individuals with hypertension or heart failure or chronic kidney disease of all causes including diabetes

Adapted from Choosing Wisely® documents published by the listed organizations

References

1. The State of Aging and Health in America. 2013. http://www.cdc.gov/features/agingandhealth/state_of_aging_and_health_in_america_2013.pdf. Accessed 30 Mar 2015.
2. Cooper JW. Probable adverse drug reactions in a rural geriatric nursing home population: a 4 year study. J Am Geriatr Soc. 1996;44:194–7.
3. McLean AJ, Le Conteur DG. Aging biology and geriatric clinical pharmacology. Pharmacol Rev. 2004;56:163–84.
4. Heidelbaugh JJ. Proton pump inhibitors and risk of vitamin and mineral deficiencies: evidence and clinical implications. Ther Adv Drug Saf. 2013;4(3):125–33.
5. NIH National Institute of General Medical Sciences. https://nigms.nih.gov/education/fact-sheets/Pages/pharmacogenomics.aspx. Accessed 19 July 2022.
6. Roskos KV, Maibach HI, Guy RH. The effect of aging on percutaneous absorption in man. J Pharmacokinet Biopharm. 1989;17:617–30.
7. Klotz U. Pharmacokinetics and drug metabolism in the elderly. Drug Metab Rev. 2009;41(2):67–76.
8. Greenblatt DJ, Sellers EM, Shader RI. Drug disposition in old age. N Engl J Med. 1982;306:1081–7.
9. Mangoni AA, Jackson SH. Age-related changes in pharmacokinetics and pharmacodynamics: basic principles and practical applications. Br J Clin Pharmacol. 2004;57(1):6–14.
10. Roden DM. Principles of clinical pharmacology. In: Loscalzo J, Fauci A, Kasper D, Hauser S, Longo D, Jameson J, editors. Harrison's principles of internal medicine 21e. New York: McGraw Hill; 2022.
11. Garg AX, Papaioannou A, Ferko N, et al. Estimating the prevalence of renal insufficiency in long-term care. Kidney Int. 2004;65(2):649–53.
12. Bennett WM. Geriatric pharmacokinetics and the kidney. Am J Kidney Dis. 1990;16:283.
13. Cockcroft DW, Gault MH. Prediction of creatinine clearance from serum creatinine. Nephron. 1976;16:31–41.
14. MedCalc: glomerular filtration rate estimation. GFR calculator using Cockcroft–Gault, MDRD equations. http://www.medcalc.com/gfr.html. Accessed 15 Mar 2015.
15. American Geriatrics Society 2019 Beers Criteria Update Expert Panel. American Geriatrics Society 2019 updated Beers criteria for potentially inappropriate medication use in older adults. J Am Geriatr Soc. 2019;67(4):674–94.
16. Gallagher P, Ryan C, Byrne S. STOPP (screening tool of older person's prescriptions) and START (screening tool to alert doctors to right treatment). Consensus validation. Int J Clin Pharmacol Ther. 2008;46(2):72–83.
17. U.S. Food and Drug Administration. Public health advisory; deaths with antipsychotics in elderly patients with behavioral disturbances. Silver Spring: U.S. Food and Drug Administration; 2005. http://psychrights.org/drugs/FDAantipsychotics4elderlywarning.htm
18. Hamilton H, Gallagher P, Ryan C, et al. Potentially inappropriate medications defined by STOPP criteria and the risk of adverse drug events in older hospitalized patients. Arch Intern Med. 2011;171(11):1013–9.
19. Lavan AH, Gallagher P, Parsons C, O'Mahoney D. STOPPFrail (screening tool of older persons prescriptions in frail adults with limited life expectancy): consensus validation. Age Ageing. 2017;46(4):600–7.
20. Curtin D, Jennings E, Daunt R, et al. Deprescribing in older people approaching end of life: a randomized controlled trial using STOPPFrail criteria. J Am Geriatr Soc. 2020;68:762–9.
21. Hsu W, Wen Y, Chen L, Hsiao F. Comparative associations between measures of anticholinergic burden and adverse clinical outcomes. Ann Fam Med. 2017;15:561–9.
22. Turró-Garriga O, Calvó-Perxas L, Vilalta-Franch J, et al. Measuring anticholinergic exposure in patients with dementia: a comparative study of nine anticholinergic risk scales. Int J Geriatr Psychiatry. 2018;33:710–7.

23. Fox C, Richardson K, Maidment ID, et al. Anticholinergic medication use and cognitive impairment in the older population: the Medical Research Council cognitive function and ageing study. J Am Geriatr Soc. 2011;59:1477–83.
24. Pagel AT, Clifford RC, Potter K, et al. The feasibility and effect of deprescribing in older adults on mortality and health: a systematic review and meta-analysis. Br J Clin Pharmacol. 2016;82:583–623.
25. Forster AJ, Murff HJ, Peterson JF, et al. The incidence and severity of adverse events affecting patients after discharge from the hospital. Ann Intern Med. 2003;138:161–7.
26. Joint Commission Center for Transforming Health Care. Project Detail. Hand-off Communications. http://www.centerfortransforminghealthcare.org/projects/detail.aspx?Project=1. Accessed 9 Aug 2022.
27. Tampi RR, Tampi DJ, Balachandran S, Srinivasan S. Antipsychotic use in dementia: a systematic review of benefits and risks from meta-analyses. Ther Adv Chronic Dis. 2016;7(5):229–45.
28. Aparasu RR, Chatterjee S, Chen H, Rajender R. Risk of hospitalization and use of first versus second-generation antipsychotics among nursing home residents. Psychiatr Serv. 2014;65:781–8.
29. Van Leeuwen E, Petrovic M, van Driel ML, et al. Withdrawal versus continuation of long-term antipsychotic drug use for behavioural and psychological symptoms in older people with dementia. Cochrane Database Syst Rev. 2018;3:CD007726. https://doi.org/10.1002/14651858.CD007726.pub3.
30. Loane PD, Tandan M, Zimmerman S. Preventive antibiotic use in nursing homes: a not uncommon reason for antibiotic overprescribing. JAMDA. 2020;21(9):1181–5.
31. Naunton M, Peterson GM, Deeks LS, Young H, Kosari S. We have had a gutful: the need for deprescribing proton pump inhibitors. J Clin Pharm Ther. 2018;43(1):65–72. https://doi.org/10.1111/jcpt.12613.
32. Helgadottir H, Bjornsson ES. Problems associated with deprescribing of proton pump inhibitors. Int J Mol Sci. 2019;20(21):5469. https://doi.org/10.3390/ijms20215469.
33. Gerstein HC, Miller ME, Byington RP, Action to Control Cardiovascular Risk in Diabetes Study Group, et al. Effects of intensive glucose lowering in type 2 diabetes. N Engl J Med. 2008;358:2560–72.
34. Duckworth W, Abraira C, Moritz T, VADT Investigators, et al. Glucose control and vascular complications n veterans with type 2 diabetes. N Engl J Med. 2009;360:129–39.
35. Bansal N, Dhaliwal R, Weinstock RS. Management of diabetes in the elderly. Med Clin N Am. 2015;99(2):351–77. https://doi.org/10.1016/j.mcna.2014.11.008.
36. AGS clinical practice guidelines for pharmacological management of persistent pain in older persons. http://www.americangeriatrics.org/files/documents/2009_Guideline.pdf. Accessed 19 July 2022.
37. McGettigan P, Henry D. Cardiovascular risk and inhibitors of cyclooxygenase: a systemic review of observational studies of selective and non-selective inhibitors of cyclooxygenase-2. JAMA. 2006;296(13):1633–44.
38. Kuehn J. FDA focuses on drugs and liver damage: labeling and other changes for acetaminophen. JAMA. 2009;302:369–71.
39. US Food and Drug Administration Medication Guides. https://www.accessdata.fda.gov/scripts/cder/daf/index.cfm?event=medguide.page. Accessed 8 Aug 2022.
40. James PA, Oparil S, Carter BL, et al. 2014 Evidence-based guideline for the management of high blood pressure in adults: report from the panel members appointed to the Eighth Joint National Committee (JNC 8). JAMA. 2014;311(5):507.
41. Agarwala A, et al. Older adults and hypertension: beyond the 2017 guideline for prevention, detection, evaluation, and management of high blood pressure in adults. ACC.org, American College of Cardiology, 26 Feb. 2020, www.acc.org/latest-in-cardiology/articles/2020/02/26/06/24/older-adults-and-hypertension.
42. Moore TJ, Conlin PR, Ard J, et al. DASH (dietary approaches to stop hypertension) diet is effective treatment for stage 1 isolated systolic hypertension. Hypertension. 2001;38:155–8.

43. Soumerai SB, McLaughlin TJ, Spiegelman D, et al. Adverse outcomes of underuse of beta-blockers in elderly survivors of acute myocardial infarction. JAMA. 1997;277(2):115–21.
44. MD+CALC. CHADS2-VASc Score for atrial fibrillation stroke risk. https://www.mdcalc.com/calc/801/cha2ds2-vasc-score-atrial-fibrillation-stroke-risk. Accessed 19 July 2022.
45. Bonanad C, Formiga F, Anguita M, Petidier R, Gullón A. Oral Anticoagulant Use and Appropriateness in Elderly Patients with Atrial Fibrillation in Complex Clinical Conditions: ACONVENIENCE Study. J Clin Med. 2022;11(24):7423. https://doi.org/10.3390/jcm11247423. PMID: 36556039; PMCID: PMC9781896.
46. Biondi B, Cappola AR, Cooper DS. Subclinical hypothyroidism: a review. JAMA. 2019;322(2):153–60. https://doi.org/10.1001/jama.2019.9052.
47. Roden DM, Altman RB, et al. Pharmacogenomics: challenges and opportunities. Ann Intern Med. 2006;145(10):749–57.
48. Andres TM, McGrane T, McEvoy MD, Allen BFS. Geriatric pharmacology: an update. Anesthesiol Clin. 2019;37(3):475–92. https://doi.org/10.1016/j.anclin.2019.04.007.
49. AMDA-The Society for Post-Acute Care and Long-Term Care Medicine. Drive to Deprescribe. 2021. https://paltc.org/drive2deprescribe. Accessed 19 July 2022.

Rehabilitation and Maximizing Function in Long-Term Care

Thomas Lawrence

Introduction

Federal nursing facility regulations require that care and services be provided to enable residents to *"attain or maintain" the highest practicable level of physical, mental, and psychosocial well-being* [1, 2]. Rehabilitation (rehab) services and overall care that promote a maximum level of function for all resident's is fundamental to high quality nursing facility care. The provision of recuperative and rehabilitative services to patients following hospitalization is among the fastest growing segment of health care expenditures in the United States. An increasing number of older adults when discharged from hospital will convalesce in a long-term care setting especially a skilled nursing facility. About 1.5 million persons receive rehabilitation in a nursing facility each year [3]. Residents in a skilled nursing represent the largest percentage of short-stay admissions. Rehabilitation is a service delivered *with* a patient, where patient motivation and participation are paramount. Engaging the individual and identifying and embracing their goals of care and goals of life should guide decision making as to the most appropriate setting and intensity of rehabilitation [4].

T. Lawrence (✉)
Geriatric Medicine and Long Term Care, Main Line Health System, Main Line Health Center, Philadelphia, PA, USA

P. Winn et al. (eds.), *Post-Acute and Long-Term Care Medicine*, Current Clinical Practice, https://doi.org/10.1007/978-3-031-28628-5_19

369

Background

The decision of *where* to receive rehabilitation therapy is dependent upon several factors
- Therapy modalities needed.
- Complexity of comorbid medical problems.
- Physical and cognitive ability to participate in therapy:

  - **Inpatient rehab facility**: Requires the patient be able to participate in **at least** 2–3 h of combined therapies daily (high intensity rehab).
  - **Skilled nursing facility**: The patient is only able to tolerate **less than** 2–3 h of combined therapies daily (lower intensity rehab).

- Site of rehab care:

  - Inpatient Rehabilitation Facility (IRF).
  - Long-Term Acute Care Facility (LTAC).
  - Nursing facility and skilled nursing facility (NF/SNF).
  - Assisted living facility (ALF).
  - Program of All-Inclusive Care of the Elderly (PACE).
  - Home Health agency (HHA).
  - Outpatient Rehabilitation Center.

- Rehabilitation services can also be provided to long-stay residents of a nursing facility if their physical functional status deteriorates due to an acute and/or chronic illness. In all these settings successful rehabilitation requires that a variety of therapeutic interventions be delivered in a coordinated and timely fashion with the goal to restore and maximize function [2, 4–6].
- Goals for rehabilitation are determined by the interdisciplinary team that includes therapists (OT, PT, ST), nurses, the attending physician, (or NP or PA) and be aligned with the preferences of the resident.
- Goals should be realistic, *attainable*, and aimed at improving resident function and independence, while respecting the individual's quality of life and dignity.
- Restoration to the level of function prior to an acute illness or event may not be an achievable goal for all residents. Instead, achieving a lesser level of functional status may be adequate for achieving a person's goals of care.
- Overall prognosis of residents may change over time and can result in the rehab plan being temporarily suspended or altered due to an acute change in status and/or changing goals of care. For example, an acute serious illness can result in the decision to forego further rehabilitation and instead decide upon a more palliative approach or admission to hospice.

Types of Therapy Services

Therapy services include three traditional rehabilitation disciples: *physical therapy (focus on mobility), occupational therapy (focus on self-care)*, and *speech therapy (focus on communication, cognition, and swallowing function)*. Other therapy complementary modalities may include *respiratory therapy*, *psychotherapy*, *cognitive therapy*, and *recreational therapy* (includes music and pet therapy); some of these modalities (e.g., psychotherapy) may be covered separately under Medicare or other insurance plans. Additional therapy services may not be separately reimbursed but instead included under the nursing facility resident per diem. All rehabilitation providers must coordinate services as part of the comprehensive assessment and plan of care following the federally mandated nursing facility resident assessment protocols (now called *care area assessments*).

- *Physical therapy* focuses on the restoration of movement and functional ability involving the extremities with particular attention to ambulation and transfer skills.
- *Occupational therapy* focuses on promoting the resident's ability to participate in basic activities of daily living such as dressing, grooming, and bathing. While physical therapy focuses on the function of the lower extremities, occupational therapy focuses on upper extremity function. Some occupational therapists have acquired additional expertise in the evaluation of patients with eating and swallowing difficulties.
- *Speech and language therapy* address disorders of speech, language, voice, communication, cognition, and swallowing. Speech therapists often provide recommendations for altered consistency diets in residents with dysphagia.

Payment for Rehabilitation Therapy

Under Medicare, the cost of rehabilitation therapy is included in the *prospective payment daily rate* paid to the skilled nursing facility. Eligibility for the SNF benefit usually requires at least a 3-day hospitalization; however this requirement was waived during the COVID pandemic. The daily rate is calculated according to the mix and intensity of rehab and nursing services needed that are to be provided. For residents whose nursing facility stay is no longer covered by the Medicare Part A benefit or private insurance, ongoing rehabilitation therapies can then be covered under the Medicare Part B benefit (during a NF stay or in the community). This coverage is contingent upon the service meeting *medical necessity* requirements as being reasonable and necessary for the resident's care. Medicare Part B therapy services are limited to an annual cap.

Multi-Morbidities and Frailty

In many cases there is a small window of opportunity to initiate rehabilitation therapy services. Older adults have an increasing number and complexity of both acute and chronic medical problems as they age—termed *multimorbidities*—that can delay rehab. Common conditions include cardiac, pulmonary, gastrointestinal, and renal disease, malnutrition, depression, musculoskeletal and neurological problems (including dementia), in addition to muscle deconditioning, generalized weakness, and sarcopenia. These conditions can interact in a dynamic and complex manner to cause further functional decline that in turn will limit the patient's ability to respond to rehab therapy and then result in less than optimal rehabilitation outcome.

Prevention During Rehabilitation

Pressure Ulcer/Injury Prevention

Residents who are undergoing rehabilitation are often at high risk for the development of a pressure ulcer/injury due to risk factors of immobility, urinary incontinence, and multiple comorbid medical conditions including diabetes. Aggressive prevention strategies must be implemented. Principles of pressure ulcer/injury prevention include: frequent total body skin inspection, frequent turning and positioning schedule (at least every 2 h), managing urinary and fecal incontinence, prevention and management of contractures, maintenance of adequate nutrition and hydration, use of offloading or pressure-redistribution devices, and proper transfer and lift techniques [7]. Worsening and delayed healing of pressure injuries can result in a prolonged and suboptimal rehabilitation outcome. Prevention and management of pressure injuries is discussed further in the chapter on Wound Care.

Prevention of Venous Thromboembolism (VTE)

Nursing home residents are frequently an overlooked group at risk for VTE [8]. Although universal application of VTE prophylaxis to *all* rehab patients is of unproven benefit, there are circumstances when prophylaxis is essential. VTE prophylaxis has proven benefit for those who have had surgery for hip fracture or knee arthroplasty. Various agents are approved for use and the duration of treatment for prophylaxis is variable but usually continues for a minimum of 4 weeks. Ongoing research will help identify other high-risk residents who may benefit from VTE prophylaxis. One clinical dichotomy that needs to be balanced as to benefit/risk is the fact that some residents, while at high risk for VTE, are also at high risk for bleeding when treated with anticoagulants [9]. Individual patient risk factors and preferences for treatment need to be considered when deciding whom to anticoagulate. Consulting a cardiologist may be needed for rehab patients with comorbid heart disease or atrial fibrillation in order to determine the most appropriate anticoagulation regimen.

Rehabilitation Approaches for Specific Conditions

Stroke

The goals of rehabilitation for stroke include
- Stabilizing and, if possible, optimizing treatment of comorbid medical and psychologic conditions (including post-stroke depression).
- Implementing stroke prevention strategies to include the treatment of modifiable risk factors (e.g., hypertension, diabetes, hyperlipidemia).
- Preventing and managing stroke-related sequelae (e.g., dysphagia, incontinence).
- Promoting recovery of neurological and physical function.

The *rehabilitation phase* is critical as up to 20% of first-ever stroke patients die within the first 30 days from pneumonia, pulmonary embolism, or cardiac complications (e.g., MI, CHF) being the most common causes of death.

Stroke rehabilitation should begin immediately upon medical stabilization. The goal should be to prevent recurrent stroke, avoid medical complications, mobilize the patient, and encourage self-care activities. Complications that require active prevention and management include pressure injuries, spasticity and contractures, bowel and bladder issues (e.g., incontinence, urinary retention, fecal impaction), and prevention of respiratory complications (e.g., aspiration, pneumonia).

Spasticity occurs in over 60% of patients following a stroke [10]. This manifests as an increase in muscle tone with exaggerated deep tendon reflexes. Although spasticity can sometimes help ambulation, it is often painful and debilitating. Management involves daily stretching exercises and avoidance of stimuli that trigger spasticity. In the elderly antispasmodic drugs are poorly tolerated due to the common side effects of sedation and confusion. For more severe spasticity, focal injections of phenol or botulinum toxin may be effective as is serial casting. Muscle contractures occur when there is permanent shortening of a muscle or tendon due to continuous and increased muscle tone due to spasticity. When severe contractures may require surgical intervention. Managing spasticity and promoting stretching and maintaining range of motion are critical to preventing contractures.

Bowel and bladder dysfunction following a stroke occurs in 50–70% of patients though in many it resolves within 3–6 months [10]. Most strokes cause a hyperreflexia bladder and uninhibited bladder contractions resulting in urinary urgency and incontinence. This is best managed with a timed voiding schedule. Monitoring urine output and post-void residual bladder volume can be helpful. Urinary retention and overflow incontinence are less common complications. Prostate hypertrophy in men, medication adverse effects on bladder function, and preexisting urinary incontinence can complicate bladder management. Urinary incontinence is a major risk factor for pressure injury development, so skin protective measures must be utilized. Bowel incontinence is less common and can be caused by fecal impaction. Risk factors include inactivity, poor nutrition, and inadequate fluid intake. A high fiber diet and adequate fluid intake can usually achieve bowel continence.

Respiratory complications are often due to stroke-related dysphagia. Aspiration usually occurs during the pharyngeal phase of swallowing and significant dysphagia can occur without clinical signs of aspiration. Up to one-third of patients with dysphagia have episodes of aspiration [10]. Formal evaluation of swallowing by a speech therapist is often needed. A video fluoroscopic swallow study can be both diagnostic and help select the most appropriate dietary consistency for the patient. The incidence of pulmonary embolism after a stroke is 10–15%, so VTE prophylaxis should be considered. Attaining ambulation of at least 50 feet per day reduces the risk of DVT and pulmonary embolism [10].

Therapy interventions can begin once neurological deficits are no longer progressing, usually within 48 h after a stroke. Initially, when the affected extremities are more flaccid, treatment involves passive range of motion and bed repositioning exercises with progressively increasing intensity. In the past the approach to the stroke patient was mostly supportive and focused on preventing complications while allowing spontaneous recovery to occur. Modern approaches now entail the use of more aggressive treatment that include compensation strategies, neurophysiologic training techniques, task-oriented retraining, as well as strengthening exercises [10].

Compensation refers to using alternate approaches to task completion such as using the *unaffected* extremity to perform a specific task or using a wheelchair to improve mobility and functional recovery. *Neurophysiologic training* involves using the *affected* side to perform tasks and to relearn normal movement. This can minimize spasticity. *Task-oriented retraining* involves intensive rehab of the affected extremity. This technique includes restraining the *unaffected* extremity in order to promote greater use of the affected extremity. *Strengthening exercises* utilize progressive resistance to improve general fitness and extremity strength. *Aerobic exercise* has been shown to improve gait speed and to decrease risk of falls.

Fracture Care

Hip fracture occurring in the community or at a nursing or assisted living facility is a common reason for postoperative admission to a skilled nursing facility. The annual mortality rate in the elderly following a hip fracture is extremely high (up to 36%) and optimal rehab outcomes require successful management of comorbidities. Up to 50% of patients do not regain their previous ambulatory function while up to 20% may become nonambulatory [11, 12]. Rehabilitation should start as soon as possible after surgery. The most important need is early mobilization in order to prevent complications such as pneumonia, deep venous thrombosis, pulmonary embolism, urinary tract infection, and pressure injuries. Other common occurrences include delirium, depression, anorexia, weight loss, and unsuccessful healing (due to nonunion, instability, or dislocation) of the hip fracture, as well as constipation, fecal impaction, and urinary retention.

A vital goal of therapy following hip surgery is to improve muscle strength and to prevent muscle atrophy on the *unaffected* lower extremity while performing isometric exercise of *affected* lower extremity at full extension. The speed of rehabilitation usually depends on the type of surgery performed, with prosthetic joint replacement progressing more quickly than after pinning. Full weight bearing can begin as soon as day 2 after surgery if the joint is replaced, followed by balance retraining and ambulation exercises beginning within 4–8 days. Stair-climbing exercises are the final stage of rehabilitation that usually can begin after 10 days. Strengthening exercise of the trunk and quadriceps muscles should be performed daily and taught to patients. Occasionally, in cases of high surgical risk, *rehabilitation without surgery* may be the best treatment approach. Here secondary disabilities such as pressure injuries, muscle atrophy, joint contractures, and general deconditioning are common and usually limit the functional outcome. *Effective pain management is essential.*

Pelvic fractures involving the pubic rami and ischium are less common than hip fractures. These are the most common sites of pelvic fracture, not the ilium. Because the ilium provides most of the weight bearing strength of the pelvis, weight bearing can usually be achieved as soon as pain eases. Isolated pubic ramus fractures often heal without causing significant long-term functional disability, with many patients able to walk short distances with a walker within a week. Early mobilization reduces similar complications as those discussed with hip fractures.

Thoracic and lumbar vertebral compression fractures are often nontraumatic and occur spontaneously during ordinary activity in the setting of preexisting osteoporosis. In thoracic fractures the vertebrae are frequently deformed into a wedge shape causing kyphosis and subsequent impairment in respiratory function. With lumbar fractures the deformity is usually narrowing of the vertebral plates. With multiple vertebral fractures, spinal deformity can result in chronic pain and a permanent gait abnormality. The goals of therapy are to control pain and restore function. Use of a brace may help in pain management but will not prevent deformity. Newer techniques aimed at vertebral fracture repair, such as kyphoplasty, may help to relieve pain and prevent deformity in selected patients. NSAIDs and/or a mixedopioid, and/or calcitonin nasal spray can provide analgesia and thus improve mobility.

Joint Replacement

Rehabilitation following total hip and knee joint replacement surgery is increasingly occurring in a skilled nursing facility. This is due to Medicare limiting payment for postoperative total joint replacement care in an acute inpatient rehabilitation facility (IRF). In contrast to hip fracture surgery, rehabilitation following total knee joint replacement must carefully balance therapy aimed at preventing deconditioning while avoiding overuse of the new joint and the contralateral limb joints. Typically, patients with cemented joints can weight bear as tolerated immediately after surgery, whereas patients with cementless joints are initially ordered to be partial weight bearing to allow bony in-growth to occur. Due to the relative uniformity of joint replacements, rehabilitation can often occur according to a highly structured therapy protocol. Pain management is often a challenge in elderly patients.

Amputation and Orthotics

The higher incidence of amputation of the lower extremity among the elderly relates to the higher prevalence of peripheral arterial disease and diabetes. Trauma and tumor are less common causes. These patients present additional challenges to therapists due to presence of medical comorbidities that include decreased cardiopulmonary capacity, neuromuscular disease, muscle weakness, poor nutrition, and visual impairment. In addition, preexisting functional decline makes high intensity prosthetic training more difficult yet challenging.

Common amputation sites of the lower limb include below the knee (transtibial), and above the knee (transfemoral) [13]. The rehab time immediately following an amputation is referred to as the *pre-prosthetic period*. During this period the rehabilitation focus is on good wound healing and initiation of therapy. Specific clinical issues include: wound management, pain control, edema control, strengthening, functional training, and maintenance of range of motion to prevent contracture.

Pain management addresses both surgical procedure-related pain and phantom limb pain. Phantom limb sensation is a perception that all or part of the amputated limb is still present. This sensation can be quite disturbing to the patient. It often improves over time and can respond to desensitization treatment. Edema of the residual limb is common. Reducing edema helps to promote healing and control pain. Management includes elastic wraps and elastic shrinker socks.

Once good healing is achieved (which can take weeks), the prosthesis can be fabricated. The components of the prosthesis include: *the socket* (interface between the residual limb and the prosthesis), the *suspension* (secures the prosthesis to the body), *joint* (such as the knee in a transtibial amputation), and *terminal device* (such as a foot) [14]. Collaboration between the patient, therapist, prosthetist, and prescribing physician is critical to successful fabrication of the prosthesis. Fit and comfort of the socket is a particular challenge. Optimal fit in the socket is accomplished by placing residual limb socks in multiple layers in the socket until a fit is achieved. Weight shifts and edema can lead to changes in fit and necessitate refitting the socket.

Prosthetic training involves significant cardiopulmonary stress as oxygen demand increases by about a third in a transtibial amputee and nearly doubles for a transfemoral amputee [13]. Thus, cardiac or respiratory compromise can limit an individual's ability to attain independent function with a prosthesis. Psychological issues often surface during this phase of rehabilitation and the services of a psychologist or counselor can be helpful.

Deconditioned State

It is common that nursing facility residents admitted from hospital suffer generalized weakness. This condition is often referred to as *deconditioning and results in generalized debility*. It is also a common complication seen in *long-stay* nursing facility residents due to an acute medical problem or exacerbation of a chronic condition that then results in weakness and functional decline. Rehabilitation interventions combined with other therapy modalities, should be implemented in order to restore strength and function. If not on skilled, this rehab therapy would be covered under the Medicare Part B benefit. Most assisted living facilities can also arrange for therapy services covered under Medicare Part B or private insurance either on-site with a contracted therapy provider or at an out-patient therapy center.

Maximizing Function

Federal regulations require nursing facilities to provide services to *attain* and *maintain* a resident *functioning at the highest practicable and achievable level of well-being*. For residents with weakness, neurological deficits, or who are convalescing from an acute illness or surgery, therapy services should be provided in a coordinated manner to achieve individual treatment goals. For those with chronic progressive decline, rehab services may need to be less intense and the frequency of treatment less often, but the goals of rehabilitation will still apply.

There is another method of long-term rehabilitation that focuses on maintaining function referred to as *restorative care*. Restorative care is a program of ongoing exercise and activities of daily living training that is individually developed for each resident by the therapy team. It is usually then carried out by the nursing staff of the facility, including nursing assistants who provide most of the daily care in the nursing home or by a designated *restorative therapy aide*. Attaining and maintaining the improvement in physical function through rehabilitation is an important goal in the care of all residents.

Pain Management

Adequate analgesia for patients is a key priority in rehabilitation. Many older adults on therapy have underlying conditions that cause pain, such as hip fracture or spasticity related to stroke, and experience pain during therapy sessions. The administration of analgesics should be provided around the clock (not only as needed) for patients with continuous pain and additional medication (as needed) be given for breakthrough pain. Because of the intensity of therapy, it has become common practice for patients to receive pain medication prior to the start of a therapy session (usually 30–60 min) to prevent excessive pain that may limit performance during the therapy session. As physical function improves, or surgical sites heal, pain frequently lessens so that reevaluation and possible gradual dose reduction of the analgesic regimen should be considered.

Depression

Depression is an extremely prevalent occurrence in excess of 50% among residents of long-term care facilities. Similarly, high rates of depression occur among those who are undergoing rehabilitation for conditions such as stroke and hip fracture. Depression among rehabilitation patients may be due to several factors including multiple medications, medical comorbidities, neuroendocrine imbalance related to the primary illness, or adjustment disorders due to psychological stress and disability. Depressed patients are at risk for slower progress in rehabilitation, longer length of stay, achieve worse outcomes, and not complete the therapy program. Practitioners should be vigilant in diagnosing depression. Treatment should be timely, comprehensive, and include both psychotherapy and pharmacotherapy (see Chapter on "Dementia, Delirium and Depression" for further discussion of depression).

Care Transitions

Rehab therapy services must be available to all residents in all post-acute and long-term care settings. Note that when residents transition from one level or site of care to another, that these services will likely need to continue. Ensuring that progress notes are available to the therapists assuming care is an important step in any care transitions. This is especially important in the transition from facility-based services to the home or outpatient setting, as well as across multiple levels of care during a period of illness. An example of this is a patient with a hip fracture who is admitted to the hospital for surgery, then transitions to a skilled nursing facility for rehab therapy, and then discharged to home with therapy provided by a home health care agency. Engaging family members to understand and support the goals of care at each transition is essential.

Outcomes Related to Site of Rehab Care

There is emerging evidence from the research literature that there may be differences in outcomes based on the site of rehabilitation in various post-acute settings [4, 15, 16]. Evidence suggests that rehab at an inpatient rehabilitation facility (IRF) may predict better functional outcomes with shorter lengths of stay, though at higher cost. This is an area of health care costs that is currently being monitored by health insurance companies and accountable care organizations (ACOs) [6].

Summary

Rehabilitation is a critically important part of health care delivery services in long-term care that is provided to all residents at some time during a nursing facility stay and many elderly in other post-acute and long-term care settings. Preserving and restoring function is an essential element of quality long-term care. Two challenges that must be addressed are:

- First, cognitive impairment is common among nursing facility residents so attaining optimal rehabilitation goals is often difficult.
- Second, resident treatment goals and the likelihood for achieving them often change so the approach to care must be frequently revised.

For long-stay nursing facility residents, who proceed toward progressive irreversible functional decline at the end of life, treatment priorities centered on maintaining the quality of life and dignity will substitute traditional rehabilitation goals.

Pearls for the Practitioner

- A skilled nursing facility is the most appropriate location for patients who are unable to tolerate the 2–3 h of daily intensive rehab therapy that is required for an inpatient rehabilitation facility (IRF).
- Physical therapy focuses on lower extremity function and ambulation while occupational therapy focuses on upper extremity tasks required for self-care.
- Interprofessional collaboration in long-term care and rehabilitation is essential [17].
- Concomitant medical conditions, referred to as medical comorbidities or multi-morbidities can interact in dynamic and complex ways to impact both the outcome and complications that can occur during rehabilitation.
- Poorly healing pressure injuries can adversely affect rehab therapy and outcome.
- Stroke rehabilitation should begin immediately upon medical stabilization of the patient—often within 48 h.
- Up to 50% of hip fracture patients do not regain their previous level of ambulation and up to 20% become nonambulatory.
- Generalized weakness following acute illness in the elderly, referred to as deconditioning, is an extremely common consequence of either a hospitalization or a stay in a long-term care facility.
- "Restorative care" is the provision of exercises and training in activities of daily living at a nursing facility following an episode of acute rehabilitation or acute illness.

- Depression among rehabilitation patients is extremely common and may involve several factors including: medication adverse effects, medical comorbidities, neuroendocrine imbalance, as well as a psychological reaction to disability.
- Short-term and long-term prognosis may change such that treatment goals of rehab must be periodically revised.

Websites
- American Geriatrics Society http://www.americangeriatrics.org
- American Academy of Physical Medicine and Rehabilitation http://www.aapmr.org
- Centers for Medicare and Medicaid Services http://www.cms.hhs.gov
- Cochrane Collaboration, Cochrane Reviews http://www.cochrane.org/reviews/
- National Institute of Neurological Disorders and Stroke, Post-Stroke Rehabilitation Fact Sheet http://www.ninds.nih.gov/disorders/stroke/poststro-kerehab.htm

References

1. Centers for Medicare and Medicaid. State operations manual, Appendix PP—Guidance to surveyors for long term care facilities, Rev. 55. 2017. https://www.cms.gov/medicare/provider-enrollment-and-certification/guidanceforlawsandregulations/downloads/appendix-pp-state-operations-manual.pdf. Accessed 22 Nov 2017.
2. Kochersberger G, Hielema F, Westlund R. Rehabilitation in the nursing home: how much, why, and with what results. Public Health Rep. 1994;109:372–6.
3. Quinn CQ, Port CL, Zimmerman S, Gurber-Baldini AL, Kasper JD, Fleshner I, et al. Short-stay nursing home rehabilitation patients: transitional care problems pose research challenges. J Am Geriatr Soc. 2008;56:1940–5.
4. Mayer RS, Noles A, Vinh D. Determination of postacute hospitalization level of care. Med Clin N Am. 2020;104:345–57.
5. Cruise CM, Sasson N, Lee MH. Rehabilitation outcomes in the older adult. Clin Geriatr Med. 2006;22:257–67.
6. Achterberg WP, Cameron ID, Bauer JM, Schols JM. Geriatric rehabilitation—state of the art and future priorities. J Am Med Dir Assoc. 2019;20:396–8.
7. American Medical Directors Association. Pressure ulcers in the long-term care setting clinical practice guideline. Columbia: AMDA; 2017.
8. The surgeon general's call to action to prevent deep vein thrombosis and pulmonary embolism. 2008. http://www.surgeongeneral.gov/topics/deepvein/.
9. Jaffer AK, Brotman DJ. Prevention of venous thromboembolism in the geriatric patient. Clin Geriatr Med. 2006;22:93–111.
10. Shah MV. Rehabilitation of the older adult with stroke. Clin Geriatr Med. 2006;22:469–89.
11. Zuckerman JD. Hip fracture. N Engl J Med. 1996;334:1519–25.
12. Bhandari M, Swiontkowski M. Management of acute hip fracture. N Engl J Med. 2017;377:2053–62.
13. Pomeranz B, Adler U, Shenoy N, Macaluso C, Parikh S. Prosthetics and orthotics for the older adult with a physical disability. Clin Geriatr Med. 2006;22:377–94.

14. Cristian A. The assessment of the older adult with a physical disability: a guide for clinicians. Clin Geriatr Med. 2006;22:221–38.

15. Herbold JA, Bonistall K, Walsh MB. Rehabilitation following total knee replacement, total hip replacement, and hip fracture: a case-controlled comparison. J Geriatr Phys Ther. 2011;34:155–60.

16. Leighton C, Sandel ME, Jette AM, Apelman J, Brandt DE, Cheng P, et al. Does postacute care site matter? A longitudinal study assessing functional recovery after a stroke. Arch Phys Med Rehabil. 2013;94:622–9.

17. Doornebosh AJ, Smaling HJA, Achterberg WP. Interprofessional collaboration in long-term care and rehabilitation: a systematic review. J Am Med Dir Assoc. 2022;23:764–77.

COVID-19 in Post-Acute and Long-Term Care: Challenges and Opportunities

Naushira Pandya, Elizabeth Hames, and Peter Winn

Introduction

The emergence of the coronavirus pandemic in early 2020 has challenged health care systems in the USA and globally and overwhelmed US nursing and assisted living facilities. As of midyear 2022, the SARS-Covid-2 virus has caused more than 152,000 US deaths among nursing home residents and over 2300 confirmed deaths among nursing home staff by early 2021. Over 1.3 million confirmed cases have occurred amid residents and staff. Weekly COVID-19 cases in US nursing facilities peaked in late 2020 and deaths in early 2021.

Despite the headway made in hospital care, COVID-19 vaccinations, the development of antivirals, and the availability of monoclonal antibodies, the continued emergence of COVID-19 variants and subvariants that are more infectious and less prevented by the original COVID-19 vaccine, present ongoing challenges in the prevention and treatment of COVID-19.

Notwithstanding these challenges, opportunities have arisen. These include:

- Improved focus on resident and family-centered care and communication.
- Better readiness in infection prevention and control.
- Adoption of telehealth and telemedicine in patient care.

N. Pandya (✉)
Department of Geriatrics, Kiran C. Patel College of Osteopathic Medicine, Nova Southeastern University, Lauderdale, FL, USA

E. Hames
UnitedHealth Group, Minnetonka, MN, USA

P. Winn
Department of Family and Preventive Medicine, University of Oklahoma, College of Medicine, Oklahoma City, OK, USA

© The Author(s), under exclusive license to Springer Nature Switzerland AG 2023
P. Winn et al. (eds.), *Post-Acute and Long-Term Care Medicine*, Current Clinical Practice, https://doi.org/10.1007/978-3-031-28628-5_20

- Initiatives to address multiple medication use and overuse (polypharmacy), such as the "Drive to Deprescribe."
- Focused state surveys on infection control in long-term care facilities.
- Structured tools for enhanced communication and care planning related to COVID-19 [1].
- Improved practitioners/clinician management of COVID-19 infections in patients with comorbid cardiovascular disease, diabetes, renal failure, and respiratory disease.

In late 2020 a consensus study report commissioned by the US Centers for Medicare and Medicaid Services was released. Written by the National Academies of Sciences, Engineering and Medicine (NASEM) it recognized and recommended the need for vast improvements on how nursing home care is delivered, financed, regulated, and quality of care measured [2]. The pandemic has presented an excellent opportunity to "re-imagine" long term care [3].

This chapter will review the presentation, clinical evaluation, precautions, and monitoring of residents with and at risk for COVID-19 infection, including a review on the general management and supportive care and pharmacotherapy recommended for nonhospitalized patients/residents afflicted with a COVID-19 infection. In addition, CDC recommendations will be reviewed on resident visitation and return to work criteria for healthcare workers (HCW) infected with COVID-19 at long-term care facilities.

Demographics and the scope of COVID-19 in LTC Facilities

- During the pandemic, nursing home residents had COVID-19 infection rates 14 times higher than older adults who lived in the community, accounting for 22% of all COVID-19 cases in the Medicare population.
- Nursing home residents diagnosed with COVID-19 had 12 times the likelihood of requiring a hospital admission as compared to adults over 65 living in the community.
- More than 43% of nursing home residents admitted to the hospital with COVID-19 died as compared to 22% among older adults with COVID-19 who were living in a community setting.
- Male and female nursing home residents had nearly equal the incidence of COVID-19 infection.
- COVID-19 infection rates among age subsets between 65 and 100 years did not show significant difference.
- Hispanic, Black, and Asian nursing home residents had higher rates of COVID-19 infection.
- There have been more than 152,000 total COVID-19 deaths in US nursing homes since January 2020, and over 2300 confirmed nursing home staff member deaths due to COVID-19 since June 2020.

- As of April 2022, an average of 30% of nursing homes continue to have shortages of direct staff, especially nurses and nurse aides.
- In the USA, over 79% of nursing home residents are now fully vaccinated and boosted for COVID-19 (as of 2022).
- According to a report by the Office of Inspector General (OIG) in June 2022, 91% of nursing home staff in the USA had received the required COVID-19 vaccine doses, 56% of staff had received a booster dose, and 6% had received a religious exemption.

Clinical Presentation of COVID-19 in Older Adults

Older adults are particularly vulnerable to severe COVID-19 infection, with advanced age being the strongest risk factor for critical illness. There is a wide range in clinical presentation, from asymptomatic to fulminant disease. Clinical presentation of SARS-CoV-2 is often atypical, and may not include common signs and symptoms such as respiratory distress and fever. Older adults undergo many physiologic changes with aging including immunosenescence. This predisposes to dysfunction of the immune system that can proceed to a cytokine storm, a multisystem inflammatory syndrome (MIS) and multiple organ failure, especially respiratory or renal failure and sepsis. Residents with COVID-19 more commonly present with fatigue, myalgias, headache, nasal congestion, shortness of breath (12% for patients >60 years versus 3% for patients <60 years), sore throat, loss of taste and/or smell, dizziness, nausea, vomiting, or diarrhea. Others may present with reduced mobility, falls, delirium (up to 28% in one multicenter study), and dysregulation of glycemic control. Falls may be a presenting symptom of COVID-19 infection in 23–32% of persons over 65 years. Anorexia has been identified as a frequent symptom that contributes to dehydration and failure to thrive, particularly in persons with advanced frailty. Studies of older adults have shown that a sore throat, new onset congestion, nausea, vomiting, or diarrhea can be more reliable diagnostic criteria than fatigue and body aches. *Up to 37% lack the classic COVID-19 symptoms of fever or shortness of breath.* In those with known pulmonary or cardiac disease, it can be difficult to determine whether a worsening cough or dyspnea is related to either COVID-19 infection or an exacerbation of pulmonary or cardiac disease or coinfection with influenza, Human respiratory syncytial virus illnes RSV, or a common cold.

Older adults with an infection may not present with fever, as the mean body temperature decreases with age and the febrile response blunted. A fever of 38.3 °C (101 °F) or higher requires prompt intervention as it can be associated with a severe infection. The Infectious Disease Society of America (IDSA) defines fever in older adults as a single oral temperature above 100 °F, repeat readings over 99 °F oral, or an elevation of 2 °F above baseline temperature. Fever may not be a reliable symptom to diagnose COVID-19, especially among frail and vulnerable residents in post-acute, long-term care and assisted living facilities. (Delirium already mentioned above) NPandya. COVID-19 may be difficult to differentiate between various

Table 1 Presenting symptoms of Covid-19, influenza, and the common cold

	Covid-19	Influenza	Common cold
	SARS-COV-2	Influenza A, B	e.g., Adenovirus, Rhinovirus
Onset	**Gradual**	**Sudden**	**Gradual**
Fever	100 and above, **2–7 days**	100 and above, **3–4 days**	**Rare**
Chills	Common	Common	**Uncommon**
Headache	Common	**Prominent**	**Rare**
Cough	Dry, **often severe**	Dry +/− severe	**Mild**
Sore throat	**Prominent**, common	Sometimes	**Common**
Runny nose	Common	**Sometimes**	Common
SHOB	Common, **severe**	Sometimes	Uncommon, **rare**
Myalgia	Common	**Usual, often severe**	**Slight**
Fatigue	Common	**Early, prominent**	Sometimes
Diarrhea	Sometimes	Sometimes	**Rarely**
V/N	Sometimes	Sometimes	**Rarely**
Loss taste/smell	**Common**	Uncommon	No
Wheezing	**Sometimes**	**Rare**	**No**

Web Sources:
1. Health Partners: "What is RSV, Symptoms, Treatment and Tips for Preventions"
2. CDC "What is the Difference Between A Cold and Flu"?
3. CDC "Flu Symptoms and Complications"
(Accessed 9 Sept 2022)

respiratory illnesses, such as influenza, bacterial pneumonia, aspiration pneumonia, and non-COVID-19 viral respiratory infections. Therefore, early testing for COVID-19 and influenza and other viruses is recommended, so that proper infection prevention, management, and control can be instituted.

Given the asymptomatic period of COVID-19 infection being 2–14 days (versus 1–2 days with the flu) and its nonspecific clinical presentation of age-related decline of taste and smell, as well as co-morbidities, geriatric syndromes of frailty, cognitive decline, falls, and polypharmacy warrant close monitoring for the emergence of COVID-19. Table 1 reviews common signs and symptoms that may help differentiate COVID-19 from influenza and the common cold.

Symptoms of COVID-19 Versus Other Viral Infections

Symptoms of COVID-19 usually occur within 5–6 days (and up to 14 days) after exposure and last up to a few days to a few weeks; while symptoms of influenza occur within 2 days of exposure and usually lasts 3–7 days; and symptoms of the common cold occur within 1–3 days after exposure and resolve within 10 days. Though these time frames may help differentiate one viral illness from the other it is not uncommon to be coinfected with COVID-19 and influenza or another virus that causes the common cold (adenovirus, rhinovirus, enterovirus, non-COVID-19 coronavirus or RSV). Coinfection with influenza or RSV can result in a more severe respiratory illness and the need for hospitalization and mechanical ventilation and increased in-hospital mortality. It is not uncommon for persons with COVID-19 to be misdiagnosed as having a common cold or worsened allergies. A comparison of symptoms of COVID-19, influenza, and the common cold are shown in Table 1.

Infection Prevention and Control Strategies in LTC Facilities

Quarantine

The CDC has previously recommended quarantine for all residents being admitted to a long-term care facility. This included residents with a known exposure to the SARS-CoV-2 virus and those who are not up to date with COVID-19 vaccination. However, quarantine is no longer needed for asymptomatic residents who have been fully vaccinated and received the COVID-19 booster or who have acquired natural immunity following infection with SARS-CoV-2 that occurred in the last 3 months.

Infection Control Program (ICP) Recommendations for LTC Facilities

The CDC recommends a robust infection control program (ICP) for long-term care facilities with ongoing surveillance and testing of residents and staff. Infection control measures such as source control and COVID-19 screening tests are dependent upon the *COVID-19 community transmission level*. The CDC's **COVID-19 Data Tracker** has two indicators that (1) determine the county level of SARS-CoV-2 for each long-term care facility, and (2) the higher level by the CDC indicator being selected as to the current transmission level (low, moderate, high).

Facilities with 100 or more residents, and facilities that provide ventilator care or on-site hemodialysis must employ a full-time infection control preventionist. The CDC has developed training courses on infection control and program management. Adequate personal protective equipment (PPE) needs to be provided to staff members as well as FDA-approved hand sanitizer (60–95% alcohol) and be available in all resident rooms and facility common areas. Training and education sessions should be provided for staff members, including health care personnel (HCP) and consultative staff such as therapists, podiatrists, hairdressers, and volunteers. Residents and family members should also attend education sessions and receive written materials on use of PPE, protocols for social distancing, and instructions on correct hand hygiene.

According to CDC guidelines, the facility should notify the local health department under the following circumstances:

- ≥ 1 residents or HCP with suspected or confirmed SARS-CoV-2 infection.
- Residents with severe respiratory infection resulting in hospitalization or death.
- ≥ 3 residents or HCP with illness compatible with COVID-19 with onset within 72-h.

SARS-CoV-2 infections, facility staffing, and point of care testing data needs to be reported to the CDC's National Healthcare Safety Network (NHSN) Long-term Care Facility (LTCF) COVID-19 Module every week. Facilities are given a secure online platform to track infections and prevention process measures. Weekly reporting to the NHSN LTCF COVID-19 Module satisfies the CMS COVID-19 reporting requirement.

All persons in a healthcare setting are recommended to use source control and practice physical distancing necessary during the provision of care. Source control (in contrast to PPE) refers to wearing well-fitting masks and respirators to prevent transmission of viral particles. PPE (masks, respirators, face shields, gowns, gloves, etc.) protects the wearer from being exposed to viral particles. This is especially important for individuals (1) not up to date with COVID-19 vaccination, (2) with current signs or symptoms of COVID-19, (3) with close contact or exposure within 10 days to a person with COVID-19, or (4) immunocompromised. Facility staff who are up to date with COVID-19 vaccination in counties with low to moderate COVID transmission rates, may *choose* to use source control in facility areas that have restricted patient access but *should* continue to wear source control in other areas that patients may frequent.

Visitation

Patient visitation recommendations from the CDC state that the safest option is wearing source control and physical distancing during *indoor visitation*. If the resident and visitor are both up to date with COVID vaccination, they can choose whether to wear source control or not, and whether to have physical contact or not. Visitors should wear source control when they are in areas with health care personnel or other residents, even if they are up to date with all COVID vaccinations. During outdoor visitation, CDC facility guidelines for source control are based on COVID-19 incidence levels in the region. During COVID-19 outbreak conditions, facilities should follow guidance from the Centers for Medicare and Medicaid Services (CMS) on visitation and encourage the use of PPE during outdoor visitation.

Consideration should be given to the fact that long-term care facilities are the "home" for long-stay residents. Specialty societies and the CDC emphasize balancing the risk of COVID-19 transmission and quality of life. Residents who are not at increased risk for severe COVID, who are up to date with COVID vaccination, and living in areas with low to moderate levels of COVID-19 infection may be allowed to not use source control in communal areas of the facility. High risk residents should continue to use source control and physical distancing. Following CDC guidelines can be confusing so request clarification from the facility staff (director of nursing, administrator, or infection preventionist) or the state survey agency.

Precautions when Providing Patient Care

Healthcare workers should follow standard precautions when caring for patients with "suspected" SARS-CoV-2 infection. Healthcare workers in areas with high number of COVID cases should wear NIOSH-approved N95 respirator or higher level respirator. A face shield or eye protection that covers the front and sides of the face is currently recommended during all patient encounters. During the hiatus of the COVID-19 pandemic the CDC recommended this due to aerosol risk to spread COVID-19 during nebulizer treatments and that multidose inhalers be used instead.

Patient Monitoring and COVID-19 Testing in Facilities

All residents need to be monitored on admission and daily for fever (temp. ≥ 100.0 °F) and COVID-19 symptoms. Oxygen saturation by pulse oximetry is recommended to be included with the standard vital signs. COVID-19 viral testing should be obtained on any resident with symptoms (including mild symptoms), even if the resident is up to date with the COVID-19 vaccine and boosters. Any asymptomatic resident who has had close contact with a person with SARS-CoV-2 should have two viral tests, one immediately and if negative, a second test 5–7 days after exposure. Testing is not necessary in asymptomatic persons who have recovered from COVID-19 in the last 3 months; however, if a test is to be performed, an *antigen test* (rather than a nucleic acid amplification test (NAAT) *should be obtained, as some persons may be NAAT positive for 3 months yet not infectious.* **Blood antibody tests should not be used to diagnosis on active COVID-19 infection**. *(www. fda.gov April 2021 communication.)*

Screening of *asymptomatic healthcare workers* without a known exposure is required. However, those who are up to date with all COVID-19 vaccines may be exempt from testing.

Pre-procedure and/or pre-admission viral testing for residents is usually decided by the center or hospital to which the resident is being sent. The CDC states that the overall yield of this testing is low. If a healthcare-associated transmission has occurred, consider expanded testing of healthcare workers **and** residents. If expanded testing detects additional infections, broad testing should be implemented, and repeated every 3–7 days, until no new cases are observed for 2 weeks. Consult the local health department or other public health government agency for guidance.

Return to Work Criteria for LTC Facility Healthcare Workers "Infected" with COVID-19

Healthcare workers infected with COVID-19 should monitor themselves for symptoms and be evaluated by occupational health if symptoms recur or worsen. Once returned to work, an antigen test or NAAT can be used, preferably the former. As noted, some persons can remain NAAT-positive for an extended period of time yet be non-infectious. *Antigen tests typically provide rapid results but are less sensitive than NAAT.* If test supplies are low, prioritize their use to diagnose new infections.

Facility healthcare workers with *mild to moderate* COVID-19 symptoms who are not immunocompromised can either return to work in 7 days since symptoms first appeared and with a negative antigen or NAAT within 48 h of return to work **OR** in 10 days since symptoms first appeared if no COVID testing was performed or a positive result was obtained on day 5–7 of symptoms—**AND** in either scenario, that at least 24 h have passed since the resolution of fever without the use of fever-reducing drugs, and symptoms have improved.

Facility healthcare workers with *severe to critical* COVID-19 who are not immunocompromised can return to work in at least 10 to possibly 20 days since symptoms appeared, and at least 24 h have passed since last fever without the use of fever-reducing drugs, and symptoms have improved. Two consecutive respiratory specimens collected ≥24 h apart (antigen test or NAAT) need to be negative.

Facility healthcare workers who are *moderately or severely immunocompromised* may produce infectious SARS-CoV-2 virus more than 20 days after symptoms appear. For these workers, an infectious disease or occupational health consult is needed to determine when to be allowed to return to work. *For immunocompromised workers who have **symptomatic** COVID-19 infection*, fever must be resolved without current use of anti-fever medications, symptoms need to be improved, and two consecutive respiratory specimens collected ≥24 h apart (antigen test or NAAT) need to be negative. *For immunocompromised healthcare workers with **asymptomatic** COVID-19*, return to work requires two consecutive negative respiratory specimens collected ≥24 h apart (antigen test or NAAT).

Return to Work Criteria for Healthcare Workers "Exposed" to Confirmed COVID-19

The CDC definition of close contact is: (1) being within 6 feet of a person with confirmed SARS-CoV-2 or (2) having unprotected direct contact with infectious body fluids of a person with confirmed SARS-CoV-2. Even distances of greater than 6 feet may still be a concern when exposures occur indoors over a long period of time. Correct use of PPE, use of source control by the infected individual, and vaccination status should all be considered when evaluating such an exposure. CDC guidance for healthcare worker exposures and PPE usage, can be found at: https://www.cdc.gov/coronavirus/2019-ncov/hcp/guidance-risk-assesment-hcp.html.

Patient Assessment and Management

A rapid and targeted evaluation is required for residents "suspected" with COVID-19 infection. In addition to managing respiratory and non-respiratory symptoms, there needs to be a heightened awareness of comorbidities and their impact on resident prognosis. Comorbidities that can worsen a resident's condition include HTN, heart failure, respiratory disease, diabetes, renal failure, and cancer. Cognitive impairment, pre-COVID mental status, and the presence of frailty also affect prognosis and outcome. Practitioners with expertise in geriatric medicine can assess and provide inclusive care to manage a residents' multidimensional health status, functional ability, caregiver involvement, and social support.

Resident evaluation and clinical assessment may be performed on site when permissible, or by telehealth with nursing staff facilitating the visit. Important factors to consider when a evaluating a resident with "suspected" COVID-19 include:

- Level of alertness, confusion, delirium, or coma.
- Respiratory effort and oxygen saturation.
- Fever.
- Hemodynamic stability (heart rate, blood pressure).
- Blood glucose level (regardless of prior diagnosis of diabetes).
- Baseline laboratory tests (CBC with differential, CMP, CRP).
- Intake of food and fluids—assess hydration status.
- Functional status and level of dependency (consider use of Clinical Frailty Scale).

Clinicians should be aware that 40% of COVID-19-positive patients can have no signs or symptoms, and 30% present atypically (in a recent study of 400 residents across four long-term care facilities). Frail individuals also have a higher risk of hospitalization and mortality [4]. In a French study of 480 residents in metropolitan nursing homes, male gender, age >85 years, diabetes, dyspnea, thermal dysregulation (hypo or hyperthermia), altered level of consciousness, and falls were associated with increased risk of COVID-19-related mortality [5]. Other studies also cite dementia and other neuropsychological conditions, urinary and bowel incontinence, chronic kidney disease, cardiovascular disease, prior pneumonia or respiratory disease, malnutrition and dehydration, as well as functional dependency as risk factors for increased mortality. Also associated with increased mortality in residents are the need for supplemental oxygen, O_2 desaturation despite O_2 supplementation, bilateral lung infiltrates, elevated C reactive protein (CRP) and/or, interleukin-6 (IL-6), a reduced lymphocyte count, low GFR, hemoconcentration, hypernatremia, and reduced serum albumin [6].

Management of COVID-19 Infection

Management of residents with COVID-19 requires good symptom control and supportive care. Pharmacotherapeutic intervention is essential. Since there are no specific guidelines for managing residents with COVID-19 in nursing and assisted living, the recommendations reviewed in Table 2 represent a consensus of professional society guidelines as well as those from the CDC. It is important to acknowledge that many facilities have been able to successfully manage COVID-19 "in house" and avoid resident hospitalization and to provide appropriate palliative care in those residents near end of life. The current pharmacological managment recommendations for non-hospitalized patients are summarized in Table 3.

Table 2 General management and supportive care

Clinical problem	Management	Notes
Fever, headache, myalgias	Acetaminophen	Daily dose not to exceed 3 g
Cough	Antitussives	Avoid preparations containing codeine
Dyspnea	Prone position may be helpful Supplemental oxygen to maintain saturation above 92%	Incentive spirometry Breathing exercises to reduce anxiety in severe dyspnea
Dehydration	Oral or intravenous fluids if necessary	Regular monitoring of vital signs and electrolyte and renal function
Weakness	Early mobilization Physical therapy	
Nutrition	Feeding assistance Reduce isolation when possible Nutritional supplements	
Identify goals of care	Initiate early discussions with patients and care partners	Formal advance care planning helpful; consider using structured tool for planning and communication
Polypharmacy	Discontinue unnecessary supplements and treatments Stop sliding scale insulin	

Sources: Centers for Medicare and Medicaid Services; Infectious Disease Society of America

Table 3 Pharmacologic management: recommendations for non-hospitalized patients [7–9]

Therapeutic agent	Suggested dose	Caveats
For patients at high risk of progressing to severe disease		
Nirmatrelvir/ ritonavir (Paxlovid)	300 mg nirmatrelvir/100 ritonavir Q 12 h × 5 days, ≤5 days from onset of symptoms 150 mg nirmatrelvir/100 ritonavir Q 12 h × 5 days, ≤5 days from onset of symptoms	If eGFR >60 mL/min If eGFR ≤60 and ≥30 mL/min Not recommended if eGFR <30 mL/min ***Evaluate concurrent medications for drug–drug interactions***
Remdesivir	200 mg IV on day 1, followed by 100 mg IV Q D on day 2 and 3	≤7 Days from onset of symptoms Expected to be active against Omicron variant If IV therapies are feasible in the facility Monitor patient during infusion and 1 h afterwards
Alternative agents for patients at high risk of progressing to severe disease		
Bebtolivamab	175 mg as single IV injection in 30 s	Observe patient for ≥1 h ≤7 Days from onset of symptoms
Molnupiravir	800 mg PO BID × 5 days, ≤5 days from onset of symptoms	Use only if nirmatrelvir/ ritonavir (Paxlovid) are not available
Other potential agents		
Dexamethasone	6 mg PO daily for duration of use of oxygen **IF discharged from ED with new or increased need for supplemental oxygen**	Not to exceed 10 days, monitor for adverse effects Continue corticosteroids if used for prior indication Equivalent doses are 40 mg prednisone or 32 mg methylprednisolone

Sources: CMS, IDSA

Medications Not Recommended, or Only in the Context of a Clinical Trial

Since the advent of the COVID-19 pandemic, many medications have been administered with varying published results. However, in the light of the current state of knowledge and results from an increasing number of larger studies, the use of *the following medications is not recommended*: ivermectin, famotidine, colchicine, and pre- and post-exposure prophylaxis with hydroxychloroquine and azithromycin. The following medications are only recommended in the context of a clinical trial: inhaled corticosteroids, and fluvoxamine.

Long-Term Consequences of COVID-19 Infection

Post-acute COVID-19 is defined as the presence of symptoms present 3 weeks after initial disease presentation, and **chronic COVID-19** as symptoms occurring beyond 12 weeks. In a telephone survey conducted by the Center for Disease Control (CDC), 47% of older adults with three or more chronic conditions reported that they had not returned to their usual state of health 14–21 days after a positive test [10]. Negative mental health outcomes have been noted in patients during the COVID-19 pandemic. These include delirium, depression, and behavioral problems. Strategies to mitigate these outcomes have included virtual visits, and increased volunteer and staff engagement of residents. After recovery from acute COVID-19 infection, patients may experience long-term effects: severe symptoms and end-organ dysfunction, altered cognition, and loss of physical function. Comorbidities may also increase in severity as usual care of conditions such as COPD and heart failure may have been disrupted. All these factors require close monitoring and prudent adjustment of treatments. Long-term effects observed in residents who have been afflicted with COVID-19 include:

- Fatigue.
- Weight loss.
- Dyspnea.
- Oxygen dependence (associated with pulmonary fibrosis, and interstitial prominence).
- Encephalopathy (white matter changes, hypometabolism, acute or sub-acute infarcts on neuroimaging) [11].
- Increase incidence of heart failure.
- Impaired circulation in the feet.
- Headache, vertigo, impaired smell, and taste.
- Myopathy.
- Peripheral neuropathy.
- Decline in function (may lead to wheelchair or bedbound status).
- Post-traumatic stress (especially in those with respiratory symptoms).
- Depression or anxiety (especially in those with respiratory symptoms).

Long COVID-19

Persistent cluster of symptoms post-acute COVID-19 can occur up to 15 months or longer, termed "Long COVID-19." These include "brain fog" (cognitive deficit, memory loss, difficulty with concentration), headaches, dizziness, tingling, blurred vision, tinnitus, and chronic fatigue. This condition may be related to the presence of increased level of autoantibodies, the presence of EBV DNA in blood, viral fragments of SARS-CoV-2 RNA in the blood, and Type 2 diabetes. Cardiopulmonary symptoms are common with persisting dyspnea, partially due to reduced lung diffusion capacity. Patients who have had more severe disease are more likely to develop long COVID-19.

Summary

The COVID-19 pandemic has precipitated a crisis in post-acute and long-term care that has challenged staff and practitioners (indeed all health care workers) to rethink and restructure the physical and people environment in the provision of care to short-stay and long-term residents of nursing, assisted living and independent living facilities. As COVID-19 shifts from a pandemic phase to an endemic phase, infection prevention and control will continue to be essential to reduce exposure risk to facility residents and staff. This will require an impetus to ensure residents have received up-to-date immunizations for the pneumococcal vaccine, annual influenza vaccination, and ongoing COVID-19 vaccination as new variant and booster vaccines are developed in order to maintain effective antibody titer levels to COVID-19. If another COVID-19 pandemic occurs that limits access to in-hospital care, it may require that staff and practitioners at nursing facilities provide hospital-level care. Readiness to meet such a challenge will be vital.

The future for post-acute and long-term care holds promise for better resident care, and better management of COVID-19 infection, better drugs, better COVID-19 vaccines, and better trained HCWs, staff, and practices as health care in facilities is "re-imagined."

Pearls for the Practitioners
- COVID-19 has transitioned from an epidemic to a pandemic and currently to an endemic phase (as of fall 2022).
- COVID-19 Omicron variant and subvariants are more infectious than the initial original/previous variants (Alpha, Beta and Delta) seen in 2020 and 2021.
- Persons are 65% less likely to die from the Omicron variant but are at increased risk to develop Long COVID.
- Be cognizant of the similarities and differences in the presentation signs and symptoms and clinical course of COVID-19, influenza, and the common cold.
- Be aware of the changing CDC recommendations for LTC facilities (testing, monitoring, isolation, cohorting, and visitation).
- CDC recommendations for infection control program pertains to all practitioners and clinicians; to understand and follow… isolation, and return to work policies applies to you!
- Follow the requirement to notify the local Health Department upon a "suspected" or "confirmed" COVID-19 outbreak at the nursing or assisted living facility.
- Practice thorough patient evaluation upon diagnosis and ongoing during active infection and during convalescence.
- Apply geriatric principles of care, knowledge and skills in geriatric syndromes that often coexist with COVID-19 in older adults.

- Keep informed of current and new pharmacotherapy including availability of convalescent plasma therapy and infusion of monoclinal antibodies.
- Support vaccination programs of residents, resident families, staff and practitioners.
- Assess all residents (COVID-19 and non-COVID-19) for the presence and need for mental health care.
- Acquire experience in the use of telemedicine with residents, staff, and care plan and family meetings.
- Recognize Long COVID-19/chronic COVID-19 signs/symptoms.
- Be alert as to the risk of a cytokine storm and coagulopathy (DVT, pulmonary emboli) with COVID-19.

References

1. Gaur S, Pandya N, Dumyati G, et al. A structured tool for communication and care planning in the era of the COVID-19 pandemic. J Am Med Dir Assoc. 2020;21(7):943–7.
2. The National Imperative to Improve Nursing Home Quality. The National Academies of sciences, engineering, and medicine. Washington, DC: The National Academies Press; 2022.
3. Abbasi J. COVID-19 crisis advances efforts to reimagine nursing homes. JAMA. 2021;326(16):1568.
4. Covino M, Russo A, Salini S, et al. Frailty assessment in the emergency department for risk stratification of COVID-19 patients aged ≥80 years. J Am Med Dir Assoc. 2021;22(9):1845–52.
5. Couderc A, Correard F, Hamidou Z, et al. Factors associated with COVID-19 hospitalizations and deaths in French nursing homes. J Am Med Dir Assoc. 2021;22(8):1581–7.
6. Dyer AH, Fallon A, Noonan C, et al. Managing the impact of COVID-19 in nursing homes and long-term care facilities: an update. J Am Med Dir Assoc. 2022;23(9):1590–602.
7. Nonhospitalized patients: general management | COVID-19 treatment guidelines (nih.gov).
8. Nonhospitalized adults: therapeutic management | COVID-19 treatment guidelines (nih.gov).
9. https://www.idsociety.org/practice-guideline/covid-19-guideline-treatment-and-management/.
10. Del Rio C, Collins LF, Malani P. Managing the impact of COVID-19 in nursing homes and long-term care facilities: an update. Long-term health consequences of COVID-19. JAMA. 2020;324(17):1723–4. https://doi.org/10.1001/jama.2020.19719.
11. Manca R, De Marco M, Ince PG, Venneri A. Heterogeneity in regional damage detected by neuroimaging and neuropathological studies in older adults with COVID-19: a cognitive-neuroscience systematic review to inform the long-term impact of the virus on neurocognitive trajectories. Front Aging Neurosci. 2021;13:646908.

Further Reading

Centers for Disease Control and Prevention, National Center for Emerging and Zoonotic Infectious Diseases (NCEZID), Division of Healthcare Quality Promotion (DHQP).
Centers for Medicare and Medicaid Services (CMS). Nursing Home COVID-19 Public File. https://data.cms.gov/covid-19/covid-19-nursing-home-data. Accessed 10 May 2022.
Centers for Medicare and Medicaid Services (CMS). The impact of COVID-19 on Medicare beneficiaries in nursing homes. 2021.

Goldberg EM, Southerland LT, Meltzer AC, et al. Age-related differences in symptoms in older emergency department patients with COVID-19: prevalence and outcomes in a multicenter cohort. J Am Geriatr Soc. 2022;70:1918.

Health and Human Services Office of Inspector General. An estimated 91% of nursing home staff nationwide received the required COVID-19 vaccine doses, and an estimated 56% of staff nationwide received a booster dose. Report No. A-09-22-02003. 2022.

Lian J, Jin X, Hao S, et al. Analysis of epidemiological and clinical features in older patients with coronavirus disease 2019 (COVID-19) outside Wuhan. Clin Infect Dis. 2020;71:740.

National Center for Immunization and Respiratory Diseases (NCIRD), Division of Viral Diseases. Interim infection prevention and control recommendations to prevent SARS-CoV-2 spread in nursing homes: nursing homes and long-term care facilities. 2022.

Saket S, Hashmi AZ. COVID-19 in older adults. Cleve Clin J Med. 2021;2021:ccc080. https://doi.org/10.3949/ccjm.88a.ccc080.

Theme Issue: Re-imagining Long-Term Care. J Am Med Dir Assoc. 2022; 23(2). Topics include articles on reimagining medical care, financing and payment, family involvement, nutrition care, post diagnostic care in dementia and nursing home design and COVID-19.

Vrillon A, Hourregue C, Azuar J, et al. COVID-19 in older adults: a series of 76 patients aged 85 years and older with COVID-19. J Am Geriatr Soc. 2020;68:2735.

Index